# Yoga Therapy for Complex Trauma

# Yoga Therapy for Complex Trauma

## Working with Child, Adolescent, and Adult Clients

**MICHELLE FURY** with
**AYALA HOMOSSANY**

Foreword by Heather Mason
Illustrated by Amanda Cordsen

SINGING DRAGON
LONDON AND PHILADELPHIA

First published in Great Britain in 2025 by Singing Dragon,
an imprint of Jessica Kingsley Publishers
Part of John Murray Press

1

A CIP catalogue record for this title is available from the
British Library and the Library of Congress

ISBN 978 1 80501 403 4
eISBN 978 1 80501 404 1

Printed and bound in the United States by Integrated Books International.

Jessica Kingsley Publishers' policy is to use papers that are natural, renewable and recyclable
products and made from wood grown in sustainable forests. The logging and manufacturing
processes are expected to conform to the environmental regulations of the country of origin.

Singing Dragon
Carmelite House
50 Victoria Embankment
London EC4Y 0DZ

www.singingdragon.com

John Murray Press
Part of Hodder & Stoughton Limited
An Hachette UK Company

The authorised representative in the EEA is Hachette Ireland,
8 Castlecourt Centre, Dublin 15, D15 XTP3, Ireland (email: info@hbgi.ie)

# Contents

## Part I: What's the Problem?

## Part II: Yoga Therapy for Complex Trauma

## Part III: Support Systems—Your Clients' and Yours

# Foreword

Trauma touches more lives than we ever imagined, and with this sobering realization comes a responsibility to seek the most effective forms of care. Research and clinical experience tell us that true recovery demands attention to the mind–body connection. Trauma isn't confined to thoughts or emotions: it imprints itself on the body, disrupting the nervous system, heightening stress responses, and creating a deep sense of disconnection within.

Yoga, meaning "union" or "connection," offers a powerful pathway to healing. Its holistic approach addresses the layered challenges of trauma, seamlessly integrating physical, emotional, and psychological care. Over the years, the yoga community has stepped forward to support trauma survivors, and the psychological community is beginning to recognize its transformative potential.

Yoga therapy, a patient-centered and evidence-informed practice, has long held the promise of transforming trauma care, but it has yet to fully step into the spotlight. Through unwavering commitment, Michelle Fury and Ayala Homossany have brought this promise to life. Their book is a masterful contribution, intricate in its insights, compassionate in its tone, and practical in its application.

Further, this groundbreaking book is the first in the field of yoga and yoga therapy to focus specifically on complex trauma (or C-PTSD), highlighting how it differs from trauma and PTSD, not only in its origins but also in its treatment approaches. By addressing the significant impact of developmental disruptions and relational wounds, the authors illuminate the unique needs of individuals with C-PTSD. They offer a thoughtful, layered approach to care, guiding practitioners toward providing support that is both comprehensive and transformative.

At its heart, this work is about meeting people where they are, especially those who have endured the complexities of trauma. By focusing on the unique developmental needs of young people, while creating frameworks that extend to adults, Michelle and Ayala have ensured that this resource is versatile, inclusive, and impactful.

As someone who has worked in the field of yoga therapy since 2007, I have seen how transformative this practice can be. Following my training in 2008 at the Boston Trauma Center, where yoga's role in trauma recovery began to take shape, I dedicated myself to exploring how yoga therapy could become a cornerstone of mental health care. Founding the Minded Institute allowed me to bring that vision forward, but it is books like this one that truly push the field to new heights. Until now, there has not been a book that brings together the many ways yoga therapy can address trauma, making this resource an invaluable contribution to the field.

What makes this book so special is its ability to weave together a multi-dimensional framework, drawing from a range of disciplines, including yogic philosophy, neurodevelopmental psychology, physiology, and somatic practices, into a cohesive and distinct tapestry not found elsewhere. By integrating yoga's ancient wisdom, the authors connect timeless yogic vistas of the gunas and the koshas, and the foundational teachings of the eight limbs, with the pressing realities of trauma care today. Simultaneously, they provide practical tools, such as fundamental movement patterns, yield, push, reach, grasp, pull, and release, helping practitioners ground these concepts in real-world application. This fusion of depth and practicality ensures that the book offers both a comprehensive theoretical foundation and actionable strategies for those working in trauma care.

The authors also guide readers through the phase-oriented approach to trauma therapy, offering clear steps for stabilization, trauma processing, and reintegration. In doing so, they provide a structure that is adaptable to each client's unique journey while emphasizing the importance of safety, care, and collaboration.

For those unfamiliar with yoga therapy, this book provides not just a guide but also a window into the field's untapped power. It demonstrates how yoga therapy can address the physical, emotional, mental, and spiritual dimensions of trauma, offering a level of care that is both holistic and precise. With practical templates for assessment and treatment planning, it equips practitioners with the tools they need to turn insights into action.

I've had the privilege of knowing Michelle and Ayala for several years and have seen first hand the dedication they bring to their work. I first connected with Michelle when I invited her to co-author a chapter on young people in my book *Yoga and Mental Health*. I chose her for her expertise in working with children and adolescents as a Licensed Professional Counselor, one of the first yoga therapists to work in a hospital, and an educator in yoga therapy for child and adolescent mental health, an area she has helped shape in meaningful ways. I came to know Ayala, an educator in yoga for children known for her creative, in-depth approach, when she trained with me as a yoga therapist. I've seen her inspire everyone she works with. Together, they've created a resource that is both deeply needed and profoundly meaningful.

This book challenges us to think differently about how we approach trauma. It urges us to embrace yoga therapy as an essential component of trauma care and recognize its capacity to foster healing. For those at the forefront of trauma work and looking for an integrated approach, this book presents a fresh lens for understanding the complexities of trauma, a framework for addressing these complexities, and a guide to navigating its challenges with insight and empathy.

*—Heather Mason*
*Founder, the Minded Institute*

# Acknowledgements

My dear friend Terri Davis told me that writing a book is like forging something out of metal. The compressive forces of hammering and rolling the raw materials into shape, then reshaping again, are required to create a sturdy tool. No wonder I kept saying, "I feel like I'm in a pressure cooker!" Like the process of yoga, we burn in the *tapas* (heat) of our *abhyasa* (practice) until some refinement emerges from the alchemical process. Hopefully, we've created a tool that you the reader find full of useful information, practical skills, and reassurance when you need support.

This book was molded and shaped by many people. First, a special thanks goes to Terri Davis, our primary reader. She read every single word with a careful eye and insightful feedback. This book would not be the same without her. Thanks to our commissioning editor Sarah Hamlin, who guided our writing process with warmth, reassurance, and confidence. Along with editing assistant Jenny Edwards, we had such a supportive publishing team through Singing Dragon. Thanks to Amanda Cordsen—you nailed our vision with your elegant illustrations!

Many thanks to Michal Orpaz-Tsipris, for her insightful comments and for offering *Anahat Bindu Dhyan* with the blessings of her teacher Dr. Bhadury. Thanks to our other readers: Rachel Krentzman, Erin Anderson, and Keira Cristobal. Thanks to our focus group: Elle Cochrane, Charm Donohue, Debs Kent, Jamie Hughes, and Keira Cristobal—we loved our conversations with you. Thanks to Mimi Felton for her inspiring leadership and tips on self-care, to Heather Kennedy for her expertise in human subjects research, to Chen Rosner Or-Bach and Adi Maron-Katz for their insights on yoga therapy and the brain, and to Rachel Bilski and Heather Mason for an exciting conversation about yoga therapy for complex trauma. To Agnes Palej-Ramirez and Emily Sledge: Our meetings during the pandemic were the incubator for this book. Thanks to my mom and stepdad, who requested "readings" of the book.

Thanks to Richard Freeman and Mary Taylor, my heart teachers. Thanks to Hansa Knox, Jeanie Manchester, River Cummings, Gary Kraftsow, and Jamie Turner Allison for showing me the depths of yoga and yoga therapy. Thanks to Gurumayi Chidvilasananda for changing my life. Thanks to my Naropa professors MacAndrew Jack and Jeff Price. Your faith in me meant more than you know. Lastly, thanks to my collaborator, Ayala Homossany, who joined me on this madcap ride. What an adventure we've had.

—Michelle Fury


With heartfelt gratitude to my dear parents—my father, a Holocaust survivor, and my mother, a second-generation survivor—who have constantly reminded me to never give up and have instilled in me a passion for learning and growth. Your unconditional love envelops me daily.

To my husband, Asaf—my rock and greatest teammate—your unstoppable support, unwavering belief in me, and endless love have been the steady wind beneath my wings. I couldn't have done it without you. To our three inspiring sons, thank you for filling my world with love and patience, and for walking beside me through it all.

To my extended family and friends, whose love and support have been invaluable, thank you for always being there for me.

To Michelle Fury, thank you for inviting me to dive with you into this project. It's been an enriching experience working together to bring this project to life.

To my teachers along my therapeutic yoga path—Jyoti Manuel, Judith Hanson Lasater, Donna Farhi, Doug Keller, Tias Little, Aadil Palkivala, Richard Freeman, Lisa Kaley-Isley, Kristin Neff, Chris Germer, Heather Mason, and Bonnie Bainbridge Cohen—thank you for opening doors that deepened my exploration of the practice.

To my ballet teachers, for holding space for my love of movement and my connection to my body, and to my design lecturers, for nourishing my creativity and inspiring me to tap into my curiosity: thank you.

To Sigalit Galron, Lilach Margalit-Shalom, Michal Yarkoni, and Deidre Opp, thank you for sharing valuable resources that enriched the work I share.

Last but not least to all the children, families, and students who have crossed my path—you have shown me the importance of hope and the strength found in community.

—Ayala Homossany

# Notes to the Reader

**About the Illustrations:** The illustrations in this book are pared down to their simplest form to reflect an inviting, inclusive, and accessible vision of yoga therapy for all ages, races, genders, and abilities. We hope you enjoy the playful elegance that graphic designer Amanda Cordsen created in the pages that follow.

In addition, minimal instruction is given for poses and sequences. This is because our book assumes the knowledge and experience of a well-trained yoga teacher. We offer alternatives to the classic poses to encourage exploration and create accessibility. And we offer more detailed instruction for poses and practices that are not as commonly known, especially ones for kiddos.

**About Pose Names:** For the most part, we label poses and sequences by their English names or child-friendly names. We include Sanskrit names in parentheses for all illustrated poses. The exception to this rule is when a pose or practice is more commonly referred to by its Sanskrit name, such as Chataranga or Yoga Nidra.

**De-identifying Clients:** All clients and case studies depicted in this book are composites, meaning personal details and histories represent a synthesis of several clients. Any resemblance to an individual is coincidental and unintentional. However, the therapy sessions that are described are factual. They are based on the authors' detailed notations of actual sessions, recollections, and experience from a multitude of clients.

**Issue of Gender:** We agree with Ruella Frank, who lamented, "It can be a struggle for writers to decide upon the most appropriate singular pronoun when referring to a general population" (2001, p. 5). We too grappled with this challenge and landed on the popular singular pronouns "they/them" whenever referring to a nonspecific individual. The caveat to this is Devin (Chapter 4) whose chosen pronouns were also "they/them."

# Introduction: How to Use This Book

## Overview

This book presents an integrative model of yoga therapy for the treatment of complex trauma. Our model integrates five key elements, with *panchamaya kosha* at the center:

1. Panchamaya kosha—the ancient yoga therapy system

2. The gunas—the yogic and Ayurvedic concept that there are three universal qualities of rajas, tamas, and sattva

3. Fundamental movements—a modern somatic psychology concept that aligns with both panchamaya kosha and Attachment Theory

4. Phase-based treatment—a trauma-informed approach to clinical care

5. Community care and self-care—we hold the value that yoga professionals (YPs) must take care of themselves to be good caregivers to others

When integrated together, these elements provide a new framework of yoga therapy (YT). Three elements in particular—panchamaya kosha, the gunas, and the fundamental movements—offer an alternative vocabulary that is strength-based, can reduce the stigma of mental health issues, and provide both yoga professionals and clients an empowering way to talk about complex trauma and its symptoms.

The book has two objectives: 1) to demonstrate the compelling and urgent need for complex-trauma-informed yoga therapy care, and 2) to present a model of safe, effective yoga therapy for the treatment of complex trauma (CPTSD; complex post-traumatic stress disorder). Part I of this book covers the first objective. It outlines the theory and rationale for CPTSD-informed yoga therapy using the five key components of our model. In Chapter 1 we define what complex trauma is (and how it differs from single-incident PTSD), and why yoga therapy is especially suited to deal with the unique symptoms of CPTSD. Since our model spans the life cycle from age 5 to adulthood, we review relevant aspects of human development for safe, effective yoga therapy treatment in Chapter 2. In Chapter 3, we explore the causes, consequences, and solutions to CPTSD. In Chapter 4, we consider one of our model's essential elements—a phase-based approach to current trauma treatment. Chapter 5 examines another core element, the fundamental movements. In Chapter 6 we present the core of our model via the gunas and panchamaya kosha. And throughout, we offer comprehensive evidence and illustrative case studies.

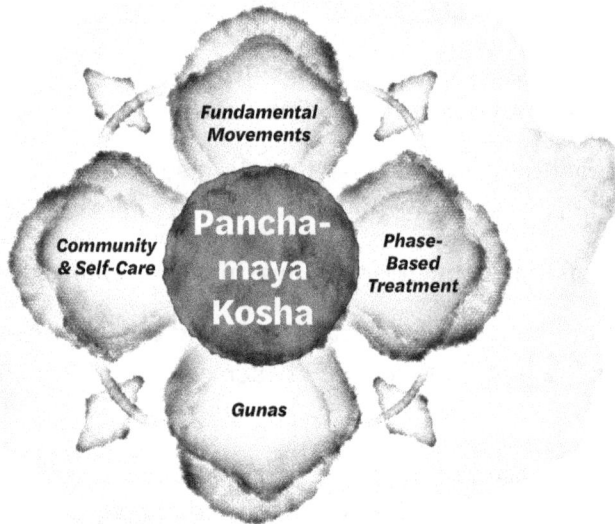

**Figure 0.1** Yoga Therapy for Complex Trauma (YTCT) Mandala
*Illustrates the YTCT Mandala, consisting of five key components, where panchamaya kosha (PMK) lies at the center of the model.*

Part II of the book is in many ways a stand-alone manual. It covers the second objective by offering yoga tools and techniques in a safe, effective, evidence-informed manner. Chapter 7 outlines our CPTSD yoga therapy model in its entirety. Chapters 8–10 demonstrate how to apply the model in a developmentally appropriate way for each of the three age groups covered (Chapter 8, 5–12 years old; Chapter 9, 13–18 years old; and Chapter 10, 19+ years old).

Part III explores support systems—those of both your clients and your own. Chapter 11 examines how to engage with clients' support systems, including family/guardians, teachers, and other healthcare providers. Chapter 12 examines the final core element of our model—community care and self-care. In this chapter, we look at the vital need for YPs to practice self-compassion for the prevention and minimization of vicarious trauma and burnout, as well as receiving support from their own caring communities.

Finally, the Appendices provide a variety of resources including an appendix of forms useful in the assessment and treatment of yoga therapy clients; and there is also an extensive reference list.

We encourage you to read this introduction fully before diving into the chapters. We recognize that any book on trauma can be triggering. Thus, the introduction starts by laying out the framework of the book. This gives you familiarity with what is coming next, so you're not blindsided or triggered by a particular section. If you notice feelings of uneasiness, discomfort, or irritation, take a break from the material.

Safety is another key concept presented throughout the book. **We define safety as the feeling of physical, emotional, and mental well-being of BOTH the client and the yoga professional.** Safety is also covered in Chapter 4. Because your sense of safety and well-being is critical to the success of yoga therapy, we offer Self-Care Practices at the end of each chapter. These are quick, practical self-care tools that correspond with the chapter they fall in.

## Why Yoga Therapy?

Complex trauma is a mental health concern that has captured global attention due to its growing prevalence. As the name suggests, complex trauma (CPTSD) is more complicated than single-incident trauma (PTSD). **Since all psychological trauma (PTSD and CPTSD) is experienced in the body, body-based approaches like yoga therapy can be enormously helpful in the treatment of trauma.** In fact, in the YouTube video "How Yoga Helps Heal Trauma," trauma expert Bessel van der Kolk (Holzer, 2022) says that yoga is well-received by traumatized individuals because it allows them to tolerate distressing feelings yet feel safe in the process.

Yoga is only truly beneficial in the treatment of CPTSD when delivered as a trauma-informed and individualized intervention. A number of training courses offer trauma-informed yoga (some are referred to in this book). While such courses are great for more generalized or single-incident trauma, the interpersonal nature of complex trauma demands that yoga tools be prescribed in an individualized manner. And when yoga tools are prescribed in this way for specific ailments or issues, it is called yoga therapy. We will address the differences between yoga and yoga therapy in detail in Chapter 6. As such, yoga professionals need high-quality yoga therapy training with a CPTSD-informed approach to offer safe, effective care.

Complex trauma often starts in childhood and is chronic, pervasive, and longstanding. However, children are not the only ones who suffer from complex trauma. Adults who have not healed childhood wounds, or as adults experience multiple traumatic events (such as war, systemic racism, or domestic violence), also contend with the fallout of what happened to them, or continues to happen to them. Regardless of age, yoga therapy clients who suffer from CPTSD may be unaware of the condition. Thus, the yoga professional benefits from evidence-informed training to identify the signs and symptoms of an increasingly pervasive issue.

## Who This Book Is For

*Yoga Therapy for Complex Trauma* assumes knowledge of yoga, so it is primarily for yoga professionals. *Yoga professional* (YP) refers to anyone with a certification or degree in yoga teaching and/or therapy, who is actively seeing yoga clients. As such, this book is for certified yoga therapists, yoga-therapists-in-training, and yoga teachers who want to integrate complex-trauma-informed skills into yoga sessions. YPs interested in pediatric mental health will also find many useful tools. In addition, a variety of mental health professionals (psychologists, psychiatrists, psychiatric nurse practitioners, occupational therapists, crisis workers, victim advocates, and first responders to name a few) looking to integrate yogic techniques with a developmental understanding into their work will find valuable resources too. The same is true for graduate students and interns entering the fields of mental and behavioral health. Lastly, teachers and caregivers may also find useful techniques in our model and book.

## What This Book Is About

This book offers yoga professionals a set of yoga tools to address complex trauma through the life cycle, focusing on three broad stages of development:

childhood (5–12 years old), adolescence (13–18 years old), and adulthood (19+ years old). It is a trauma-informed manual that recognizes *when* a client has experienced trauma matters as much as *what* the trauma itself is. This volume offers a unique combination not found in many other books or resources on the topic of yoga for trauma, including: 1) a global view of the problem, 2) how to work with children and adolescents, 3) a focus on complex trauma, and 4) a focus on yoga-specific tools. Simply put, it offers a comprehensive introduction to yoga therapy for complex trauma. As such, it is also recommended that you seek further training, especially in-person training, for this subject matter whenever possible.

*Yoga Therapy for Complex Trauma* consists of four "golden threads": 1) the definition and exploration of CPTSD, 2) yoga therapy, 3) human development, and 4) self-care. The book is further divided into four sections: Part I illuminates the problem of CPTSD globally and current treatments for it. Part II introduces our method and the practical application of it throughout the life cycle. Part III discusses both the client's and your own support systems. The Appendices contain all the forms, handouts, and important resources covered throughout the book.

## Part I: What's the Problem?

Chapter 1 defines the global problem of CPTSD and current treatments. We explore the symptoms—the ones in common with PTSD and ones unique from it. We discuss the importance of knowing one's scope of practice and of creating safety (emotional and physical) for your client and you. In addition, the authors offer our personal (and very different) experiences of complex trauma and how yoga helped each of us transform our wounds into healing for ourselves and others.

In Chapter 2 we consider another fundamental topic of this book: human development. We describe the three main age groups mentioned above as well as four types of human development (musculoskeletal, social/emotional, cognitive, and neurobiological). We will return to the important topic of human development in Part II, when we apply yoga therapy to each of the three age groups.

Chapter 3 brings these concepts together—how CPTSD impacts a child's development, giving special consideration to the ground-breaking ACEs study and subsequent test. Chapter 4 examines three evidence-based phases to consider when treating clients with CPTSD. Considering a client's phase of treatment is critical to delivering safe, effective yoga therapy care.

Chapter 5 introduces the somatic psychology concept of the fundamental movements, which ties our very first movements with the way we attach to our caregivers. And in Chapter 6, we review the two most essential parts of our model: the gunas and panchamaya kosha. We examine how yoga in general, and these two concepts in particular, offer an alternative vocabulary of healing that can reshape and recontextualize how we talk about trauma, approach our clients from a strength-based perspective, and offer healing on a more integrated, holistic level.

## Part II: Yoga Therapy for Complex Trauma

Part II explores the application of yoga therapy for the three age groups. In Chapter 7, we introduce our model in its entirety through the lens of assessment, treatment planning, and course of treatment. We offer a flow of treatment that YPs are welcome to use and adopt in whatever ways work for their current practice. As clinicians ourselves, we encourage you to use what works for you, and nothing more.

Chapter 7 also demonstrates the importance and usefulness of *case conceptualization*, a communication tool used globally in healthcare. Understanding and utilizing this tool allows YPs to communicate effectively and efficiently about an individual client's needs. It also provides a forum to ask vital questions about care and best practice.

Chapters 8–10 cover the practical application of our method tailored to each of the three age groups. These three chapters are structured as follows:

- Case study for age group

- Evidence and rationale of YT for age group

- Pictorial sequences tailored for age group

- Self-care tools for yoga professionals working with this age group

## Part III: Support Systems—Your Clients' and Yours

When working with adults, a YP may not interact with any other members of a client's support system. But when working with youth, yoga professionals will invariably need to interact with caregivers, and possibly teachers and other providers. Chapter 11 explores the myriad kinds of support systems clients may have. We consider the legal matters regarding minor clients, including consent to treat, age of majority, and mandatory self-guarding of minors and vulnerable persons. We also explore how to collaborate in meaningful and impactful ways with the client's support system.

Chapter 12 then turns the spotlight on your support system. We explore community care—the need to receive from and provide support to your own support system. Who do you go to when you are feeling stressed? Self-care receives its own section because it is essential for any caregiver working with those impacted by CPTSD. We know how powerful yoga can be in healing the wounds of complex trauma, because we ourselves are survivors. But it can be taxing on the YP, as well. Learning and regularly practicing self-care skills allows you to have better boundaries with clients, which reduces vicarious trauma and burnout.

## Appendices and References

The Appendices consist of all the sample forms we cover in this book, plus details on special practices like Sa Ta Na Ma, PMK self-assessment for yoga professionals, and background and contact information on the powerful Concentration on the Heart Point (*Anahat Bindu Dhyan*). Our extensive reference list is a great place to find further resources on complex trauma, yoga therapy, and any other topic covered in this book that you'd like to explore in more depth.

## One Final Note

Simply reading about complex trauma can feel overwhelming. As you read this book, take a break whenever you need. Do not try to "power through it." Also, it can be helpful to know that overwhelm is experienced differently by different people. For instance, you may feel spacey and unable to take in the material. If that happens, have a drink of water and take a walk. Or perhaps you start feeling antsy and irritable. The water and a walk will probably do you good. But you may also consider taking some deep breaths, moving the body, or chatting with a friend.

Overwhelm can show up too as thoughts like, "I'll never get this! I don't have what it takes. This is too much / too advanced / above my level. I should just give up." But take heart and do not give up. Take baby steps. You don't have to know it all now. That's why you're reading this book. We are going to take it step by step. Absorb what you can. Let the rest go. Start where you are.

# Part I

# WHAT'S THE PROBLEM?

## CHAPTER 1

# Complex Trauma Is a Global Issue

## Why Yoga Therapy?

**Complex trauma commits identity theft (Greenberg, 2022). Yoga therapy heals and restores that identity.** Yoga therapy is the perfect complement to complex trauma treatment for two reasons: 1) it is a mind–body treatment that offers an integrated model to address the symptom cluster unique to complex trauma (CPTSD; complex post-traumatic stress disorder). First and foremost, among these symptoms is the loss of one's sense of self. Yoga therapy restores a person's identity through a gentle, mindful approach that empowers clients to increase somatic awareness with intention and at their own pace.

The second reason yoga therapy is an important complement to CPTSD treatment is that it is highly relational. Yoga therapist Amy Wheeler (2021) says that traditional schools of yoga therapy such as the Krishnamacharya Yoga Mandiram prioritize the therapeutic relationship. "Without a strong, compassionate connection between the client and the yoga therapist… the yoga therapy process will not produce the intended healing effects" (Wheeler, 2021, p. 60). This statement mirrors current CPTSD experts, who agree that effective treatment must be relational in nature (Courtois & Ford, 2016; Schwartz, 2021). As psychologist and yoga teacher Arielle Schwartz (2021) puts it, "the greatest predictor of meaningful change in clients with C-PTSD is the quality of the therapeutic alliance" (p. 49).

Complex trauma is one of the silent issues fueling a global mental health crisis. **CPTSD is not the same as single-incident trauma (PTSD).** We will define and differentiate these two diagnoses throughout this book. But the takeaway for now is that yoga professionals (YPs) are currently not equipped to adequately deal with CPTSD, even though it is increasingly common.

Yoga is evolving to be an evidence-based therapeutic approach for mental health issues. Trauma-sensitive approaches are at the forefront of this evolution. These trainings are often tailored to PTSD or single-incident trauma. Yet yoga clients may more frequently present with complex trauma that stems from pervasive, oftentimes childhood, traumas that persist into their adult lives. Given this, YPs will benefit from learning how to identify and work with CPTSD. Not only is this important for the compassionate care of the yoga client; it also helps the YP guard against vicarious trauma. While trauma-sensitive yoga trainings are on the rise (some of them even cover CPTSD), there is a critical piece missing. None of them covers how to work with child or adolescent clients specifically.

## What Is CPTSD?

Survivors of complex trauma think they're damaged, defective, and unlovable. These beliefs result in feelings of shame, doubt, and unworthiness that can cause them difficulty in relationships and life (Courtois & Ford, 2016; National Health Service [NHS], 2022b).

To get a sense of how complex trauma emerges, imagine a family who immigrates from Afghanistan to the United States. (All case studies and examples in this book are *composite cases*, that is, amalgamations of many different clients' histories and symptoms.) Their immigration will likely entail several stressful events: the violence and social unrest that caused the family to flee, destabilization of their home and income, possible racial and ethnic discrimination, loss of identity, to name a few. These stressors can then impact parents' treatment of each other and of their children. This example shows how an entire family may be impacted by complex trauma. Not surprisingly, the younger the individual the more they are impacted. Courtois and Ford (2016) point out that "infants are traumatized more readily and by less-intense events than are older children or adolescents" (p. 15). Similarly, children and adolescents are more readily traumatized by less-intense events than adults are.

This case example demonstrates that adult onset of CPTSD is also possible. "Complex trauma is not always the result of childhood trauma. It can also occur because of adults' experience of violence in the home, family, neighborhood and workplace" (Blue Knot, 2021, "As an adult" section). However, in this book we address childhood-onset CPTSD almost exclusively. We will also address how to provide trauma-informed yoga therapy to adult clients, since CPTSD at any age will most likely affect the individual into adulthood.

In his webinar video *Surviving at the Heart of the Storm*, clinical psychologist and internationally recognized trauma and disaster expert Dr. Rony Berger explains the different levels of stress that lead to trauma in his chart Progression of Stress Symptomatology (2023, 16:34–19:40). With each progressive stage of stress, the severity of symptoms increases. Notice the inverse relationship between the period after a single-incident trauma and the percentage of people who suffer these symptoms.

**Table 1.1** shows Rony Berger's Progression of Stress Symptomatology (2023, 16:34–19:40), reprinted with permission.

| Stress Level | Symptoms | Time Period | % |
|---|---|---|---|
| Acute stress reactions (ASR) | Anxiety, nervousness, mild flashbacks, sleeping problems, and some avoidance | Hours–days after a single traumatic event | 70–85 |
| Acute stress disorder (ASD) | Flashbacks, avoidance, mood swings, and hyper-arousal | 2–4 weeks after event | 25–35 |
| Post-traumatic stress disorder (PTSD) | Re-experiencing, numbing, avoidance, enduring sleep problems, hypervigilance, and outbursts | 4+ weeks after event | 15–20 |
| Chronic PTSD | Personal, relational, and occupational problems | Months–years after event | Unknown |

After a highly stressful event like a terrorist attack, Berger (2023) says most people (70–85%) experience *acute stress reactions* (ASR), while a much smaller percentage of people (25–35%) experience *acute stress disorder* (ASD). Berger (2023) adds that only about 15–20% of people will go on to develop PTSD. And an unknown percentage, according to Berger, will develop chronic PTSD, which includes symptoms almost identical to those of CPTSD.

Now let's consider the modern definition of psychological trauma. Psychiatrist and trauma pioneer Judith Herman transformed our current understanding in her ground-breaking book *Trauma and Recovery: The Aftermath of Violence—From Domestic Abuse to Political Terror* (1992b). In it, she said that the root of all traumatic reactions is the inability to act. "When neither resistance nor escape is possible, the human system of self-defense becomes overwhelmed and disorganized" (Herman, 1992b, p. 34).

Herman was also one of the first to propose a new diagnostic term beyond single-incident PTSD in her article "Complex PTSD: A Syndrome in Survivors of Prolonged and Repeated Trauma" (1992a). She and other mental health experts around the world campaigned for a new diagnosis that captured this more complex form of trauma. And in 2018 the World Health Organization (WHO) added complex trauma to its International Classification of Diseases (ICD-11).

The ICD-11 defines complex trauma as "a disorder that may develop following exposure to an event or series of events of an **extremely threatening** or horrific nature, most commonly **prolonged or repetitive** events from which **escape is difficult or impossible**" (ICD-11, 2018; emphasis added). **Interpersonal trauma** is also an important feature of CPTSD (Courtois & Ford, 2016; Schwartz, 2021). These four conditions are the main culprits that knock an individual's nervous system off balance and out of rhythm. They also offer the keys to restore balance and healing rhythm in CPTSD survivors' lives.

The most vulnerable in our communities are at greatest risk for complex trauma (Courtois & Ford, 2016; National Child Traumatic Stress Network [NCTSN], 2023). The NCTSN website (2023) lists multiple populations commonly impacted by CPTSD: LGBTQIA+ youth; immigrant children and families; military soldiers, personnel, veterans, and their families; trauma and substance abuse survivors; individuals with intellectual and developmental disabilities; those who are unhoused; and those with economic stress. This is not an exhaustive list, and there are caveats. For instance, simply because a yoga client identifies with one of these groups does not mean they have complex trauma. Many individuals show incredible resilience in the face of adversity and overcome the wounds of their past (Courtois & Ford, 2016). Conversely, a client with none of these demographic markers may present with complex trauma symptoms.

Having considered what complex trauma is and whom it impacts, let's explore the symptoms a person may experience. Experts agree that CPTSD includes all the symptoms of PTSD, plus a few more (Cleveland Clinic, 2023; Courtois & Ford, 2016; NHS, 2022b; PsychCentral, 2021; Schwartz, 2021). Below is an amalgamated list of symptoms in common with PTSD and unique to CPTSD (both sets of symptoms are covered in detail in Chapter 3):

*Symptoms in common with PTSD:*

- Re-experiencing

- Avoidance and emotional numbing

- Hypervigilance

*Symptoms unique to CPTSD:*

- Emotional dysregulation

- Negative self-view

- Relationship problems

While this book should not be used to diagnose a yoga therapy client with CPTSD, it is a helpful reference guide and manual for creating CPTSD-informed yoga therapy treatment. In addition, given the complexity of complex trauma, yoga professionals should avail themselves of in-person training whenever possible. This book does not replace in-person, synchronous training.

As the list above shows, PTSD and CPTSD share many of the same symptoms. The ICD-11 refers to them as "sibling" diagnoses (2018). As such, it is important to understand their differences. One of the biggest differences is that survivors of CPTSD often struggle with identity and relational issues to an extent not seen in PTSD survivors. In fact, someone suffering from CPTSD may have multiple issues impacting on their mental and physical health. Why does this matter to a yoga professional? It matters because whether or not you specialize in yoga therapy for mental health, yoga therapy can uncover the symptoms of CPTSD in a way that other therapies may not. As a mind–body intervention, yoga can unlock body sensations, memories, and triggers. **Yoga *therapy* (meaning yoga used therapeutically to treat an individual's symptoms) can increase a client's awareness in ways that conventional talk therapy and/or allopathic medicine may not.** (The distinctions between yoga and yoga therapy are covered in detail in Chapter 6.)

What's more, a client may have no idea they have complex trauma. While this is often true of PTSD survivors, it's even more true of CPTSD since it is such a new diagnosis—one that both clinicians and clients may not recognize. If CPTSD is suspected, the yoga professional should refer the client to a behavioral health professional who is licensed to diagnose and treat CPTSD.

## The Yoga Professional: Caring for Others and Yourself

Working in a caring field such as yoga therapy means that clients entrust their well-being to you. The International Association of Yoga Therapists (IAYT) has created guidelines to help YPs follow the highest standards of conduct. We look to the standards that IAYT has created, as they are comprehensive and easily accessible.

## Scope of Practice

Thus far, we have alluded to a key concept in yoga therapy—scope of practice. *Scope of practice* defines the boundaries of a YP's training, experience, and knowledge base (Downie et al., 2023). Borrowed from the medical community, this term is equally important in yoga therapy. Knowing one's scope of practice helps you examine and stay within the boundaries of your skills and experience. This ensures the safety of both you the YP and your clients. You can find IAYT's definition of scope of practice at this link: https://cdn.ymaws.com/www.iayt.org/resource/resmgr/docs_certification_all/2020_updates_scope_ethics/2020-09_sop_v2.pdf

Think of your own set of skills. What are you certified and trained in? Have you received training, supervision, and a formal release to work with a particular population? For instance, perhaps you are certified to work with individuals with sensory integration issues, developmental disabilities, and/or attention deficit hyperactivity disorder (ADHD). Do you have a particular set of skills, such as reiki or experience working as a yoga teacher in a school setting? These are all specialized skills and experience to consider.

Let's consider some specific examples. Perhaps you are a yoga teacher who specializes in yoga for youth in schools or other educational facilities. You may have students from a wide variety of different backgrounds. You observe that many of your students exhibit a lot of anxiety and depression, and you suspect CPTSD in a few. You know you can't prescribe yoga techniques for individual students' symptoms. But without further yoga therapy training, you *can* use almost all the yoga tools presented in this book within the group yoga setting. In addition, when correctly followed the teaching methods in this book ensure a trauma-sensitive approach for PTSD and CPTSD.

Let's say instead that you are a licensed social worker and yoga therapist in training. You have recently decided you want to work with refugees. (As the earlier example about an Afghani family illustrated, simply being a refugee or immigrant puts an individual in harm's way and can easily lead to CPTSD.) With the supervision of a certified yoga therapist from your yoga therapy school, you can use this book as an invaluable resource and reference manual to learn and practice CPTSD-informed yoga therapy. When in doubt, consult the yoga teachers who conducted your highest level of training to determine what is within your scope of practice.

## Code of Ethics

A *code of ethics* is a set of standards that guide the behavior of a group of professionals (National Association of Social Workers, 2024, "Read the code of ethics" section), such as YPs. Whether or not you are a certified yoga therapist, following a clear code of ethics ensures the safety and well-being of not only your clients, but you as well. For instance, practicing ethical behavior means holding healthy boundaries with clients, which benefits clients and YPs alike. You can find IAYT's code of ethics at the following link: https://cdn.ymaws.com/www.iayt.org/resource/resmgr/docs_certification_all/2020_updates_scope_ethics/2020-09_code_of_ethics_v2.pdf

## Community Care and Self-Care

We care as much about your safety and well-being as that of your clients. Likely, you have heard the airplane metaphor: the flight attendant tells you the caregiver to put the oxygen mask on yourself before you help vulnerable others. The same applies in yoga therapy. You must take care of yourself to be truly caring toward others. Equally important is having a strong social network, also known as *community care* (Kim, 2024, "Community care" section). Chapter 12 covers this in detail.

In addition, we offer Self-Care Practices at the end of each chapter. The theme of the practice coordinates with the chapter it is in. We invite you to practice it right after reading the chapter or save it for later reference. It is good to get in the habit of regularly practicing self-care in any helping field. Use these self-care practices whenever you need them.

In this chapter we offer Mindful Transition, a technique Michelle created to help YPs practice healthy boundaries with their clients. You can use Mindful Transition as a "bookend" before and after the session to ensure you don't "take on" clients' emotional baggage. Here, the practice bookends the beginning of the next section and the end of this chapter.

## Mindful Transition

In this moment, we invite you to notice your thoughts, feelings, body sensations, and state of mind. The next section features the authors' trauma narratives. They may be triggering for some, so pause now to reflect on your internal state. What are your thoughts, feelings, body sensations, and state of mind? Do you feel equipped to read about the authors' complex trauma? Is there a calming technique you need to do before continuing to read? Take some deep breaths, shake your limbs, or walk around the room for a moment. Though neither Michelle nor Ayala's stories are explicit, the suggestion of war or childhood trauma can be triggering. Take care of yourself.

## Eye Level: The Authors' Lived Experience

The best way to understand CPTSD, and how yoga therapy can aid in its healing, is to understand the lived experience of it. Although this book is evidence-informed and meant for a professional audience, we feel it is important to give faces and names to this issue that impacts so many people around the world. Both Michelle and Ayala came to the practice of yoga (unknowingly at first) to heal trauma. We know firsthand the power of yoga in creating safety and stability, empowering one's sense of self, healing relationships, and cultivating lasting peace.

We also want to highlight the vastly different contexts in which complex trauma can arise. The authors' stories are very different from each other. We come from two different cultures and countries, halfway around the world from each other. We endured different kinds of trauma. Ayala has suffered the trauma of war and political conflict. Michelle endured chronic interpersonal traumas over the course of her childhood. You will also notice a difference in writing style that reflects our unique "voices," and is intentional. Despite these differences, we both experienced anxiety (hyper-arousal), avoidance, shame, and negative self-views.

Note: To protect the confidentiality of others, Michelle refers only to her own experience and feelings in the following narrative.

## Michelle's Story

It was 1993, and one minute I was balancing in Dancer's Pose, the next I had collapsed sobbing on my yoga mat. I was alone in my apartment, observed by no one, thank God. But what had just happened?

In the two years I'd been practicing, I had learned that yoga could bring up body memories and deep emotion. I'd had some experience of it, but this grief was more intense. As I allowed myself to cry, I noticed feelings of rage, sadness, guilt, and shame.

Growing up I felt like an outsider and "less than," though I consistently received high grades in school and had a solid group of friends. In fact, I strove for good grades because I felt damaged and unworthy but had no idea why. Now in my early 20s, yoga was helping me unearth those grief-rage-shame feelings. They scared me a little.

Luckily, yoga elicited in me a calming confidence that helped me face those big feelings. Yoga also helped me cultivate rhythm in my life through breath, heartbeat, movement, and regular practice. This new rhythm was a safe haven I returned to daily. It gave me trust in myself and the process of yoga that felt unshakable.

At the time I was working on my bachelor's degree at Florida Atlantic University. As luck would have it, the university's psychology department was brimming with courses on neuropsychology and human perception, as well as research opportunities. I volunteered for research in Betty Tuller's lab on the human perception of speech, as well as Bibb Latané's research on the bystander effect.

But one of the most memorable experiences was attending Dr. Steven Bressler's course on neuropsychology. During one lecture, he said something about how being in a calm, relaxed state increases one's ability to focus (Bressler, personal communication, 1994). This matched my newfound ability to find a relaxed state in yoga that gave me laser focus. Learning that modern neuropsychology validated my experience fueled my love of yoga even more.

After graduating with a bachelor's in psychology, I moved in 1996 to Colorado to study with Richard Freeman, one of the great yoga masters in the United States. During his teacher training in May 2001, he said something surprising about anger. He said that we don't have to act out or suppress our anger (R. Freeman, personal communication, May 8, 2001). I was confused. What else can we do then? He said we simply acknowledge it and use it as fuel for doing good. This was novel to me. See, along with the peace and confidence I was cultivating through yoga practice, I became reacquainted with the well of rage within me. It was confusing to feel both things—peace and anger.

To uncover the roots of my anger (and all those other uncomfortable feelings) I sought out psychotherapy. Yoga had shown me that I could handle vulnerable feelings and body sensations. The addition of therapy helped me understand their origin. In the safe space of my therapist's office, I began to recall unsettling episodes early in my life. Throughout childhood I witnessed high conflict and abusive relationships. In one situation when I was little more than a toddler, I was the direct victim of abuse. These experiences left me feeling helpless, weak, and like I didn't belong.

Therapy taught me that my feeling of unworthiness was a sign of trauma. It was the adaptive strategy of a young child who was deeply hurt. It was hard to sit with these feelings. I would leave my therapy session feeling as if I was physically in pieces. But then my daily yoga practices seemed to free me from that disjointed feeling, like taking flight away from the lonely, frightening aspects of my childhood.

Yoga philosophy also gave me a different view of myself—one of self-compassion and self-acceptance to face the shame and unworthiness I felt. Yoga taught me that no matter what traumas had befallen me, at my core, I was whole, stainless, and shameless.

When it comes to trauma, Bessel van der Kolk and Pat Ogden say that far more important than the detail of the traumatic memory is the way they become organized into meaning (Ogden & van der Kolk, 2023). The way my developing brain made sense of my chaotic childhood was to conclude that I must be defective. This is a negative self-view that many (if not all) trauma survivors adopt, especially when the traumas are chronic, pervasive, and acute. While this self-view no longer served me as an adult, it had been an adaptive strategy when I was a child.

In September of 2001, the same year I completed my teacher training with Richard, two planes collided with the World Trade Center in Manhattan. Like every other American watching their TVs on that awful Tuesday morning, I was dumbfounded to see the Twin Towers vanish in an enormous puff of smoke. It was like watching a Hollywood movie, not reality. But even as I watched, something shifted in me. I was tired of feeling helpless. Instead, I felt suddenly mobilized to help others. It was time to act. I wanted to share the art and science of yoga with others who, like me, were suffering from trauma and mental health issues.

In 2003 I went to graduate school to become a psychotherapist with the goal of combining yoga and psychotherapy. In my third and final year of graduate school, I was accepted to two internships—one at the Rape Assistance and Awareness Program (RAAP, which has been renamed the Blue Bench) and one at Children's Hospital Colorado (CHCO). These two internships proved to be a powerful combination that laid the foundation for the rest of my career.

My internships of 2005–2006 coincided with the growing global consensus in the mental health community to rethink and redefine trauma. This new understanding was reflected in my training at RAAP, where we read the new trauma classics from Herman, Levine, Rothschild, and van der Kolk.

Even in my interview, I was asked to differentiate between trauma early in life and trauma as an adult. Intuitively, I answered that early trauma would have a more harmful impact on a child, whose developing brain could not process harmful events the way an adult brain could. My supervisors at RAAP emphasized this point throughout the internship.

My RAAP supervisors also recognized the importance of including the body in trauma therapy. They encouraged me to use my yoga skills and mindfulness techniques in concert with the trauma therapy skills under their supervision and guidance. I stayed with RAAP the year after I graduated as a contract therapist, conducting both individual and group therapy sessions. One of my favorite groups to lead was Trauma Therapy for Teens. This group allowed me to integrate mindfulness and gentle yoga techniques even further with traumatized adolescent girls.

Yet I thirsted for more training to bolster my understanding of how to integrate yoga into trauma treatment. There were no trauma-informed yoga trainings at the time, so I sought out as many relevant courses and conferences as possible. I studied with Gary Kraftsow (founder of the American Viniyoga Institute) in weekend courses and at Mount Madonna in California; and I attended weeklong workshops with Marsha Linehan on dialectical behavioral therapy and Steven Hayes on acceptance and commitment therapy.

In my other internship at CHCO, a brand-new Creative Arts Therapy Program had been created in the behavioral health department. I was thrilled that they wanted yoga to be a part of this pioneering collaboration and was asked to combine my yoga and counseling skills into something new called *yoga therapy*. To enhance my own skills as a pediatric yoga therapist, I became certified in YogaEd©, one of the early children's yoga teacher training programs created by Leah Kalish and Tara Guber.

I received my master's degree in May 2006, and days later I was hired as the first ever yoga therapist in a hospital setting according to the International Association of Yoga Therapists (J. Kepner, personal communication, 2014). During my nearly 15 years at CHCO, I co-created and ran the yoga therapy program. I led weekly groups and saw individual patients in our mental health units and clinics, such as the Adolescent Psychiatric Unit (APU), Child Psychiatric Unit (CPU), Eating Disorder Unit (EDU), Neuropsychiatric Special Care Unit (NSCU), Medical Day Treatment (MDT), Intensive Outpatient Program (IOP), and the Partial Hospitalization Program (PHP).

I often received referrals for patients whose needs and issues were outside the scope of treatment as usual. These were youth who had unique or per-plexing symptoms, like stomach migraines brought on by stress, tantrums that caused a child to rip a sink out of a wall, psychotic episodes that caused another adolescent to scream incessantly at staff, and several clients who complained of acute derealization and depersonalization (symptoms that we now know are related to trauma). I found that ensuring that I was well-reg-ulated—meeting my youthful patients wherever they were at, and using whatever combination of psychotherapeutic and yogic skills worked for a patient—yielded promising results.

During my time at CHCO, I was involved in various pilot studies and proj-ects. None was directly related to trauma, but each one increased my under-standing of how to integrate yoga for pediatric mental health in clinically safe and effective ways.

The first of these was a pilot study of a structured yoga intervention for adolescents with comorbid medical and mental health diagnoses. Our results showed clinically and statistically significant reductions in anxiety, depression, and somatization, as well as improved cardiovascular health. The study was eventually published in the *Journal of Yoga and Physiotherapy* (Wamboldt et al., 2019).

The second was a manualized yoga protocol I created with Hansa Knox's guidance for the Integrative Headache Clinic. For six years in our monthly clinic, I conducted this 60-minute yoga intervention aimed at reducing head-aches in youth 5–18 years old. In a retrospective chart review, we found clin-ically and statistically significant reductions in both headache pain and stress related to the headaches. We presented this at a national conference, but did not publish our findings.

Lastly, I had the opportunity to create several instructional recordings. We created a Yoga Nidra audio recording that anyone could listen to from the CHCO website. It helped many youth right before surgery! I also created an instructional yoga video for NSC, our unit for patients with neurodiver-sity. And I created two instructional yoga videos for the EDU (eating disor-der) patients. EDU patients who were discharging and loved yoga could not simply go to their local yoga studio. They needed a yoga therapy resource tailored to their special needs. We created these videos as a parting gift.

Over the years, I have continued my education with as many thera-peutic yoga courses as I could find. In 2012–2013, I took the *Children's Yoga Teacher Training* by psychologist Bethann Bierer at Hansa Knox's PranaYoga and Ayurveda Mandala. As a licensed psychologist, Bethann integrated invaluable psychological tools with our study of yoga. It was from Bethann that I learned "kids are not just small adults" (B. Bierer, personal communication, November 30, 2012).

In 2015 my first book was published, *Using Yoga Therapy to Promote Mental Health in Children and Adolescents* (2015). And then in 2018 I co-wrote the chapter "Children and Adolescents" with Lisa Kaley-Isley in *Yoga for Mental Health* (2018). They say the final stage of healing is when we help others through the same crisis we ourselves have been through. Without meaning to, my work at CHCO meant I worked with children and adolescents, the ages when my own trauma occurred.

One of the most enduring lessons I have learned on this journey is that rhythm heals trauma. Bessel van der Kolk (personal communication, April 3, 2020) says that rhythm is an essential component to a child's healthy development, especially during early attachment. It is expressed through the child's interactions with their caregiver through rocking, feeding, reciprocal sounds, facial gestures, and movements, and so much more. On the other hand, trauma is the lack of rhythm and human connection.

Yoga helped me heal my trauma through the rhythm of breath, heartbeat, regular practice, and connection with caring teachers. The combination of yoga and talk therapy allowed me to transform my trauma into healing wisdom for myself and others.

## Ayala's Story

"Ayala, I am with you; it is all going to be okay." I held my father's wrist and followed him to the shelter.

Just five minutes prior, we were seated at a restaurant, waiting for our food. This place, nestled in Israel next to one of Tel Aviv's beaches, is a favorite of mine. Growing up by the seaside, the sea is a haven for me where I consistently find comfort. The rhythmic sound of waves, people strolling along the beach, even the distinct scent of seaweed—all make my heart sing, even in the winter of 2024.

As we waited, a siren pierced the air, signaling a missile attack. This familiar sound sent shivers down my spine. My breath quickened, my body tensed, and fear gripped me. I looked at my brother across the table, caring for his daughter. My 14-year-old niece stood up, ready to go to the shelter, a thin veil of worry on her face but attentive and task-oriented. In contrast, I felt a paralyzing shame. My chest tightened; my legs felt anchored. A critical voice in my head questioned why, after two decades of therapeutic yoga, couldn't I stop this immobilizing freeze response? Peter Levine (1997) says that the freeze response occurs when our human brain "overrides the instinctual responses that would initiate the completion" (p. 101) of our survival instincts. When the freeze response takes over, we experience trauma.

Meanwhile, people quietly left the restaurant for the safety of the shelter. My brother went outside with his daughter, while my father urged me to follow. Despite his encouragement, my body succumbed to paralysis. I thought, even if something terrible happened, at least I was with my father. This time, I wasn't leaving him.

When I was 10 years old, living in Northern Israel, my parents planned a visit to my grandmother in Central Israel. During a missile attack warning, I resisted changing my commitment to be my friend's dance partner. My parents eventually allowed me to stay at my friend's house. That night, a missile attack struck close to the shelter we occupied. My parents weren't with me. The details of the moments following the explosions remain hazy, but my mother recalls that for weeks after the attack, I clung to her hand, a silent testimony to the profound impact of that harrowing experience.

Now at 52, back at the restaurant during a missile attack, I held onto my father, tears streaming down. My father, a Holocaust survivor and a retired orthopedic surgeon, remained calm. Holding his wrist, I walked with him to the shelter. A missile exploded nearby, and past and present blurred. My father's voice broke through, "Ayala, I am with you; it is all going to be okay."

At the shelter, the air was thick with anxiety. The metallic taste of fear lingered on my tongue, and my heartbeat roared in my ears. Each breath was a struggle. My father's reassurance melted the paralysis, grounding me momentarily.

This situation reminded me of the power of co-regulation, a concept central to the book *What Happened to You? Conversations on Trauma, Resilience, and Healing* (Perry & Winfrey, 2021). Perry and Winfrey's insights into how supportive relationships can aid in managing intense distress resonate deeply with my own journey.

I clutched my father's wrist, seeking solace in the warmth of his steady pulse. And with that, the spell of frozen fear broke. The warmth of my father allowed me to tap into the wisdom of my yoga practices: I whispered my Sanskrit mantra, which became a lifeline and a rhythmic chant amidst the dissonance.

With that, the shelter transformed into a cocoon of shared humanity. I suddenly noticed the people around me and was amazed at their calmness. A mother's comforting words to her daughter, a couple soothing their baby, and the quiet strength radiating from those around me. The tingles in my palms reduced, and the involuntary clenching of my fists—the body's dance between fear and resilience—softened.

Walking back to the restaurant a few minutes later, I could move independently. Each step carried the weight of collective resilience. Seated again, my legs gradually shed the burdens of fear. A vocal sigh escaped my lips, both a release and a proclamation of triumph over an ancient fear. My body, now an instrument of healing, rejoiced in its newfound lightness. I massaged my wrists, upper arms, and face. I shook my arms and legs. It was not just a physical release but a symbolic shedding of the past.

As I sat, I directed self-compassion toward the lingering shame. I acknowledged the impact of over 20 years of practice, a journey empowering me to navigate the present challenges. This internal shift allowed me to emerge from a frozen state and relish in the simple joy of enjoying my lunch. I marveled at the resilience my yoga practices had brought me. My brother, who sat opposite me, was amazed at how quickly I managed to literally shake it all off.

At 29, I discovered the resilience that yoga offers when I took my first yoga lesson. It was then I began to convert the physical, mental, and emotional imprints of trauma into strength. Guided by a friend who sensed yoga's potential resonance with my ballet background, I quickly fell in love with the practice. For the first time in years, a profound quietness enveloped my thoughts, silencing the mental chatter. However, the instructions on the breath during that first class confused me. When I followed the teacher's direction to place my hands on my belly, I discovered an incongruence—my belly contracted on inhalation and expanded on exhalation. This realization unveiled a pattern of *reverse breathing*, also known as paradoxical breathing. This type of breathing causes the chest to contract during inhalation and expand during exhalation, contrary to normal breathing patterns (Villines, 2017), and can be a manifestation of unresolved trauma. It restrained my breath and elevated my stress and anxiety.

In 2003, by studying with Jyoti Jo Manuel of Special Yoga, I continued my yoga journey by becoming a yoga teacher specializing in yoga for children as well as children with special needs. As a result of my trainings with Jyoti Jo Manuel, I expanded my offering and started working in mainstream schools, yoga studios, and community centers in London, UK. I shared yoga with children, adolescents, and families, some of whom suffered from domestic abuse, bullying, and rejection.

Through my work during this period, I identified the gap that children with special needs and mainly ADHD and autism spectrum disorder experience in the mainstream educational system. As such, I started incorporating specific yoga tools with these audiences. In retrospect, I realize now that my intuition to work in a trauma-informed way was a result of my own self-work over the years, which helped me better understand the needs of my students and provide a supportive environment for their healing and growth.

One of the most important ways I have supported children and adolescents in my yoga classes is by prioritizing physical and emotional safety and using invitational language. This approach stemmed from my belief that fostering creativity and self-expression begins with creating a safe space for participants to be seen and heard—just like the banks of a river contain and guide the flowing water. By using invitational language and empowering children to make decisions, I aim to allow the river of creativity and self-expression to flow freely within the physical and mental safety I have established. Judith Herman (1992b) emphasizes that trauma-informed teaching involves creating a safe environment and offering choices to help individuals feel more secure and in control.

In 2015 I co-created and published the *Enchanted Wonders A–Z Cards: Inspiring Yoga Activities to Elevate Your Child's Self Expression*, with illustrator Dikla Calo-Henkin. It is a set of yoga cards for children that became a bestseller on Amazon and won several awards. These cards bridged my work as a visual communication designer and my career as a yoga teacher. Along with the cards, I developed a children's yoga and mindfulness teacher training. This program included creativity tools for children to help manage anxiety, and self-compassion tools for teachers.

The creation of my yoga toolbox didn't happen overnight. It was shaped by a constant inner voice whispering to my heart that yoga is more than just poses. To deepen my knowledge, I constantly sought out trainings and courses that complemented my knowledge and deepened my understanding. I studied Tantra Yoga for over a decade with Parayoga of the Himalayan Institute, where the practices of mantra, meditation, and Yoga Nidra became inseparable parts of my practice and sharing. This journey into Tantra Yoga helped me understand the profound connection of body, mind, and breath and paved my way into exploring the power of therapeutic yoga with yoga therapist Doug Keller, and yoga for anxiety and depression with yoga therapist Lisa Kaley-Isley. Additionally, yoga masters Donna Farhi and Tias Little expanded my understanding of somatic yoga, reinforcing the idea that the body and brain retain the memory of our experiences (van der Kolk, 2014).

When my mother suddenly passed away in 2013, I was overwhelmed with deep grief. I grappled with an overpowering sense of failure, accompanied by shame and guilt, feeling as if I had failed my mother by not being able to do more for her despite my yoga practices. I couldn't see that it was in no way my fault. At that time, I believed the knowledge I had accumulated on my yogic path was useless. With my mother—my anchor—gone, I felt exposed and vulnerable. The trauma I carried since childhood resurfaced fully. I realized that the knowledge and experience I had up until then needed another layer of support.

In the year following my mother's death, I devoted myself to various self-help practices, determined to find a way to smile again. I studied self-compassion meditation and restorative yoga from teachers like Judith Hanson Lasater, Kristin Neff, and Chris Germer. These practices became the cornerstones of my healing, transforming my self-perception and helping me embrace all emotions, including unworthiness, shame, and guilt. They also provided a gentler, nurturing approach that helped me address emotional pain and grief directly. These practices allowed me to cultivate a deeper sense of inner kindness and acceptance, which was essential in healing the silenced and untreated trauma I held. As I continued to navigate the co-existence of sadness and happiness, I became fully aware of the transformative power of integrating these new practices into my life and work.

The natural next step for me was to become a yoga therapist. I enrolled in and graduated with the yoga therapy diploma program at the Minded Institute under the guidance of Heather Mason in London, UK. There, I finally acknowledged that the symptoms of hypervigilance, anxiety, guilt, shame, and unworthiness that I grappled with were the result of my childhood growing up in a conflict zone in Israel.

My toolbox of coping methods and healing practices has grown significantly, helping me support myself and others. It also led me to develop and deliver, both during and after graduating from Minded, yoga therapy programs for adolescents with ADHD and autism spectrum disorder at schools in London. These experiences have reinforced my commitment to integrate trauma-informed practices into my work, ensuring that I can provide my students and clients a safe and supportive space for healing.

These tools, while not preventing the initial body reaction to a triggering event, could help me to swiftly return to a more peaceful, regulated version of myself. The restaurant incident was a testament to the efficacy of these practices. Despite being unable to prevent the event, the tools I have acquired facilitated a rapid reconnection with my center, enabling me to navigate the aftermath with resilience.

## Self-Care Practice: Mindful Transition

After reading one or both authors' trauma narratives, we highly recommend practicing Mindful Transition again. Pause to notice your internal state. How do you feel after reading these stories? What are your thoughts, feelings, body sensations, and state of mind? Take some deep breaths, shake your limbs, or walk around the room for a few moments before transitioning to your next activity.

## Other Resources

There are now other high-quality yoga resources for trauma and youth. Some of our favorites include the Trauma Center's Trauma-Sensitive Yoga through the Justice Resource Center, founded by Bessel van der Kolk; Fierce Calm, an international organization founded by Dr. Lee Watson that offers free yoga classes in shelters and community spaces across the world; and the online course Trauma-Informed Yoga for Children and Adolescents through PESI, a US-based organization that offers a variety of trainings for healthcare professionals. One youth-specific training is Jennifer Cohen Harper's online course *Teaching Trauma-Informed Yoga for Children* through Yoga International. Lastly, Michelle teaches a yearly online synchronous course called *Yoga Therapy for Child & Adolescent Mental Health* through the UK-based Minded Institute.

## Chapter Summary

- CPTSD-informed yoga therapy allows you the YP to make a bigger difference in clients' lives that is safe, effective, and age-appropriate.

- This book offers a unique combination not found in many books or resources on the topic of yoga therapy for traumatized youth, which: 1) includes working with children and adolescents, 2) focuses on complex trauma, and 3) focuses on using yoga-specific tools.

- This book is a helpful reference guide and manual for creating CPTSD-informed yoga therapy treatment. It is NOT a diagnostic manual. In other words, one cannot diagnose clients using this book.

- You the yoga professional should avail yourself of in-person training whenever possible. This book does not replace in-person, synchronous training.

- Self-Care Practices are offered at the end of each chapter. The theme of the practice coordinates with the chapter it is in. You can practice it right after reading the chapter or save it for later reference. It is good to get in the habit of regularly practicing self-care in any helping field. Use these self-care practices whenever you need them.

- Your yoga therapy clients may discover old wounds and traumas in yoga sessions before they're uncovered in traditional talk therapy. The body-based tools of yoga can help clients re-regulate. This book will show you how to help clients do just that.

- Research now backs up the importance of body-based therapy for the healing of trauma. This book is full of evidence-based support for the yoga tools we offer. But no amount of research replaces the human experience. We hope that in remembering the human connection that you and your client share you will feel inspired and empowered to use your yoga therapy skills to help them find their rhythm and heal.

## CHAPTER 2

# Human Development

"I am still every age that I have been."

As author Madeleine L'Engle (1972, p. 443) suggests in this quote, each of us holds within us the history—a record, if you will—of everything we've experienced in our lives. But where exactly is this record? Research tells us it is our bodies that record the history of what we have been through (Schwartz, 2021; van der Kolk, 2014), a core tenet of complex trauma treatment.

As a mind–body practice, yoga can unlock and uncover the body's history in a way that talk therapy alone does not. "The body's intelligence is largely an untapped resource in psychotherapy" (Ogden & Fisher, 2015, p. 13). Thus, whether you're a yoga professional who works with youth or adults only, a basic understanding of human development helps you better understand a client at any age.

## Case Study: Teresa

At 45 years old, Teresa is a highly successful head of a renewable energy start-up living in the US. She has lots of charisma and drive, three young boys, and an orange cat. She is also in the throes of a recent messy divorce. She identifies as a woman of color—her mother is Senegalese and her father German. Despite her outward success, she struggles with feelings of inadequacy. She left the 15-year marriage in which she felt undervalued. Yet she continues to feel "unseen" in a culture that also devalues women of color, despite her accomplishments. The way she combats this systemic racism is to excel at everything she does and be extra hard on herself.

Teresa was first referred to Michelle as a psychotherapy client (e.g., for talk therapy) to help her decrease anxiety, including perfectionism and a tendency to put others before herself. Despite being divorced for a little under a year, she notices she worries about what her ex-husband thinks of her. This frustrates her, and she wants to be free of this worry. But she says she cannot think her way out of what she feels. She said she liked that Michelle offered yoga therapy as part of her services, because she does yoga herself on a regular basis. "I've been told I over-intellectualize, so I think yoga may help me get out of my head and into my body and emotions more." As treatment progresses, they have used yoga therapy more and more in her sessions.

In yoga therapy, Teresa has been working on a yoga sequence for several weeks that helps her learn and practice self-compassion. She has her own yoga practice and naturally gravitates to active poses and vinyasa, avoiding relaxing ones. The exception is Child's Pose, which she says she finds calming and regulating (in yogic terms, *sattva*) most of the time.

Despite her preference for a challenging, active practice, Teresa notices that it brings up aggravation and self-aggression in her. She says she feels attached to those challenging poses and wants to push to do more and get better in a way that does not feel balanced to her. "I push in Chataranga the way I push at work. I used to feel strong and accomplished in tough poses—in fact, I still do. But sometimes it feels less like strength and more like a compulsive aggression, especially toward myself."

Yet as she stated, poses like Relaxation Pose (savasana) feel barely tolerable to Teresa. "I feel suffocated. If I'm in a yoga class, I'll just daydream to distract from how uncomfortable I am. If I'm at home doing yoga, I just don't do savasana." Before starting yoga therapy, she attempted a yin yoga workshop, and "felt like I was going to scream" because it was so hard for her to move slowly and relax. She also judges herself for not being able to relax.

Michelle suggested that she start where she is, rather than force herself into a relaxing yoga practice that is not in fact relaxing for her. Since she mentioned she liked Child's Pose (balasana), Michelle used this as the "center" of a vinyasa flow called the Wave. The Wave Vinyasa starts with Child's Pose, moves into Wave Pose, followed by Table Pose, and finally back to Child's Pose.

Because the Chataranga brings up feelings of self-aggression, Michelle suggested Table Pose where her arms press strongly into the floor (as in the push-up position) but her belly and legs can relax more, since the knees are holding some of the weight of her body. In the first round she said she felt strong but continued to feel some low-level aggravation that she deemed tolerable. She said she wanted to keep this pose in the sequence to see what happened. She also noticed some "floaty" feelings (a sign of *dissociation*, a trauma symptom that will be explored in Chapter 3) in Child's Pose in the first repetition. She said the floaty feeling diminished after practicing the vinyasa four times.

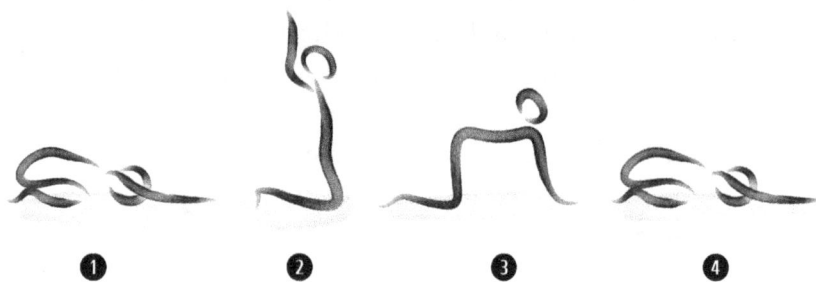

**Figure 2.1** Wave Vinyasa

*Depicts the Wave Vinyasa, which is useful for clients who prefer moving rather than stillness when they want to feel calm.*

During this same yoga therapy session, in each consecutive vinyasa, Teresa reported feeling less dissociation and aggravation, and more clarity. She said doing the Wave Vinyasa helped her explore what felt like two different parts of herself: a feisty, aggravated part of herself triggered in active poses like Chataranga, and a vulnerable self that she only barely became aware of during relaxing poses. She recognized that this vulnerability felt so unworkable that she had to "zone out" or dissociate. Yet when she alternated between these two poses in the vinyasa, she reported that she could tolerate the vulnerability and relax her usual armored, aggravated self. Through yoga therapy, she has begun to allow these two parts of herself to co-exist.

Throughout her sessions, Teresa has spoken of dualities she holds within her—the duality of her Senagalese-German heritage, the duality of code-switching from her home environment to that of her British school environment, and the duality of her vulnerable part and strong, armored part. Michelle suspects all this duality has created trauma for Teresa. As a "traditional" psychotherapist, Michelle suggests they also used the trauma treatment of "parts work" to help Teresa explore this. (*The Complex PTSD Treatment Manual* by Arielle Schwartz, 2021, offers an excellent mind–body approach to trauma and offers description of parts work.) Teresa recognized not only the split of her strong, protective self and vulnerable self, but also her cultural heritage split. As a woman of mixed race, she says she is often caught between two identities and struggles to reconcile them. "When I'm with my Caucasian relatives, I don't feel White enough. When I'm with my African family I don't feel Black enough. It's so frustrating."

Between the integrating movements of yoga therapy and the more cognitive process of psychotherapy, Teresa began to find some balance and synchronization with these different parts of herself. She says she is still a work in progress, but she feels more peace with her unique identity—whether or not others do. Though she says she was engaged in talk therapy by itself years ago, it did not feel totally effective on its own. She said it helped, but also felt incomplete. She says that the addition of yoga therapy helps her address her own internalized aggression about her race and body on a direct, physical level that feels more integrated and complete.

Teresa's childhood experiences of being a mixed-race girl in a white society informed her adult awareness of herself. Teresa's case gives us a window into how complex trauma can arise in the absence of war, sexual assault, or other overtly gruesome events. The day-to-day micro- and macro-aggressions of systemic racism, and the crisis of identity they cause for individuals, can be overlooked not only by others but also by the individual subjected to them.

Teresa's case shows too how important childhood is in the creation of one's sense of self. Now let's explore human development, examining it in terms of stages and types of development.

## Human Development Overview

Human development is one of the four golden threads, or building blocks, of this book. It is a big topic to tackle—entire books and college courses are dedicated to it. In this book we offer a general overview, detailing only those aspects that are most pertinent to yoga therapy. For simplicity, we divide human development into two sections: *Stages of Development* defines the three age divisions covered in this book, whereas *Types of Development* covers human development in four areas—musculoskeletal, social/emotional, cognitive, and neurobiological.

One unique feature of Chapter 2 is that it is a stand-alone reference guide. Throughout the chapter we consider the specific developmental tasks and changes for each of the three age groups. Summary tables are provided at the end of the chapter to help you distill the essential points covered.

We as authors have found that understanding human development and working with youth have given us a better appreciation of working with yoga clients at any age. Whether you work with youth or not, we hope that integrating developmental awareness into your own practice benefits you too.

## Stages of Development

First, let's consider three general stages of human development:

1. Childhood (5–12 years old)

2. Adolescence (13–18 years old)

3. Adulthood (19+ years old)

### Childhood

Childhood represents a period of rapid growth in all areas of development. Children's bodies grow quickly during this period, and they gain social skills by learning to follow rules. Cognitively, they are in the midst of language acquisition and learn through stories and games. Most children at this age don't understand metaphors just yet. Because this period is sometimes also referred to as "primary school age," we will use this term interchangeably throughout the book.

We start with the age of 5, because strategies used for children under the age of 5 years old tend to be less like yoga and more like play. In addition, we as authors have little experience working with infants and children below the age of 5 years and believe in staying within our scope of practice.

### Adolescence

In adolescence, musculoskeletal development continues but not at quite the same rapid pace as before. One of the biggest physical changes is secondary sex traits as puberty begins. In addition, major brain changes occur during this period of development (Eagleman, 2017; Siegel, 2014) that can impair an adolescent's judgment and make them prone to relational trauma (Schwartz, 2021). Cognitively, adolescents understand metaphors. Socially, they become attuned to their peers and may test boundaries and rules set by adult authority. Lastly, adolescents begin to develop their identities.

### Adulthood

Internationally the age of majority (when we are considered an adult) is between 18 and 20 years old, varying slightly from country to country. During this period of life, the body reaches its final stature, our cognitive and social/emotional skills are fully developed, and our personality structure is for the most part stable. By the time we're 25 years old, all major neurological development is also complete (Eagleman, 2017). Yet throughout life, we retain *neuroplasticity,* or the brain's ability to continue growing and changing in response to life (Eagleman, 2017; Psychology Today, 2024).

## Types of Development

Four areas of human development that are important for assessing and creating safe, effective yoga therapy treatment are:

1. Musculoskeletal

2. Social/emotional

3. Cognitive

4. Neurobiological

These four domains are vital for YPs, because they impact how we teach yoga to each age group. This includes (but is not limited to) how we relate to clients, the way we word instructions, length of pose "holds," duration of entire sequence, and what yoga techniques are appropriate.

All four types of development occur simultaneously as an individual develops, and there is a lot of overlap among them. Yet it is helpful to separate them to better understand some of the discrete changes of the developmental process that impact yoga therapy treatment for clients at each age and stage. During the initial assessment phase of yoga therapy, obtaining the individual's *current* level of development in each of these four areas is crucial for assessing a client's current skills. For both youth and adult clients, obtaining a *history* of development in these four domains is also crucial. This history helps the YP understand a client's overall functioning. And it is in the historical record that the YP may uncover a client's potential complex trauma.

We have provided a sample intake form appropriate for all ages in Appendix 1 for your review. All forms provided in the Appendices are ones we use in our own clinical practice, in teacher trainings, or both. These forms are simply offered for your consideration. In the following sections, examples are provided to illustrate how each domain of development relates to yoga therapy.

## Musculoskeletal Development

At birth, we are a fraction of our ultimate stature. Our proportions also change as we grow. These proportional differences from childhood into adolescence and finally into adulthood greatly impact an individual's center of gravity. For instance, a 5-year-old's head is a sixth of her height, whereas an adolescent's head is a little over a seventh of her height, and an adult's is a mere eighth of her height. This means the child's center of gravity is higher than that of an adolescent, whose center of gravity is also slightly higher than that of an adult. Understanding these proportion changes helps the YP better meet the physical needs of their youthful clients.

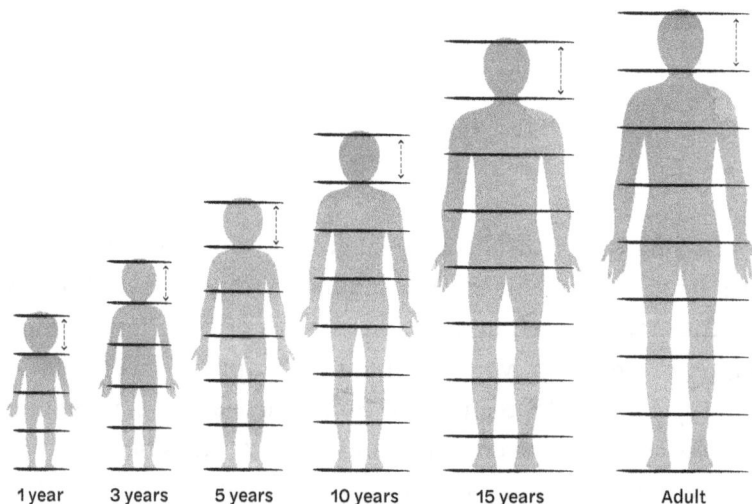

**Figure 2.2** Body Proportions

*Illustrates how the proportion of the head changes from one-fourth of a child's body at one year old to one-eighth of an adult's body.*

Let's consider how body proportions impact a common balancing pose like *Tree Pose*: of the three age groups presented in this book, a child will have the least ability to balance and may need a chair or wall for support. For instance, an 8-year-old child can hold the pose an average of 3–5 counts on each side. An adolescent can hold Tree an average of 5–10 counts, often without support. And a well-balanced adult can hold it freestanding for 30 seconds or so per side. From the musculoskeletal perspective, adolescents and adults differ greatly in their ability to balance, depending on how active and athletically engaged they are. In addition, growing limbs and torsos also impact children's and adolescents' strength, mobility, and endurance. In turn, these factors impact length, duration, and difficulty of physical activities for each age group.

The YP assesses a client's musculoskeletal needs during the intake process through a range of motion (ROM) assessment. If you do not already have a ROM assessment in your clinical yoga therapy practice, we recommend reading *Structural Yoga Therapy* (2012) by Mukunda Stiles, an expert in the field of anatomy and physiology of asana. Below are further musculoskeletal considerations for youth and adults.

## Musculoskeletal Considerations for Youth

Occupational and yoga therapist Mary Hallway teaches the musculoskeletal portion of one of Michelle's trainings, and offers the following musculoskeletal considerations for 5–19-year-olds (personal communication, 2022):

- Joint structure, ligaments and soft tissue are more flexible in children than in adults (Mirtz et al., 2011).

- Bone is still growing via epiphyseal growth plates up through the end of puberty (Mirtz et al., 2011).

- Physical activity and exercise support bone growth in children.

- Excessive and extreme activity can cause injury and damage in growth plates (Mirtz et al., 2011).

- **Formal pranayama should only be taught after the age of 8 years**. This is because the alveoli of their lungs have not yet fully developed before this age (Narayanan et al., 2012; Saraswati, 2003).

Hallway's recommendations demonstrate the "Goldilocks principle" of being "just right" when working with youth: regular physical activity is important for growing bodies, but not too much.

## Musculoskeletal Considerations for Adults

As noted above, the YP should conduct a ROM assessment during the intake process. For adult clients, the YP can also use Mukunda Stiles' *Joint-Freeing Series: Pavanamuktasana* (2000, available at https://guthrie.tricare.mil/Portals/67/4-%20Structural%20Yoga%20Therapy.pdf) as part of the ROM assessment.

## Social/Emotional Development

We are not merely smaller at birth. While most animals have some degree of mobility and functioning early on in development, humans are helpless for quite some time. We cannot walk, talk, feed ourselves, or even go to the bathroom on our own when we're first born. While this might seem like a disadvantage, it is by design. "Baby animals develop quickly because their brains are wiring up according to a largely preprogrammed routine" (Eagleman, 2017, p. 6).

For humans, being so unformed at birth allows our environment to shape us in a way that almost no other species does. We are molded by and adapt to the family we are born into. Neuroscientist and psychologist Lisa Feldman Barrett calls this our *cultural inheritance* (Corrigan, 2022, 9:07), because it is the way that information is passed from one generation to the next. So from a socially adaptive lens, our dependency actually helps us fit into our social environment.

## Attachment

Due to this initial dependency, the bonds we form early in life matter greatly. In the 1950s, British psychologist John Bowlby created Attachment Theory, which posits that humans are born with a need to bond with others (Ackerman, 2024). *Attachment* is the lasting emotional connection between two people (Ackerman, 2024; Sincero, 2012).

The need to bond with others is so great that when we do not receive it early in life, it impacts our relationships throughout life. Attachment Theory codifies four styles of attachment (Ackerman, 2024; Flaherty & Sadler, 2011; Sincero, 2012):

- Secure—a baby cries when the caregiver leaves and is comforted upon their return.

- Anxious—when a baby is anxiously attached, it cries when the caregiver leaves but then is difficult to comfort when the caregiver returns. Sometimes this style of attachment is called "resistant," because the infant resists comfort (Ackerman, 2024).

- Avoidant—a baby shows avoidant attachment when it barely recognizes that the caregiver left or has returned.

- Disorganized—a baby who shows unpredictable behavior when a caregiver leaves and returns is said to have disorganized attachment.

Secure attachment evolves when a caregiver is responsive and nurturing toward the child most of the time. This doesn't mean caregivers need to get it right all the time. What's more important is being a "good enough" parent (Winnicott, 1953, p. 94). This means a caregiver makes the child their priority but is at peace with making mistakes (Cavell & Quetsch, 2023).

Attachment Theory helps us understand how and why early relationships with caregivers play such an outsized role in a child's development, self-concept, and later relationships. In this way, Attachment Theory plays a major role in how we assess and treat clients with complex trauma.

## Somatic Psychology's Take on Attachment

One exciting development in the theory of attachment is the role that movement plays in healthy development, and healing from trauma. Part of our model includes a concept from somatic psychology called the fundamental movements. In Chapter 5 we will explore how the first movements we make are in service of forming and sustaining those crucial early attachments (May, 2022). In this sense, our movements also play an important role in our development and relational health.

## Social Learning

Lev Vygotsky said that the social environment is also crucial to a child's cognitive development (McCleod, 2024). School-age children can cooperate with others and take others' points of view. As mentioned earlier, they learn from and like rules. If you forget one of your own rules while leading a children's yoga therapy group, one of the children will likely remind you! Rules help children learn the social norms of their society. School-age children are socially attuned to adults and are eager to please. They tend to like group activities and show friendliness and generosity toward others. They also show persistence and focus when learning new skills. We will explore how social development is linked to cognitive development in the next section.

Demonstrating poses for one another in a group yoga setting is excellent for children's social/emotional development. *Student demonstration* is when a child demonstrates a yoga pose to the rest of their peers using an age-appropriate yoga flashcard to guide their instructions. When a YP invites child participants to demonstrate yoga poses, it teaches them a wealth of social skills: how to follow rules, how to take turns, how to lead, and how to show respect and kindness to others.

By contrast, adolescents are more attuned to their peer group. They may test rules and limits. Adolescents are also developing secondary sex traits, so they are often self-conscious. As a result, peer demonstration of yoga poses is *not recommended* in the adolescent group setting. In addition, it is important to be mindful of how adolescents' yoga mats are positioned in relation to one another so that their backsides are not facing each other. A good strategy to engage this age group is to invite adolescents who have a positive view of yoga to share with the group what they like about it. Adolescents not only cooperate with and take others' views; they also have an increased ability to empathize (compared to their younger peers).

## Cognitive

Cognitive development is defined as "the development of knowledge, skills, problem solving and dispositions, which help children to think about and understand the world around them" (Huang, 2021, p. 28). It includes neurological and psychological development, though for our purposes we will discuss neurological development separately.

Moving increases cognitive development (Mualem et al., 2018), so physical activities like yoga are great for children and adolescents. A child learns better and more fully when a physical movement is tied to a cognitive concept (Bidzan-Bluma & Lipowska, 2018). For example, if children learn a song about the Sun Salutation while practicing it, they will learn the movements and the concepts in the song better. The Sun Salutation movements and the song about them reinforce one another.

The most widely used theories of cognitive development were created by Swiss psychologist Jean Piaget (1896–1980) and Russian psychologist Lev Vygotsky (1896–1934). While there is a lot of overlap in their theories, Piaget focused more on a child's self-initiated discovery, whereas Vygotsky emphasized the social environment's influence on a child's cognitive development (McCleod, 2024).

Vygotsky (1978) said that adults are the *More Knowledgeable Other* (MKO) in a child's life. (Note: Vygotsky's book *Mind in Society* was translated from Russian in 1978 after his death.) The MKO can be a teacher, parent, or even peer who "provides guidance and modeling to enable the child to learn skills within their *zone of proximal development* [ZPD] (the gap between what a child can do independently and what they can achieve with guidance)" (McCleod, 2024).

One small study examined the effectiveness of learning through the ZPD (Vygotsky's theory) versus self-initiated discovery (Piaget's theory). In this study, Freund (1990, as cited in McCleod, 2024) found that children learn better when guided by an adult (an example of learning through the ZPD) than on their own (self-discovery learning). Student demonstration of yoga poses is an example of learning through the ZPD because the child demonstrating the pose has the support, guidance, and encouragement of the YP (the MKO).

When working with youth, both Vygotsky's and Piaget's models are helpful to know because many pediatric professions use them—from teachers to school counselors to medical providers. Piaget's model is especially convenient because it is divided into four distinct stages. The YouTube channel Sprouts created a handy video of the stages: www.youtube.com/watch?v=IhcgYgx7aAA

The following is an amalgamated summary of Piaget's stages (Fishman, 2023; Practical Psychology, 2023; Sprouts, 2018). It includes notes from the authors about how each stage relates to yoga therapy.

## Sensorimotor Stage (0–2 years old)

In this first stage, a child learns about the world through sensation and movement. They also learn through cause and effect. For instance, if they squeeze a dog toy it makes a squeaky sound. The main goal of this stage is to understand *object permanence,* "the concept that objects exist even if you can't see them" (Fishman, 2023). If mom leaves the room, a child of this age believes that Mom ceases to exist.

As noted earlier, this book addresses yoga therapy for persons 5 years and older. Postnatal and early childhood yoga therapy and practices are outside the authors' scope of practice. Yet a general understanding of this stage gives the YP an appreciation for the importance of movement and sensation from the very beginning of life.

## Preoperational Stage (2–7 years old)

In this stage, a child develops memory and imagination, learns to imitate others, and begins to engage in make-believe or pretend play. (If a child at this age does not engage in pretend-play and does not seem to imitate or reciprocate with others, they may benefit from a neurodiversity assessment.) Children at this age are *egocentric,* meaning they think everything is connected to them.

This is also the stage of *magical thinking,* "the idea that a person's thoughts, wishes, or sometimes actions may influence the course of our world" (Practical Psychology, 2023, "What is magical thinking?" section). Common through to the age of 10 years old, magical thinking is the reason children believe in Santa Claus or the tooth fairy. The main goal of this stage is symbolic thought, and magical thinking is a natural manifestation of this. Incorporating stories and make-believe play into yoga therapy increases a child's interest and facilitates their learning.

If a child has a diagnosis of autism spectrum disorder or other neurodiversity, they learn yoga best through visual learning. For instance, a YP can use colorful yoga flashcards, demonstrate the pose, and offer clear, simple instructions for these children.

### Concrete Operational Stage (7–11 years old)

At this stage, a child can think logically and begins to understand the *law of conservation*. For example, if water is poured from a wide vessel into a tall, thin vessel the child understands that the amount of water is the same. The child also develops an understanding that their feelings are unique, and not necessarily shared by others. This is the beginning of empathy. The main goal of this stage is operational thought. Children at this stage are very literal, and do not understand metaphors.

Because children are curious and excited about learning at this stage, they like to learn new things. They respond well when a YP relates what they have learned in school to yoga. For example, if they have learned in science that trees give off oxygen and humans need oxygen, the YP can tie this scientific fact to instructions on full yogic breathing. As mentioned previously, children at this age love stories. They learn best when yoga is presented in stories and interactive games.

### Formal Operational Stage (12+ years old)

Adolescents can think abstractly, make hypotheses, and understand theories. In addition, they develop self-awareness and morality, which leads to compassion and understanding for others. Sometimes adolescents get a bad rap for being self-absorbed. Interestingly, this stage of development does mirror that of the defiant, egocentric 2-year-old. While adolescents may challenge rules and question authority, most are usually open to adults who take the time to explain things, as well as take them and their questions seriously.

Adolescents benefit from understanding how their interests relate to yoga. For instance, if an adolescent likes football, let them know what popular teams do yoga as a regular part of practice. Because adolescents can think abstractly, many enjoy the philosophical teachings of yoga. When presented in a secular way, yoga philosophy can help adolescents think about their lives and choices in meaningful ways.

## Neurobiological Development

Neurobiological development describes how brain structures develop. By contrast, cognitive development is "what we do with what we got" (Berude, 2018, "Definition" section). Whereas Piaget and Vygotsky postulated their theories of cognitive development in the field of social science in the early 1900s, current understanding of neurobiological development has evolved significantly in the last few decades, giving us a more robust understanding of human development.

In this book, we draw upon several contemporary brain science resources such as Daniel Siegel, Lisa Feldman Barrett, Bruce Perry, David Eagleman, and others. In Chapter 4, we use Bruce Perry's Sequence of Engagement model (2020a) to explore the role of neurobiological dysregulation in CPTSD. While Stephen Porges' Polyvagal Theory (2011) is often used for this purpose in yoga therapy and mind–body circles, we have chosen to focus on Perry's work. The Sequence of Engagement aligns well with both Attachment Theory and our own model, and we feel it is best to stick with one theory. It is important to point out that *all* models are oversimplifications of the complex processes that occur in the brain (C. Rosner Or-Bach & A. Maron-Katz, personal communication, June 17, 2024).

For now, let's consider neurobiological development through life. When we are born our brain is a quarter of the size of a mature brain. By the time we are 6 years old, the brain has grown to be 90% of its final size (Casey et al., 2008). That is a lot of growth in a short amount of time.

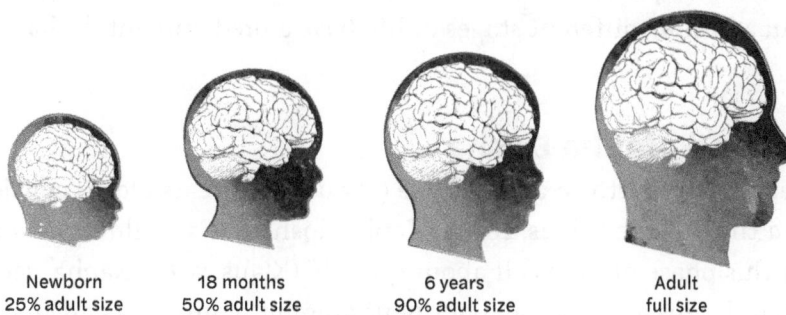

| Newborn | 18 months | 6 years | Adult |
| 25% adult size | 50% adult size | 90% adult size | full size |

**Figure 2.3** Head Size
*Depicts brain growth and head size from birth to adulthood*

The Centers for Disease Control and Prevention (CDC) in the United States (2023) says three factors are most important to a child's brain development: proper nutrition, avoidance of exposure to toxins, and the child's experiences with people and its world. This last factor is crucial for YPs: being a caring, reliable adult in a child's life can bolster positive experiences. It is an example of a *protective factor*, or a positive condition that supports a child's healthy development and protects them from stressful events. For now, the most important point is that when offered in a developmentally appropriate way, yoga therapy can be a protective factor that bolsters a child's positive experiences thereby reducing the negative impact of stressors in other areas of their life.

There are two critical periods of brain development: 1) early childhood (birth to 8 years old) when children are building their primary attachments to caregivers (CDC, 2023; Schwartz, 2021), and 2) adolescence (13 to 18 years old) when brain changes cause an increase in emotionality and impulsivity (Ford, 2020; Schwartz, 2021; Siegel, 2014).

Understanding these brain changes and how they impact a child's behavior, learning, and affect are crucial to offering safe, effective yoga therapy. For instance, a 10-year-old who initially loves the rules of their yoga therapy sessions may start to question them when they are 12 years old. Rather than take this change personally, we as the YP can recognize that their brain has probably developed and changed, which in turn changes their behavior.

Let's consider these two developmental windows in terms of Ayurveda and neurobiology. Ayurveda posits three *doshas*, the constituents of humans' biological existence (Frawley, 1999) that relate to the five elements: *kapha dosha* (earth and water), *pitta dosha* (fire), and *vata dosha* (ether and air). While all living beings possess all three doshas, individuals have differing ratios of each. In addition, different stages of life have a predominant dosha.

## Childhood: Kapha Dosha

The period from birth to adolescence (about 15–16 years old) is considered a *kapha* time of life (Klaus, 2023). "Kapha dosha has a building quality to it, and this phase of life is all about growth" (Klaus, 2023, "Kapha" section). Children's brains are doing an enormous amount of growing and changing.

From birth to 2.5 years old, *neurons* rapidly build connections (*synapses*) with the help of another type of brain cell called *glia*. During this time, children build approximately one million new connections every second (Zerotothree, 2024). Then suddenly, at around 2.5 years old, this process reverses. From 2 to 10 years old, *synaptic pruning* takes over. Synaptic pruning is "the process by which extra neurons and synaptic connections are eliminated in order to increase the efficiency of neuronal transmissions" (Santos & Noggle, 2011, p. 1464). Tohoku University researchers in Japan found (2022) that microglia may assist in synaptic pruning, which may enhance learning and memory.

## Development of Self-Regulation

Around the same time of life (birth to 3 years old), a child's interactions with a stable, safe, and nurturing environment allows them to develop the first stage of *self-regulation* in the form of flexible attention—that is, the ability to shift attention internally or externally (Ford, 2020). From toddlerhood through early primary school years, normal brain growth leads to the development of the *learning brain* (Ford, 2020, p. 43), which allows a child to exercise beginnings of self-control. For instance, a healthy 5-year-old can problem solve to handle frustration and disappointment.

Ford (2020) says that by primary school a child's ability to control emotions allows them to actively engage in learning and develop social competence. Thus, when a child is well-regulated (they have control over their emotions) they can learn and socialize.

## Adolescence: Pitta Dosha

Ayurveda says that adolescents transition into a pitta stage of life around 15 or 16 years old (Klaus, 2023). Pitta dosha relates to the element of fire, and this period from adolescence through adulthood is marked with identity formation, skill acquisition, ambition, competition, and achieving goals.

Recall Teresa: as an adult she was very competitive and hard on herself. She told her YP Michelle that she learned to be this way as an adolescent, playing competitive sports like field hockey. She received a lot of praise for her skill and strategy in the game. When she felt self-conscious about being the only girl of color on the team and in school, she leaned on her newfound identity as a capable competitor. This was a positive adaptation that helped her deal with her white friends' gaffes, such as when one friend marveled at how dark her face looked after being flushed in the heat of a game. "I think I started to over-rely on this image of myself as strong and capable at the expense of allowing softer, more vulnerable feelings."

The fiery quality of pitta in adolescence also presents as impulsive behavior and mood swings (Ford, 2020; Siegel, 2014), which are often blamed on hormones. While hormones play a role in adolescents' behavior (Corrigan, 2022), child psychiatrist and best-selling author Daniel Siegel (2014) says that another culprit is a "remodeling state" of the brain that explains the challenges adolescents experience in cognitive control, emotion regulation, and susceptibility to peer influence. Let's consider these three domains in more detail.

## Cognitive Control

First, the prefrontal cortex undergoes a total reconstruction that temporarily causes disruption in connectivity with other parts of the brain (Siegel, 2014). Like a messy construction site, the prefrontal region loses access to other brain areas throughout the remodeling process. Even physical actions like coordination and balance are affected during this stage.

In addition, *myelination* starts in adolescence. Myelin is a fatty layer that covers the remodeled synaptic connections (Siegel, 2014). A myelinated synapse fires 3000 times faster than an unmyelinated synapse. The result is that the individual can think more globally and generalize in ways they could not before.

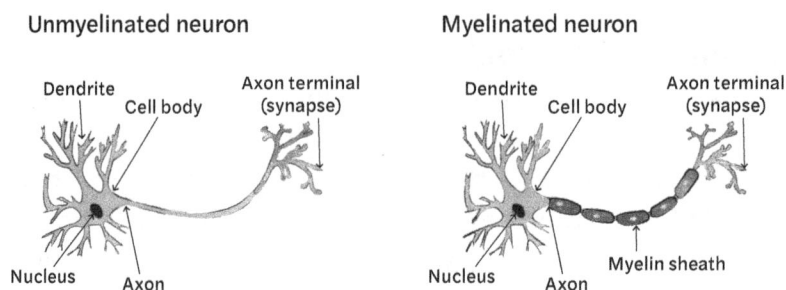

**Figure 2.4** Unmyelinated and Myelinated Neurons
*Depicts an unmyelinated and a myelinated neuron, which fires 3000 times faster than the unmyelinated neuron.*

*White matter* is a term used to describe *myelinated axons* (the tail of a neuron that connects and delivers impulses to other neurons). White matter (that is, the result of myelination) steadily increases from childhood through early adulthood (Deoni et al., 2016), and progresses from the back of the brain (brainstem) to the front (prefrontal cortex) (Konrad et al., 2013). This means that brain areas such as the prefrontal cortex mature later than the cortical areas associated with sensory and motor tasks (Konrad et al., 2013). As a result, adolescents feel and act before they think (Perry & Winfrey, 2021).

## Emotion Regulation

Second, adolescents experience emotions more strongly than either their younger counterparts or adults. While there is controversy in the neuroscience world about exactly *why* this is the case (Feldman Barrett, 2017), there seems to be agreement that all the brain changes in adolescents can cause emotional dysregulation. Along with experiencing strong feelings, adolescents are also prone to *naive realism*, the belief that the way they see the world is objective reality rather than their own biased, personal perception (Corrigan, 2022).

## Susceptibility to Others' Influence

Arguably the most significant vulnerability in adolescence with regards to complex trauma is their susceptibility to others' influence.

Feldman Barrett points out that all humans regardless of age are susceptible to others' influence, because we are "context-driven animals" (Corrigan, 2022, 16:14) who are influenced by many factors including who we are with. But as noted earlier, adolescents tend to rely less on family members and adults, and more on the emotional support and advice of friends, who are at the same stage of life as they are. When coupled with impaired judgment (a tendency to act before they think) and strong emotionality, it is no wonder that adolescents are particularly vulnerable to relational trauma (Schwartz, 2021).

## Adolescence: A Second Chance

Despite the vulnerabilities and upheaval of adolescence, it is also a period of second chances. Siegel (2014) says we move from the generalized potential of childhood to the specialization of adolescence. These changes collectively enhance the brain's integration and efficiency, equipping adolescents with the cognitive tools that can benefit them in various aspects of life.

Repeated practice of a skill lays down myelination (Siegel, 2014). The more an adolescent practices yoga, the more it becomes a habit and a skill. Feldman Barrett (Corrigan, 2022) points out that **moving the body is one of the most effective ways to increase emotion regulation because movement changes perceptions**. In this way, yoga and yoga therapy offer adolescents powerful ways to take control of their experience and regulate their emotions.

## Adulthood: Pitta and Vata Doshas
### Pitta Dosha Stage of Adulthood

Ayurvedic medicine practitioner Jo Formosa (2017) says that the pitta stage of life extends through the age of 50. From the Ayurvedic point of view, this is a time of life when many are juggling multiple responsibilities from work to children to householder duties (Formosa, 2017). For many of us, early and middle adulthood is a time when we are still figuring out who we are and what we want.

As a 45-year-old, Teresa was living in the pitta stage of adulthood when she sought out yoga therapy. Her divorce had brought her internal identity struggle to the surface. She could feel she'd become over-reliant on her self-image of being strong and capable. Now she was ready to expand her identity to include a more vulnerable side. With the help of yoga therapy, she learned how to slow down—not all at once, but little by little. By progressively staying in Child's Pose longer and longer with each round of her Wave Vinyasa, she was able to relax and "soften," as she put it.

### Vata Dosha Stage of Adulthood

By the age of 50 and beyond, many of us have learned valuable lessons from life, and know who we are. On the other hand, whatever ways we have neglected our health or well-being also show up. It is harder to recover from injury and illness at this stage. So it is also an optimal time to create healthy habits.

Vata is the final stage of life, which includes qualities of light, cold, dry, and more flexibility (Formosa, 2017). Vata shows up as dry skin, brittle bones, arthritis and joint pain, digestive issues, as well as decreases in mental flexibility. But by staying physically active, and learning new things, one can enjoy a healthy life.

One of Michelle's yoga therapy clients, Joe, is a 53-year-old Mexican American man, who sought talk therapy to treat debilitating anxiety. Early on in his treatment, it became clear that he had symptoms of complex trauma because of a near-drowning experience as a toddler, systemic racism as a man of color, and prolonged stress when his wife was diagnosed with breast cancer 10 years ago. (She has now been in remission for 9 years.) When these CPTSD issues came to light, Michelle and Joe agreed it would be best to incorporate yoga therapy to increase his "toolbox" of coping strategies. We will learn more about Joe's journey in Chapter 3.

For now, let's fast forward to Joe's current status to get a sense of how yoga therapy can facilitate the vata stage of life. In his fourth year of yoga therapy, he has made many health gains that position him to age gracefully. By using deep breathing that he learned in yoga therapy, he calmed his anxiety and panic attacks. By consulting a dietician, Joe learned healthier eating habits and minimized stomach irritation that often flared up when he was stressed. He took up doubles tennis with his youngest daughter to bond with her and to learn a new skill. And currently in his yoga therapy sessions, he has become fond of lying over a yoga bolster while Michelle leads him through Yoga Nidra. "When I lie on the bolster, and extend my limbs out, I feel like the stress is draining out my fingers and toes like water out of one of those CamelBak bags you take on hikes!" Joe and Michelle had a chuckle about that apt image.

## Self-Care Practice: Happy Moment

We invite you now to consider a happy memory from your own childhood. Pick a memory that evokes playfulness, childlike wonder, and/or connectedness with someone special. Maybe it was a summer vacation or time spent with a grandparent or best friend. Perhaps learning to ride your bike brought a sense of awe or freedom in your life that you had not experienced before. Not everyone has happy memories of childhood. Alternatively, you may visualize a favorite animal, color, scent, mastering of a skill, or person from any stage of your life who evokes feelings of calm and connection.

Once you have your memory in mind, you may want to close your eyes to visualize it fully. Use your five senses to recall it. What do you see? What can you hear? Do you smell anything? How do you feel? Is anyone with you?

As you recall this happy moment in time, bring your attention to your body. What body sensations do you notice? Is there a light smile on your face? A feeling of warmth or lightness in your chest? Do you feel like laughing? Allow yourself to fully feel where this memory lives in your body.

You may want to take some deep breaths in and long, slow breaths out. Allow yourself to fully feel where this memory lives in your body. Stay with this body scan practice as long as it feels natural for you.

## Chapter Summary

- Humans develop more slowly than any other animal on earth. Our relatively "slow" development allows our environment to shape us. It also allows us to adapt to the unique circumstances we're born into.

- The first three years of life are critical to an individual's overall development.

- A child's school age years are a window of opportunity to bolster protective factors and minimize risk factors.

- Yoga therapy is an excellent practice to introduce to school age kids, who naturally attune to stable, caring adults who offer them consistent rules and boundaries.

- Adolescence is a second window of opportunity when the brain is being remodeled through both synaptic pruning and myelination.

- Adolescents are developing a sense of self- and social identity, which includes adopting their core values. This age group can benefit from learning about yoga philosophy as they develop their values.

- Yoga therapy can teach clients of all ages to develop healthy body image and habits, confidence, good judgment, and positive coping skills that will last a lifetime.

## CHAPTER 3

# CPTSD—Causes, Consequences, and Solutions

The subject of complex trauma is... complex. In this book we examine its complexity one facet at a time. In Chapter 1 we looked at complex trauma from the widest lens—its definition and its global prevalence. In Chapter 2, we considered four domains of human development that are essential in pediatric yoga therapy. Now in Chapter 3 we combine these two broad topics together to explore the impact of complex trauma in childhood. We'll investigate the **causes** of CPTSD through the lenses of adverse childhood experiences, the timing of those experiences, protective and risk factors, and epigenetics; we'll consider the **consequences** of CPTSD by viewing the roller coaster of symptoms that result; and we'll examine **healing solutions** that integrate yoga therapy with the latest treatment modalities.

## Yoga, Ayurveda, and Complex Trauma

Complex trauma is a loss of rhythm—the very rhythm that makes life safe, stable, and enjoyable (Chapter 1). It throws life out of balance—or homeostasis, in scientific parlance. One of the reasons yoga is so effective for complex trauma is that it aims to restore balance, which is also the aim of its "sister science" of Ayurveda (Frawley, 1999). Ayurveda shares many understandings and concepts with current research, especially epigenetics (Sharma & Keith Wallace, 2020).

Throughout Chapter 3, we offer Ayurveda as a conceptual framework. Ayurveda means "life science" (Feuerstein et al., 1995, p. 212). Feuerstein and colleagues (1995) note that Ayurvedic concepts were part of the Vedic canon as far back as 150–350 AD, and its surgical techniques remained ahead of European techniques until the 18th century.

Yoga and Ayurveda evolved together and have influenced each other throughout their shared history (Frawley, 1999). Yoga is the "science of Self-realization" (1999, p. 5): it addresses the needs of the body *first* to transcend awareness to one's true nature, which is said to be joyful and full of awe. On the other hand, Ayurveda is the "science of Self-healing aimed at relieving diseases of body and mind" (Frawley, 1999, p. 5). In this sense, Ayurveda is ready-made for the treatment of CPTSD symptoms, which also impact body and mind.

## The Gunas

In the Ayurvedic system, the mind—and the experience of consensus reality—is made up of three qualities, or *gunas*: sattva, rajas, and tamas (Feuerstein et al., 1995; Sullivan, 2020; Wheeler, 2021). *Sattva* is a state of harmony and lucidity (Feuerstein et al., 1995); *rajas* is the principle of change, high energy, and "dynamism" (1995, p. 213); and *tamas* is its opposite with qualities of stability, low energy, and lack of movement.

Derived from the five-element theory of Samkhya philosophy, the gunas are the "constituents of reality" (Wheeler, 2021, p. 66). Many traditional medicines including Ayurveda, shamanism, and Native American practices base their philosophy and application on the five elements. Even quantum physics shares some foundational ideas with Samkhya philosophy (Wheeler, 2021). In the *Yoga Sutras*, Patanjali narrows the five elements into the three mental states of the gunas, according to Wheeler.

The gunas are a very important component of CPTSD-informed yoga therapy, because they are key to understanding the *psychology* of yoga (Mohan & Mohan, 2004, p. 10). Yoga therapist Marlyssa Sullivan (2020) points out that the gunas "create the myriad manifestations of thought, emotion, physiological state, and experience" (p. 64).

### First Law of the Gunas

The gunas are present in all aspects of life from the external environment to the physical body to the inner workings of the mind (Sullivan, 2020). Their constant and dynamic interplay creates the manifest world. This is the first law of the gunas, the *law of alternation* (Frawley, 1999). Ayurvedic and yoga scholar David Frawley (1999) likens this interplay to the times of day: "Night as darkness belongs to tamas, sunrise and sunset as transitional periods relate to rajas, and day as light corresponds to sattva" (p. 28).

## Second Law of the Gunas

The second law of the gunas is the *law of continuity* (Frawley, 1999). Continuing with the movement of time metaphor, Frawley (1999) notes that much like night and day last for a length of time before transitioning to the next phase, so each guna endures for a time before transforming into the next. And just as day and night last longer than sunrise and sunset, so too do sattva and tamas tend to last longer than changeable rajas.

When the gunas are in balance, health and well-being abound. They create a harmonious flow embodied by the ever-changing rhythm of life, also known as homeostasis. For instance, Sullivan (2020) says that in a healthy body sattva is vitality, rajas is the body's movements like digestion and repair, and tamas is the skeletal and structural stability (p. 60). In a balanced psychological state, Sullivan says tamas provides stability and boundaries; rajas provides the energy and momentum for needed change and growth; and sattva provides the equilibrium and equanimity to accept one's life as it is. The three are intertwined, interdependent parts of the whole, as shown in Figure 3.1.

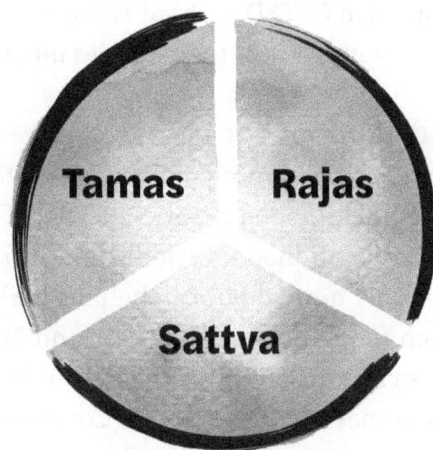

**Figure 3.1** The Gunas
*Infographic depicts the interdependent and holistic nature of the three gunas—sattva, tamas, and rajas.*

At time of press there are not many well-designed studies showing Ayurveda's overall efficacy (National Center for Complementary and Integrative Health, 2024). In this sense, we are not inferring that any Ayurvedic concepts mentioned here have been proven by the scientific method. Yet given

Ayurveda's longevity over the millennia, it clearly has stood the test of time. We hope more rigorous research is eventually done on Ayurveda, because of its parallels to yoga and modern scientific study.

## Causes

The causes of complex trauma include abuse, neglect, interpersonal violence, community violence, racism, discrimination, torture, kidnapping, slavery, and war (UK Trauma Council, 2024). As previously noted, the four key features of CPTSD are extreme threat, repetition of that threat, little or no escape possible (lack of control), and interpersonal trauma (Courtois & Ford, 2016; NCTSN, 2023; Schwartz, 2021). Complex trauma most often occurs in childhood or adolescence but can happen anytime throughout the lifespan (Courtois & Ford, 2016; Schwartz, 2021).

Because the circumstances and events that give rise to complex trauma vary greatly, some experts suggest that complex trauma should be sorted into different categories (Ford, 2020; Liberzon, 2018). For instance, the symptoms resulting from complex trauma that includes sexual assault or exploitation are often more extreme than CPTSD without it (Keith & Skidmore, 2024). At press, though, CPTSD encompasses both categories into one diagnostic label.

### Adverse Childhood Experiences

Since complex trauma is often synonymous with childhood trauma, it is useful to consider adverse childhood experiences. All of us experience some degree of adversity in our childhood. Periodic and infrequent amounts of stress in youth are not only normal but can help us build distress tolerance for life. However, when the frequency, duration, and intensity of adversity tip the scale, trauma can result. And when that adversity is chronic, extreme, and longstanding it becomes complex trauma (Courtois & Ford, 2016; Ford & Courtois, 2020; Schwartz, 2021). In the US, the Centers for Disease Control and Prevention (CDC) and Kaiser Permanente (an American insurance company) conducted a study from 1995 to 1997 that explored the types and frequency of adverse events that can lead to childhood trauma. Surveying over 17,000 patients, this study was "one of the largest investigations of childhood abuse and neglect and household challenges, and later-life health and well-being" (CDC, 2021, "About the CDC-Kaiser ACE study" section).

This study coined the term *adverse childhood experiences* (ACEs), which refers to "potentially traumatic events that occur" before a person turns 18 years old (CDC, 2024, para. 1). The ACEs framework and its resulting self-report questionnaire has received some well-founded criticism: the questionnaire is not standardized, and it is very general (Kelly-Irving & Delpierre, 2019; Pondisco, 2020). This means the ACEs questionnaire is not a diagnostic tool and can be "misappropriated" as if it were used as such a screening tool (Pondisco, 2020, para. 5). Despite these critiques, the invention of the term adverse childhood experiences is quite useful with regards to complex trauma and is used ubiquitously in schools and mental health settings.

## Timing
### Childhood Onset of CPTSD

The ACEs study highlights the important role that timing plays with regards to adversity and trauma over the lifespan. Courtois and Ford (2016) point out that the younger the child is, the more readily traumatized they are by less severe events. As highlighted in Chapter 2, there are two critical periods in a child's life: 1) early childhood—the first eight years (CDC, 2023; Schwartz, 2021)—when children are building their primary attachments to caregivers, and 2) adolescence, when brain changes cause an increase in emotionality and impulsivity (Ford, 2020; Schwartz, 2021).

If a child does not have a safe, nurturing environment and caregivers, and "the child is exposed to traumatic stressors or complex trauma, their attention will become selectively focused on threat" leading to an over-emphasis on the *survival brain* (Ford, 2020, p. 44). Adolescents are particularly vulnerable to relational trauma (Schwartz, 2021), because of major reorganization in the brain.

### Adult Onset of CPTSD

Adult onset of CPTSD is different than an adult who is suffering the lingering effects of CPTSD that occurred in childhood. We are referring specifically to adults who did not experience trauma in childhood but develop it due to events that occur as an adult. Causes for adult-onset complex trauma may include interpersonal violence (such as domestic abuse), war, kidnapping, community violence, genocide, slavery, repeated sexual assault and/or exploitation, and systemic racism. While this book focuses primarily on child-onset CPTSD, complex trauma can and does occur in adulthood (Blue Knot, 2021).

## Protective and Risk Factors

Whether or not a child develops CPTSD depends greatly on the protective versus risk factors (CDC, 2024) at these critical periods of development. As mentioned in Chapter 2, *protective factors* are positive aspects of a child's life that can counterbalance negative stressors. Conversely, *risk factors* increase the likelihood of trauma or complex trauma. Each set of factors can be categorized into individual, family, or community aspects. Table 3.1 shows some examples of both protective and risk factors.

**Table 3.1** lists protective and risk factors that influence a child's overall well-being.

| Protective Factors | Risk Factors |
|---|---|
| *Individual* | |
| Does well in school | Does poorly in school/requires frequent redirection or consequences |
| Positive friend or peer group | Isolation from friends or peers |
| *Family* | |
| Caregivers with steady income | Caregivers with low or unsteady income, food, or other resources |
| Families who create safe, stable, and nurturing relationship | Caregivers who are abusive and/or have mental health issues |
| *Community* | |
| Safe community environment with lots of natural supports | High rates of crime and violence (due to war or other factors) |
| Access to good healthcare, schools, and community resources | Limited or no access to healthcare, schools, or nutritious food |

Another important risk factor not mentioned in the ACEs study is social media (most likely due to the timing of the study in the late 1990s before social media had taken off). In a 2023 report, the US Surgeon General expressed deep concern about the negative impact of social media on youth, noting how scrolling social media can increase the risk that a child will isolate from friends, become anxious and/or depressed, develop negative perspectives of diverse groups, and increase polarized views (US Department of Health and Human Services, 2023).

YPs can be a protective factor by being one more stable force in clients' lives. In fact, we as YPs may be the only adult who recognizes the child or adolescent in a positive way. In addition, when we recognize that a client is struggling with risk factors, we can refer them to additional mental health or community resources that further bolster their protective factors.

## Epigenetics and Intergenerational Trauma

Epigenetics offers another important perspective on the timing of trauma. *Epigenetics* (also *epigenomics*) is "the science of how the environment—both social and biologic—impacts the gene" (Brockman, 2024). We are born with a fixed set of DNA that doesn't change, but the epigenome can turn genes on or off (Foo, 2022). Ford (2020) says that internal and external stressors can activate certain genes that lead to all levels of trauma.

Epigenetics also reveals that trauma can be passed down. In her book *What My Bones Know: A Memoir of Healing from Complex Trauma* (2022), journalist and podcast producer Stephanie Foo offers a powerful account of how epigenetics informs current understanding of intergenerational trauma: "There is real scientific evidence that the traumas we experience can be passed on to our children and even grandchildren... Both the genome and epigenome are passed down generationally" (2022, p. 200).

*Intergenerational trauma* is defined as trauma experienced by a group of people that negatively impacts the health and well-being of future generations (Ullah et al., 2023). It is caused by a multitude of factors including socioeconomic instability, poverty, natural disasters, genocide, war, migration, refugee status, racism, oppression, and domestic violence, to name a few (Foo, 2022; Isobel et al., 2019; Ullah et al., 2023). Like CPTSD, intergenerational trauma is often transmitted through the attachment relationship (i.e., the parent–child relationship) and can lead to further relational trauma (Isobel et al., 2019).

The most effective approach to intergenerational trauma is prevention. This includes 1) trauma-focused interventions for caregivers and adults, and 2) relational-focused interventions for children and families (Isobel et al., 2019). "Preventative strategies need to target individual, relationship, familial, community and societal levels, as addressing and preventing trauma requires a multipronged, multisystemic approach" (Isobel et al., 2019, "Conclusions" section).

Part of a multipronged approach is creating repair where damage has already occurred. At the level of society, communal repair is needed (Isobel et al., 2019; Jeyasundaram et al., 2020; Ullah et al., 2023) through such actions as financial reparations (Ullah et al., 2023), restorative justice, and psychosocial repair in the form of trauma-informed therapy (Jeyasundaram et al., 2020). At the level of family, relational trauma therapy among family members is needed (Isobel et al., 2019).

A global groundswell of yoga professionals are pioneering trauma-informed yoga programs at the community level. A small sampling of these exciting programs includes Jessica Barudin's "culturally adapted" yoga program for Indigenous adolescent girls (2021, p. 21); Beth Shaw's YogaFit Yoga for Intergenerational and Collective Trauma (YogaFit, 2024); Nityanda Gessel's Trauma-Conscious Yoga Method (the Trauma Conscious Yoga Institute, 2024); and Lee Watson's Fierce Calm (Fierce Calm, 2024).

On the yoga therapy front, pioneers are also emerging. One such pioneer is Mimi Felton, owner and founder of Mimi's Yoga Kids (www.mimisyogakids. com). In 2018 Felton started her community yoga and wellness space near Atlanta, Georgia, after discovering the healing benefits of yoga with her young grandson. She recalled that she was the only woman of color when she'd go to yoga classes. She wanted to share this great resource with her community, and when she couldn't find what she was looking for, she created her own.

Her next challenge was that many people in her own community were resistant to yoga. "Black people don't do yoga!" Felton recounts with a laugh (personal communication, July 11, 2024). She said people made every excuse why they didn't want to try yoga—they weren't flexible, they didn't have money for a yoga mat. She realized she needed to join her Black community members where they already were, such as after-school programs, senior centers, and festivals.

Of all the strategies Felton tried, she said the most effective was "starting with the babies" (personal communication, August 5, 2024). She offered yoga to children in schools and other community settings and saw how open they were to learning new things. Children turned out to be the best ambassadors, because they shared what they learned with their parents. When parents and other adults saw how effective yoga was for their children, she said they were more open to trying it themselves.

Having surmounted those early hurdles, Mimi's Yoga Kids has been offering free yoga and wellness classes to the Atlanta metropolitan area since 2018. Felton and her dedicated staff have literally changed the lives of the children and families with whom they work. Felton herself was the Africa Yoga Ambassador for 2023, as well as the 2023 recipient of the International Association of Yoga Therapists' Seva award. At time of press, she is in the midst of applying for her yoga therapist certification.

On the individual level, epigenetic research suggests that making life-style changes can improve one's overall health outcomes (Alegría-Torres et al., 2011). Thus, incorporating yoga therapy into one's lifestyle can be a pow-erful adjunctive therapy in the amelioration of intergenerational trauma and its transmission. Positive changes in behavior, nutrition, stress, and environ-ment can lead to better health outcomes, and are the same as those recom-mended by Ayurveda (Sharma & Keith Wallace, 2020). Notice the striking similarity between these factors and the protective and risk factors listed above. In the final section of this chapter, we explore the specific mecha-nisms that foster balance and lead to healing after CPTSD.

Great resources for learning more about yoga therapy for intergenera-tional and racial trauma include Gail Parker's books *Restorative Yoga for Ethnic and Race-Based Stress* (2020) and *Transforming Ethnic and Race-Based Traumatic Stress with Yoga* (2021).

## Consequences

The consequences of childhood adversity and trauma are as unique as the individuals who endure them. Some individuals are scarred for life, struggle with addiction, are unable to sustain jobs or relationships, and can remain unhoused for much of their adult lives. Others suffer silently and feel the need to mask, especially those with neurodiversity. Still others are forced to code switch, such as minorities who need to change their behavior and patterns of speech to match the culture of "majority." (See the Window of Tolerance section of this chapter for a full description.) Some individuals coast seemingly unscathed by all they have been through. And many, many others exist somewhere in between, suffering in some areas of life while finding a degree of success and stability in others.

### A Flexible Nervous System Is a Healthy Nervous System

Before we consider the sequelae of trauma, let's establish a baseline of what a healthy nervous system looks like. Consider Ayurveda's view of optimal health (both physical and mental/emotional): far from being static, opti-mal health is an ever-shifting balancing act among the three gunas, or uni-versal qualities. In fact, the first law of the gunas is the *law of alternation*, which states that "the three gunas are ever in dynamic interaction" (Fraw-ley, 1999, p. 28). This means that a healthy nervous system flexibly adapts to our needs in each situation, as shown in Figure 3.2.

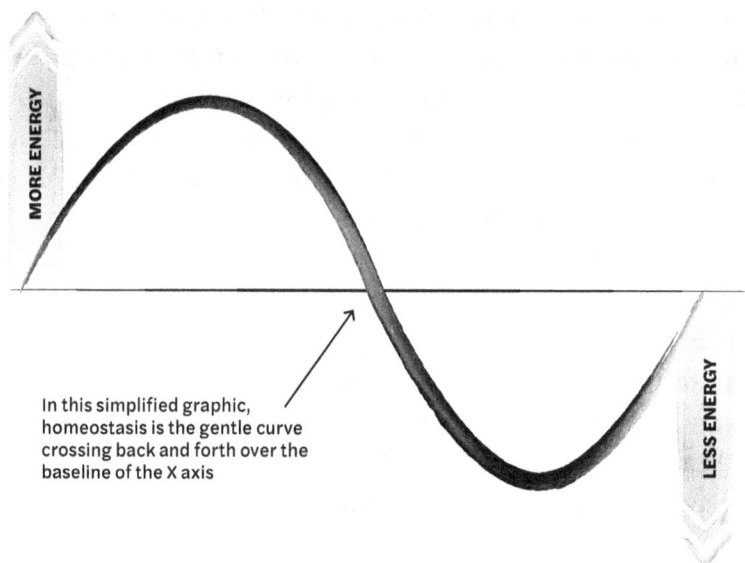

**Figure 3.2** Homeostasis

*The graph depicts a nervous system in homeostasis—throughout the day our energy waxes (depicted by the upslope of the curve) and wanes (depicted by the downslope of the curve).*

Given this, we can see that the emotional dysregulation after trauma is an attempt by the nervous system to find balance. From this yogic lens, the imbalances are unsuccessful yet hopeful attempts to heal (Figure 3.3).

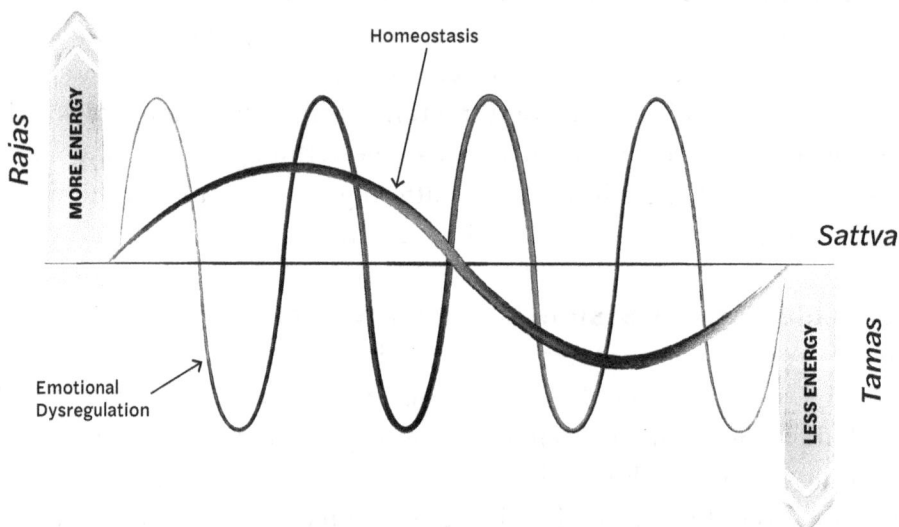

**Figure 3.3** Emotional Dysregulation Versus Homeostasis

*The graph depicts the longer, smoother wavelengths of a nervous system in homeostasis as compared to the short, steep, choppy wavelengths of a dysregulated nervous system.*

To be clear, acute trauma, including CPTSD, can damage all aspects of a survivor's life—relationships, employment, sense of meaning, physical health, and even mortality—in extreme and permanent ways. We are not suggesting that yoga therapy is a cure-all or an easy fix for such pervasive symptoms. What we are saying is that health and well-being occurs when the dysregulation of the nervous system is restored to a fluid, calm, responsive rhythm. When balance is cultivated in the nervous system, the repetitive, rigid, and acute emotional dysregulation and behaviors of CPTSD subside.

## Neurobiology of Dysregulation

In trauma, our responses become rigid. Clearly, all the factors mentioned previously play a role in how well someone survives the wounds of childhood trauma. Neurobiology helps explain the physical and emotional reactions an individual experiences (Ogden & Fisher, 2015) that keep them on a roller coaster of dysregulation. To begin, let's first explore how single-incident PTSD develops before considering CPTSD.

### The Roller Coaster of Emotional Dysregulation

The image of a roller coaster is often used to describe what happens in the nervous system during and after trauma. Picture this: riders board the roller coaster cars that climb to a peak before plummeting down the track to a valley only to once again be whisked up another harrowing peak. Think about the surge of energy you feel from a roller coaster. If you *choose* to get on the roller coaster willingly to feel that rush, you can discharge it afterward. If you feel pressured to go on it, you may not be able to shake it so fast. The meaning we place on the surge of energy makes all the difference.

Or consider another example: imagine taking a hike in the woods on a beautiful spring day, when you spot a snake. The hair rises on the back of your neck. You hear the snake hiss and see it recoil. Without conscious awareness, your nervous system kicks into gear. Your attention constricts to focus on the closest escape route. With superhuman speed, you flee as fast as possible. Everything will appear to move slower than usual not because time has slowed but because your reaction time has sped up substantially. You stumble several times as you run back to the trail head. If you've been bitten, you can't tell because now you have other bumps and bruises.

The surge of energy that mobilizes you to escape is thanks to a highly coordinated effort in your *autonomic nervous system* (ANS), which controls bodily functions like heart rate, breathing, blood pressure, and body temperature (Ogden & Fisher, 2015; Schwartz, 2021). This system is activated unconsciously, because our conscious mind would take too long to decide what to do (Levine, 1997). The exact same process is activated in the ANS during a roller coaster ride. But once again, **how you interpret and process that surge of energy will determine whether the event is or isn't traumatic to you**.

Your nervous system may return to baseline if you're able to do three things:

1. Move: shaking, pacing—any instinctive movements that allow the body to discharge the energy

2. You tell a caring person your terrifying tale

3. Review the timeline of the trauma, which allows you to recognize the event has ended

Engaging in these activities changes the context and meaning of the event. While not identical, this list closely aligns with neuroscientist and psychologist Lisa Feldman Barrett's advice about how to "master feelings in the moment" (Corrigan, 2022, 50:20–50:23). Feldman Barrett recommends that you move your body, change your location or situation, and re-categorize how you feel. Her suggestions mirror the idea of sharing your experience with a caring person, which can help reframe what happened. Then you'll retell this exciting and dangerous story to all your friends like any other memory in your life.

Imagine instead that you're whisked away by an emergency vehicle. At the hospital, you sit immobilized in a hospital room as medical staff assess your injuries. Just as the staff announce you haven't been bitten, they're called away to attend to other patients. You don't have an opportunity to review the events with a caring person now that the staff have left. The combination of not moving, not sharing this scary experience with a caring person, and not reviewing the event timeline is a formula for trauma. The surge of energy may stay locked in your nervous system. Your "memory" of the event will be less like a memory and more like a reliving of the experience (Herman, 1992b). You may develop a fear of snakes you didn't have before. Your fear may generalize to a fear of the woods, and you may feel suspicious of beautiful spring days. In contrast to the flexibly adaptive nervous system in homeostasis pictured in Figure 3.2, a traumatized nervous system is rigid and reactive, such as Figure 3.3.

This almost snake attack is an example of an event that can turn into a single-incident trauma—classic PTSD. Let's look at how trauma can arise in more urban settings. Recall Joe (Chapter 2), the Mexican American man whose wife had cancer 10 years ago at Christmas time. Now he can barely stand to be in a hospital setting. Though his wife has been in remission for years and says she has few memories of it, for Joe this time was excruciating. He sat for hours and days in hospital waiting rooms, worried he would lose his wife and partner, the mother of his children. He feels panicky if he hears the beep-beep of medical equipment, and he said he feels nauseous when he smells the sterile cleanliness that often permeates hospital environments. This is an example of *re-experiencing*, a topic we will cover shortly.

"Sometime in early November—about three weeks before the anniversary of her surgeries—I get this sense of foreboding." He says he vacillates between feeling depressed and numb to panicky and irritable. Sometimes he has panic attacks when he has too much to do during the week. Other times, especially on weekends, he feels like he can barely move. He said he feels like a tire that's lost all its air. Even though his wife is healthy, and life has returned to "normal," Joe's nervous system hasn't.

When he first learned of his wife's diagnosis, Joe said he went into "fix it" mode. He researched her condition extensively and they visited countless specialists. He took the kids to all their extracurricular activities to let his wife rest and made dinner for months. These actions not only helped his family but helped him feel a sense of agency. He couldn't stop her from having a brain tumor, but he could engage in these other activities to help.

But when it came time for his wife's surgeries, all Joe could do was sit in a hospital waiting room and hope for the best. Though he was not in mortal danger, his wife was. And as he sat for hours in the waiting room, he ruminated. He said all his actions of the previous months felt futile—even though these had been fruitful, necessary acts of love. He said he felt a numbness or fatigue come over him. "I'd just zone out." Joe's dissociated fatigue was a state of hypo-arousal.

## Shared Symptoms of PTSD and CPTSD

- Hypervigilance

- Avoidance/emotional numbing

- Re-experiencing

Using Joe's case example, let's take a closer look at the three symptoms that PTSD and CPTSD share: hypervigilance (hyper-arousal), avoidance/emotional numbing (hypo-arousal), and traumatic re-experiencing (such as flashbacks and intrusive thoughts). For reference, "hyper" means high. Thus, hyper-arousal is heightened arousal or reactivity beyond what would normally be expected. For instance, if one flinches when a person calmly says "hi" or calls their name, this is hyper-arousal. In contrast, "hypo" is low, and thus hypo-arousal is a lower-than-normal reaction. In the above example, a hypo-aroused response to one's name being called might be no response or a delayed and muted response.

## Hypervigilance (Hyper-Arousal)

*Hypervigilance* is a state of hyper-arousal and anxiety. In yogic terms, it is an expression of *rajas guna*, meaning it has the quality of frenetic energy and movement. An individual may experience tingling, shaking, and/or trembling when implicit or explicit memories of the trauma arise. Other symptoms of hyper-arousal include increased heartbeat and breathing, anxiety, panic, nightmares, flashbacks, or restlessness (Levine, 1997; Ogden & Fisher, 2015; Schwartz, 2021). Clients may overreact, have emotional outbursts, have difficulty concentrating, or feel rage. They may engage in risk-taking or impulsive behavior, or even self-harm (Schwartz, 2021).

Each year around Christmas, Joe notices an increase in nightmares, panic, and irritability toward his family. He said he finds it hard to concentrate and jokes about losing his keys a lot.

## Constriction

A key component of the initial hyper-arousal during a traumatic event is *constriction*, when the nervous system narrows our focus and effort to ensure the best possible chance of survival (Levine, 1997). Recall that snake in the woods. When you first spot it looking your way you won't notice the charming trill of birds or the piney scent of the forest. Instead, your senses will zero in on the snake, and your body will react in a "maximally optimal way" (Levine, 1997, p. 135) to get you out of there. This constriction is part of the energy surge that can become locked in the nervous system and later becomes trauma (Figure 3.4).

Hyper-arousal

*Rajas*

MORE ENERGY

Homeostasis

*Sattva*

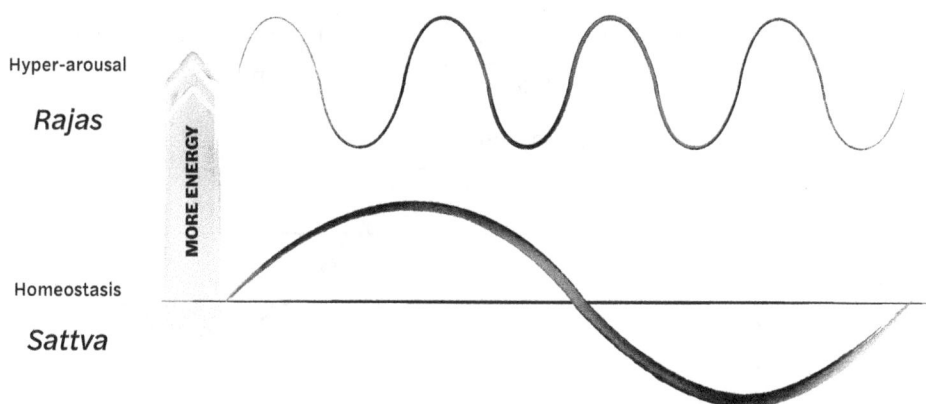

**Figure 3.4** Hyper-Arousal

*The graph depicts a nervous system in hyper-arousal (upper, choppy wavelength) compared to a nervous system in homeostasis (lower, smoother wavelength).*

## Avoidance/Emotional Numbing (Hypo-Arousal)

On the other hand, *hypo-arousal* is a state of depleted energy. It is an expression of *tamas guna*, which has the qualities of inertia, darkness, and lack of activity. Clients in this state say they feel empty, lethargic, numb, unable to move, depressed, despair, hopeless, and/or helpless (Ogden & Fisher, 2015; Schwartz, 2021). They may complain of feeling stuck, or of not finding interest or enjoyment in things they used to love.

Joe does a lot of volunteer work for his church, including taking meals to sick parish members. But when his pastor asked him to take a gift basket to a parishioner in the hospital, Joe made excuses. He said he couldn't bring himself to go. There are too many scary reminders in a hospital. For Joe this avoidance behavior was also coupled with numbing—he said he would usually feel guilty for saying no but instead he feels nothing.

### Dissociation and the Sense of Self

A key component and type of hypo-arousal is *dissociation*, which is the experience of detaching from thoughts, feelings, and a sense of self (Beutler et al., 2022). Daydreaming or focusing on a book are normal, everyday forms of dissociation. However, it is also the "essence of trauma" (van der Kolk, 2014, p. 66). During the traumatic event, dissociation helps protect the individual "from the pain of death" (Levine, 1997, p. 136). The problem is that the enormous energy mobilized by the ANS is often not able to discharge, and traumatic dissociation becomes avoidance and emotional numbing

(Figure 3.5). Peter Levine gives an excellent description of dissociation in his ground-breaking book *Waking the Tiger: Healing Trauma* (1997).

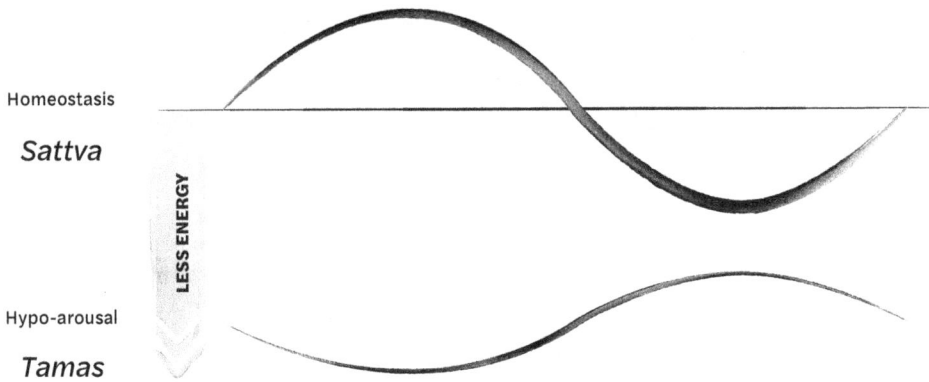

**Figure 3.5** Hypo-Arousal

*The graph depicts a nervous system in hypo-arousal (lower wavelength) compared to a nervous system in homeostasis (upper wavelength).*

In more acute forms, clients with unresolved trauma (whether PTSD or CPTSD) report feeling as if they themselves are not real (*depersonalization*) or that nothing around them feels real (*derealization*). In the most extreme case, a person's traumas may cause them to dissociate from a single sense of self in a diagnosis known as dissociative identity disorder (DID). What this shows is that trauma can cause this sense of disconnection from a sense of self.

One important area that neuroscience has pinpointed in relation to our sense of self is the *default mode network*, which is "an array of brain structures that extend across the entire brain" (Ford, 2020, p. 50). When a person is traumatized, the connectivity in the default mode network can be disrupted, leading to a disruption in the sense of self (Lanius et al., 2020). Trauma survivors say things like "I do not know myself anymore" (Lanius et al., 2020, "Abstract" section), indicating a shift in survivors' sense of self.

## Traumatic Re-experiencing

The result of all this constriction and dissociation (hyper- and hypo-arousal) is *traumatic re-experiencing*. The dissociation of trauma cuts the aversive experience off from ordinary awareness. Then it comes flooding back in. For Joe, the smells and sounds of a hospital take him right back to the dreadful moments of sitting in the hospital, waiting to hear whether his wife would live or die. Like being on a roller coaster, the trauma survivor is yanked around unbidden by emotional dysregulation. But unlike willing amusement park riders, trauma survivors don't have a choice. Brain changes after trauma cause victims to become triggered easily, and to feel as if the trauma is happening in the here and now (Ogden & Fisher, 2015; van der Kolk, 2014). "Traumatic memories lack verbal narrative and context; rather, they are encoded in the form of vivid sensations and images" (Herman, 1992b, p. 38). Today, we call this *traumatic re-experiencing* (NHS, 2022b).

Some clients report spending more time in either hyper- or hypo-arousal. Other clients may report see-sawing between the two. Regardless of individual symptoms, the emotional dysregulation and behaviors that result from re-experiencing are often out of proportion or out of alignment with the person's current life. Some survivors consciously recognize that their reactions are out of proportion. This often causes embarrassment and shame that maintains the trauma. For instance, a client may apologize profusely for not wanting to practice a yoga technique that makes them feel self-conscious, such as repeating a mantra out loud. As YPs, we can help dispel this self-conscious shame by reminding them that this is *their* therapy, and we want to respect and stay within the bounds of what feels comfortable to them.

Conversely, other clients may truly believe that they are in danger even when they aren't. For example, Michelle's client Devin had a deep fear of savasana, because it mirrored the acute dissociation they had experienced during childhood trauma. As such, Devin was encouraged to stay away from any yogic practice that felt similar, including meditative practices that called for silence or closing his eyes. It is very common that meditative or mindful practices are triggers for trauma survivors who experience frequent dissociative symptoms. Before starting any yogic or body-based practice, it is vital to assess a client's *window of tolerance* (covered in the next section) to create safe, effective treatment planning.

## Symptoms Unique to CPTSD

- Emotion dysregulation
- Negative self-view
- Relationship problems

In response to normal stressors, the nervous system returns to a state of homeostasis after the stressor or threat passes (Ford, 2020). But when the four key features of complex trauma are present (extreme threat, repetition of that threat, no escape possible, and the threat is interpersonal) returning to homeostasis is more challenging. This state of perpetual threat is called *allostatic overload*, when the "stress response capacities are exceeded" (Ford, 2020, p. 37). Allostatic overload is when the body and nervous system remain in a chronic state of stress, causing the individual to be more prone to exhaustion and illness. Let's review the three symptoms that distinguish CPTSD from PTSD, which are as follows (Schwartz, 2021): emotion dysregulation, negative self-view, and relationship problems.

## Emotion Dysregulation

The roller coaster metaphor used in the last section illustrates *emotion dysregulation*. While PTSD sufferers experience some degree of this, survivors of CPTSD experience more acute, chronic, and entrenched forms of dysregulation. As discussed, another defining feature of CPTSD is extreme threat that is often chronic and inescapable. Over time the ANS becomes habituated to responding to threat, even when it's not there.

When Michelle first started working with Joe, she assumed his trauma around his wife's cancer was single-incident PTSD. While yoga therapy combined with traditional psychotherapy helped regulate his mood to some degree, many of his symptoms persisted. As we'll see in the next section on symptoms unique to CPTSD, there was more going on for Joe than this one trauma.

## Negative Self-View

*Negative self-view* refers to the "impaired sense of self-worth" (Schwartz, 2021, p. 5) that many CPTSD survivors experience. Individuals develop a chronic sense of guilt, responsibility, and "intense shame" (Courtois & Ford, 2016, p. 48). Experts agree that this shame occurs especially for children, who feel like they've failed when they are unable to flee the abuser or traumatic situation (Courtois & Ford, 2016; Schwartz, 2021).

To understand the impact that negative self-view has on CPTSD survivors, let's differentiate between guilt and shame. Guilt is the statement, "I did something bad." Shame is the statement, "I am bad." For example: if I accidentally run over my Basset Hound's enormous ear with my office roller chair, I might feel guilty. Because this is an errant action, I can apologize and make it better by allowing him a few extra minutes in my lap before I return to writing. If instead I feel shame when I run over my dog's ear, I will undoubtedly feel like a bad person, and it will wreck my day. Also, I may forgo spending time making it up to him because it's a foregone conclusion that I'm a bad person.

## Relationship Problems

*Relationship problems* refer to an individual's avoidance of and difficulty with maintaining relationships. The root of the relational issues stems from the interpersonal trauma that creates lack of trust (Courtois & Ford, 2016; Schwartz, 2021). Consider this: children are in the midst of forming attachments to primary caregivers, and they depend on those caregivers for survival. "When (caregiver) relationships are unstable or unpredictable, children learn that they cannot rely on others to help them" (NCTSN, 2023). The NCTSN website goes on to say that someone with a complex trauma history can have lifelong problems in all manner of relationships, including romance, friendship, and with authority figures.

In Chapter 2, we explored the four styles of attachment: secure, anxious, avoidant, and disorganized. The interpersonal wounds that a survivor carries are sometimes collectively referred to as *attachment trauma* (Schwartz, 2018). Clients with CPTSD may develop a combination of secure, insecure (anxious, avoidant, or anxious-avoidant), and disorganized strategies, depending on their circumstances and the fact that they may have had different relational styles with different caregivers.

## Healing Solutions

Healing from complex trauma is a process. The process is highly individual and can feel messy or uneven. Effective treatment requires bravery, time, consistency, and a safe, stable rapport with the YP and other care providers. The goal of treatment is that the client not only *is* safe but *feels* safe. Through the nurturing support of the yoga therapy practices and YP, a client's nervous system comes back into balance. The client finds a sense of self and feels the rhythm of their own life again (or for the first time).

Let's consider the four key conditions of CPTSD: extreme threat, repetition of the threat, no escape possible (lack of control), and interpersonal trauma. From a yogic perspective, we restore balance by reversing these conditions. To remedy the threat and its repetition, we offer safety and repeated opportunities to find that safety. To heal the lack of control and feelings of helplessness, we empower clients to make decisions and exercise agency. And to heal interpersonal trauma, we provide safe, stable, nurturing care that engenders trust and connection.

When a CPTSD survivor feels safe, empowered, and connected to others their nervous system relaxes. The following section gives an overview of how current psychological understanding can be integrated into yoga therapy to help reduce and relieve the six CPTSD symptoms.

**Table 3.2** summarizes the four key conditions of complex trauma, as well as the type of remedy that works best with each.

| CPTSD Condition | Symptom | Remedy |
| --- | --- | --- |
| Extreme threat | Hypervigilance | Safety |
| Repetition of threat | Re-experiencing | Bottom-up approach |
| No escape possible | Dissociation | Energize; cultivate agency |
| Interpersonal trauma | Disengage from social system | Create trust and connection (attachment) |

## Window of Tolerance

Due to CPTSD, survivors have a narrow window in which they feel calm and emotionally regulated. This can make it hard for a client to tolerate stressors outside this window without becoming dysregulated. Yet therapy—including yoga therapy—requires clients to work at the boundaries of or just outside their comfort zone. In response to this conundrum, Dr. Daniel Siegel created the concept of the *window of tolerance,* which is the "**optimal zone of 'arousal' for a person to function in everyday life**" (National Institute for the Clinical Application of Behavioral Health [NICABM], 2019). You can find a helpful window of tolerance graphic at www.nicabm.com/trauma-how-to-help-your-clients-understand-their-window-of-tolerance

In the first few yoga therapy sessions, the YP and client work together to assess the client's window of tolerance. Through gentle yoga techniques, the client gets to know what movements and areas of the body generate rajasic, tamasic, or sattvic states. For instance, Teresa (Chapter 2) reported that Child's Pose made her feel sattva—calm and well-regulated. But she said she could barely stand savasana, and "zones out" when she does it. This meant that savasana elicited a tamasic, dissociative state. To lessen the dissociation, Teresa was invited to try the Wave Vinyasa that incorporated a relaxing pose (Child's Pose) into a temporal flow of other poses. In this way, Teresa was staying within her window of tolerance during yoga therapy practice.

## Distress Tolerance

This case vignette illustrates the power of CPTSD-informed yoga therapy to help clients build distress tolerance. *Distress tolerance* is a "person's ability to manage actual or perceived emotional distress" (Tull, 2024, para. 1). By working with Michelle to mindfully incorporate poses that elicited low levels of hyper- and hypo-arousal, Teresa was able to tolerate uncomfortable body sensations and feelings.

## Bottom-Up/Top-Down Approaches

*Bottom-up* approaches to therapy and treatment are body-based interventions like yoga therapy. Top-down approaches are cognition-based interventions like talk therapy. Bottom-up approaches interrupt the physical reactions of traumatic dysregulation and can be especially useful when the nervous system reacts "as if what happened in the past is still occurring in the present" (Ogden & Fisher, 2015, p. 183).

Mindfulness is a good example of using both bottom-up and top-down approaches. For instance, doing a body scan or practicing mindfulness of the body is using both our felt-sense (bottom-up) as well as our conscious awareness (top-down). In this book we recommend an integration of both top-down and bottom-up approaches for the most effective CPTSD-informed treatment.

**Collaborating with the yoga client allows them to take charge of their experience, thereby giving them back their power.** Remember: complex trauma breaks a client's rhythm. It creates an imbalance in the form of emotional dysregulation that makes them feel helpless, because the dysregulation is automatic and out of their conscious control. When instead a client learns they can tolerate mild forms of dysregulation through yoga tools, they gain a sense of agency and empowerment. "Yoga makes it safe for you to experience yourself even though your experience may not be that great" (Holzer, 2022, 4:13–4:19).

## Self-Care Practice: Finding Sattva

This chapter focused on the ways clients get out of balance through rajas (hyper-arousal), tamas (hypo-arousal), or the roller coaster between the two. But as Frawley points out, the gunas are not static or rigid, but are constantly in interplay with one another.

Which style did you relate most with? Yoga tells us the way to find balance (sattva) is to practice a counterbalancing technique. If you found yourself relating more with anxious hyper-arousal, what calming practice would help counterbalance this state? If you found yourself relating more with the stupor and numbness of hypo-arousal, what energizing practice would gently restore your vitality? And if you related most with the roller coaster between the two, what practice could restore harmony in your system?

## Chapter Summary

- As more and more people seek out yoga therapy as an integrative approach to all mental health issues, YPs will work with more clients who have CPTSD. **Thus, yoga professionals need to learn how to identify and work with CPTSD.**

- When yoga therapy is combined with traditional "talk" therapy it can maximize the benefits of both.

- Exciting advances in epigenetics suggest that lifestyle changes in behavior, nutrition, stress management, and environment can improve health outcomes. Yoga therapy can be an invaluable tool toward these outcomes.

- **Re-experiencing symptoms (e.g., flashbacks and intrusive thoughts):** CPTSD survivors re-experience their trauma through bodily sensations, flashbacks, and intrusive thoughts. Yoga therapy helps clients increase interoceptive awareness, a bottom-up approach. Ogden and Fisher (2015) say bottom-up interventions help clients interrupt the physical reactions that keep their nervous systems stuck in the past.

- **Avoidance/emotional numbing (tamasic state of hypo-arousal):** Yoga therapy helps clients tolerate distress and decrease avoidance strategies. Yoga helps heal trauma because it makes the body safe for clients (Holzer, 2022). Once the body becomes a safe space, the client increases their window of tolerance.

- **Hypervigilance (rajasic state of hyper-arousal):** On the other end of the spectrum, clients can become flooded with traumatic re-experiencing and have a hard time relaxing. Yoga therapy helps clients develop incremental ways of staying present to the distress of hyper-arousal. Over time they can tolerate more anxiety without becoming flooded.

- **Emotional dysregulation:** Yoga therapy can help clients reframe the painful roller coaster of emotional dysregulation. Once a client understands body sensations as impulses of energy that won't hurt them, they observe them with more equanimity. When clients help create yoga sequences and practices, they become empowered. This felt sense of agency further increases their window of tolerance.

- **Negative self-view:** As the body sensations that were once triggering become neutral, clients increase their window of tolerance, and they stop associating with a negative sense of self. Body sensations become transient states, rather than permanent states. "I feel bad" versus "I am bad." In addition, yoga therapy helps clients develop calming skills, self-compassion practices, and a sense of empowerment—all of which challenge the negative self-view.

- **Relationship problems:** Yoga therapy helps clients develop a positive sense of self that leads to greater trust in themselves. The therapeutic rapport with a caring, stable YP also creates a template of what the client should expect in other relationships. This is foundational to changing their relationships with others.

## CHAPTER 4

# Phases of CPTSD Treatment

## Case Study: Devin

When Devin, a White American transgender male (they/them), was 16 years old they were referred by their psychologist to Michelle for debilitating anxiety and depression. Early on, Devin emphasized that their transgender status was just one aspect of who they were.

"I don't like the way some people make my gender a defining factor," Devin said. Some family members and friends focused on their gender to the exclusion of other aspects of their life, they said, while others seemed to ignore them as a person because of it. But Devin had more pressing issues that brought them to therapy.

Despite being a high-achieving student in advanced courses, Devin became so overwhelmed by the pressures of school that they stopped socializing with friends and dropped out of extracurriculars like theater and choir. One of the most challenging symptoms was a feeling of paralysis when doing homework that led to a trance-like state. When they "came to" hours later, Devin reported that they'd cut on their legs (a form of self-harm) with no recollection of it.

Devin had been in and out of therapy since childhood. Over the years, they'd acquired a patchwork of diagnoses from general anxiety to panic disorder to major depression with other severe symptoms thrown in. This put Devin's treatment team in the unenviable place of trying to piece together an effective treatment plan. It was about this time that the psychologist recommended yoga therapy with Michelle.

Michelle recognized that this was a complex case. All the diagnoses had left not only the treatment team, but also Devin and their family, flummoxed. Michelle could see that Devin wanted to feel included and empowered in treatment and wanted relief. Devin didn't want to cut anymore, so the first order of business was to help them feel safe enough not to go into that trance state where the cutting occurred.

To begin, Michelle introduced the *window of tolerance* (Chapter 3). She explained that in sessions together, they'd stay within Devin's own personal window of tolerance where they felt relaxed and comfortable. Devin joked that they didn't know what "relaxed and comfortable" felt like. Michelle said they'd figure this out together.

Devin then shared that calming techniques like deep breathing and savasana tended to make them dissociate. Hearing this, Michelle suggested yoga practices that emphasized present-moment body awareness like massaging the soles of the feet with a tennis ball or massaging the neck and back with a foam roller. The tennis ball massage can help clients who dissociate by increasing awareness in the feet, thereby increasing their connection to the ground. Devin immediately reported liking both practices, because they felt more aware of their body in the present moment while also feeling relaxed. Michelle pointed out that they were learning what relaxed and comfortable was, to which Devin replied, "Wow! Yes!"

In the first few months of yoga therapy treatment, Michelle noticed Devin "zone out" from time to time during sessions, something that Devin said occurred frequently. But as Devin learned to increase awareness of body sensations through the tennis ball massage and other active yoga practices, their ability to stay present increased and their tendency to zone out decreased. Michelle told Devin that in this first phase of treatment, the focus was on learning skills to calm the nervous system and guard against moving into that dissociative state. Though at the time she wasn't aware of it, Michelle was initiating phase-based treatment with Devin.

## Introduction to Phase-Based Treatment

Evidence shows that the best course of treatment for those who suffer from both PTSD and CPTSD is a phase-based approach (Courtois & Ford, 2016). Within these phases we find the remedies to the four key conditions of CPTSD (extreme threat, repetition of the threat, no escape possible, and interpersonal trauma). The literature has outlined three distinct phases (Courtois & Ford, 2016; Ford & Courtois, 2020; Schwartz, 2021):

- Phase 1: Build safety, stability, and engagement

- Phase 2: Process trauma

- Phase 3: Integration of new skills and knowledge

If a client is currently in treatment for CPTSD, obtain a release of information to discuss the client's case, including what phase(s) of trauma work they are currently working on. Many, if not all, clients with trauma shift back and forth among the phases. So, establishing a regular line of communication with the trauma treatment team, especially the primary therapist, is vital to effective care.

A client may also suspect or know they have trauma but not have a formal diagnosis. If this is the case, advise the client to seek mental health counseling, and stick with yoga therapy interventions that bolster safety and stability (in other words, assume Phase 1 of treatment).

In still other cases, a client has no idea they show symptoms of CPTSD. As such, this individual will not identify as a trauma survivor, so it's important to bear in mind several important factors. First, consider that surviving trauma and/or complex trauma can cause an individual to armor up and resist the self-concept of being a victim. Hearing that you suspect they have trauma may deviate from their self-concept and cause them not to trust you. Or a client may become identified with the label of trauma even though they have not received a formal assessment.

Most importantly, if diagnosis is outside your scope of practice, it is unethical to suggest or hint at a potential diagnosis. The optimum way to handle this is to refer to specific symptoms or behaviors (like panic attacks, dissociation, negative self-talk, to name a few) that you think therapy could help the client with and suggest therapy for those reasons without mentioning trauma.

Finally, children and adolescents may continue to live in a traumatic home environment from which they cannot leave. Recall from Chapter 4 that it is your obligation to learn your country's laws regarding vulnerable clients. Stay within your scope of practice when discussing your clinical impressions with a client. Understanding and staying within the bounds of your scope of practice can be a very empowering practice for you the YP, because doing so keeps you safe. You can validate a client's current life stressors (that you suspect may be traumatic) and mental health challenges without using diagnostic labels.

## Levels of Trauma Care

Related to the topics of phases of treatment (the client's current stage of healing) and scope of practice (the YP's skillset and experience) is the level of trauma care the YP can provide. The possible levels include trauma aware, trauma sensitive, trauma-informed, and trauma-focused (Employee

Assistance Program Association—South Africa [EAPA-SA], 2023; MindRe-mapping Academy, 2023). These terms apply to all levels of trauma, including PTSD and CPTSD. In the list of bulleted descriptions, we have bolded "trauma-informed care," which is the level of care offered and described in this book.

- Trauma aware—The most basic understanding of trauma and its potential impact on a person. This approach recognizes that many people have experienced trauma, and that clients may have potential sensitivities to sound, light, or other stimuli.

- Trauma sensitive—This approach takes awareness one step further by using skills and practices that foster an atmosphere of safety and trust, such as clear boundaries and open communication.

- **Trauma-informed**—This approach integrates an understanding of trauma into all aspects of care, including the prevention of retrauma-tization. For instance, at this level of care the YP provides a trauma-informed intake (that potentially incorporates trauma screening tools) and provides resources and referrals for trauma-specific treatment options. The approach introduced in this book offers this level of care.

- Trauma-focused—This is trauma therapy. At this level of care, the trauma therapist works with the client to "understand the impact of specific traumas" (EAPA-SA, 2023, "Trauma-focused care" section). For example, Michelle's internship at RAAP (Rape Assistance and Awareness Program) taught her to be a trauma therapist where she guided clients through evidence-based stages of processing their sexual trauma.

## The Initial Intake: A Roadmap for Safe, Effective Treatment

In the case of Devin, Michelle knew she needed to proceed slowly. This meant building trust in the therapeutic rapport, helping Devin become aware of their internal state, and helping them feel empowered to use coping skills rather than cutting or dissociating. To start, she conducted an initial intake. The intake highlighted the need to start Devin's treatment plan with yoga tools that were energizing to keep them out of a dissociative state. While the initial intake session helps you capture a lot of important information right from the start, it's not uncommon for clients to share more vulnerability later in treatment once they've established trust with you. For instance, eight months into therapy Devin shared that their stepfather had been very emotionally abusive to their mother and them. This abuse had been reported by their past therapist, which meant that Michelle didn't need to report it to authorities. Even though they now understood that the way their stepfather treated them was abusive, they said they didn't always connect how it impacted them.

Now they became aware of how trapped and scared they felt while living with him. This gave both Devin and Michelle insight into their tendency to dissociate. As a child (10–13 years old) they couldn't escape their stepfather's abuses. Dissociating had been an adaptation to this traumatic home environment. The fact that this took a while to surface is normal. It takes time to establish a healthy rapport—there's no shortcut. The process of establishing safety and trust in relationships is multifaceted, individual, and must take cultural differences into consideration (Qina'au & Masuda, 2020). Even if *you* the YP suspect CPTSD, your client may not be able to look at it for a while. Be patient with your client, and yourself.

## Phase 1: Safety, Stabilization, and Engagement

To offer a safe, nurturing, therapeutic environment for clients, the YP must offer at least a trauma-informed level of care. Trauma-informed care not only acknowledges the impact of trauma on a client, but also actively seeks to avoid re-traumatization (MindRemapping Academy, 2023). We devote much of this chapter to Phase 1 of treatment, since this book is a trauma-informed approach.

### Safety

Phase 1 of CPTSD treatment entails creating safety by teaching the client calming and regulating skills. Building safety in the therapeutic rapport and in yoga therapy sessions consists of three components: decreasing danger, building boundaries, and cultivating self-regulation. Let's consider each of these components in detail.

### Increase Safety

It is brave work to uncover the deep wounds of trauma. As such, clients need to be and feel safe before they can look meaningfully at their traumas. That means that the trauma is over, and not ongoing. "Only with a decrease in danger or its ongoing threat can the client begin to disengage the 'survival brain' to engage the 'learning brain' in therapy and outside life"

(p. 123, Courtois & Ford, 2016). Decreasing danger in a client's life happens in three domains (Courtois & Ford, 2016; Schwartz, 2021): a client's environment (home, community, and yoga therapy space), their personal behavior and habits, and their physical and mental health and well-being.

First and foremost, a client ideally lives in a safe environment, free from emotional and physical abuse, as well as community violence. The client has a roof over their head, a safe place to sleep, and their home feels emotionally stable. For instance, Devin confirmed that they felt a lot safer since their stepfather had left three years ago. However, we know that many times our clients live in suboptimal environments. When this is the case, work with the client and their care team to ensure they are as safe as possible.

## CAUTION: PROTECTING AGAINST TRIGGERS

Yoga therapy can be a very powerful tool in a CPTSD survivor's healing journey, especially with regards to helping a client feel safer in their body and more able to access body awareness. However, because yoga therapy *is* a body-based practice, it also has the potential of triggering one's trauma. The YP must proceed with an abundance of caution and care, especially if a client shares that they have suffered from sexual trauma (or the YP suspects it). Importantly, clients who have been victims of complex trauma may not feel like they have a voice to speak up about their needs. Thus, it is essential that the YP learn the client's needs and preferences with regards to poses, other yoga practices, and touch.

During the initial intake, the YP needs to find out what poses, positions, and other yoga tools should be modified or avoided altogether. Backbends and other yoga poses and practices that place the client in an open and vulnerable position can be triggering. For instance, if the YP thinks a client may benefit from a backbend, they may suggest Baby Cobra or Sphinx instead of a pose like Wheel. In fact, any pose where the chest is facing upward and the client is in a prone or upward-facing position may be contraindicated.

Other practices that clients may find triggering include closing their eyes, lying down, and meditation (for those who dissociate or ruminate on negative self-talk). Each client is unique, so the YP should take care to find out what kinds of practices may be triggering and steer practice away from these practices and movements.

Lastly, touch can be triggering for a client. This is another area to highlight during the initial intake. Talk to the client (and their family if present) about the importance of them feeling empowered to make a choice about touch that feels comfortable and safe for them. In place of touch, the YP may hone their verbal skills to give adjustments and directions in poses to help keep the client's joints safe. If a client requests touch in the form of a hug or physical adjustment, use an abundance of discernment and caution. For instance, a child client may request a hug, which shows their trust in you and the level of safety they feel in the therapeutic rapport. In this case, you may want to offer what is called a "side hug," in which you hug them side to side.

As the YP your comfort matters too. If you do not feel comfortable with touch or showing a client a particular pose (even if they are comfortable), you have every right not to.

The YP provides safety for a client by conducting an age-appropriate intake and range of motion assessment at the beginning of yoga therapy treatment. Another way to increase a client's safety is by providing a yoga therapy space that is safe and free from danger. This means that sessions are held in a private space (e.g., a door that closes and windows with coverings) and that is free of hazards that could cause harm, such as the pointy end of a table or other furniture. If a client reports they are actively suicidal or engaging in self-harm, be sure to secure (that is to say, put away) items they could harm themselves with, such as straps. For instance, securing all yoga props in a locked cabinet or drawer allows the YP to have necessary props at ready disposal without putting vulnerable clients at risk.

A client's personal behavior and habits also need to be safe. Many survivors adopt unhealthy coping such as self-harm (cutting, eating disorders) or compulsive behaviors (drug or other addictions). Devin admitted they started cutting about six months before their stepfather left, when fights between their mom and stepfather had escalated. Even after the stepfather left, Devin said they kept cutting as school became more stressful.

Clients should develop safety plans with their primary therapist to decrease and eliminate these behaviors (Courtois & Ford, 2016). A safety plan is a formal document created by therapist and client with input from caregivers and other important providers (like teachers or counselors) that a client agrees to follow when they feel unsafe. If a safety plan has already been created, request written permission to obtain it. If they do not have one, request that they start the process with their primary therapist, and then share it with you.

Devin had a safety plan, first developed by the psychologist and then updated by Michelle, Devin, and their mother. The original plan recommended that Devin use an app on their mobile phone to track their impulses to cut, which Devin found very useful. The updated plan included prompts to use the tennis ball massage or foam roller if they noticed feelings of spaciness and zoning out while doing homework. This plan helped to eventually eliminate the cutting behavior.

Survivors of complex trauma struggle with health issues (Schwartz, 2021). Checking in on their physical health and well-being on a regular basis helps clients feel seen. Devin complained of migraines that sometimes lasted for days. By periodically asking about them, Michelle learned that Devin's migraines often corresponded with their monthly cycle. This not only was painful and disruptive to their life, but also caused them a lot of gender dysphoria. Michelle suggested they consult their gynecologist. As a result, Devin went on birth control that simultaneously curbed their menses and decreased the headaches. This in turn relieved some of their gender dysphoria.

As important as safety is, Courtois and Ford (2016) emphasize that we as providers are not responsible for removing danger from our clients' lives. When determining the safety threshold that a client needs to work with you, consider some factors: your scope of practice and risk tolerance, the recommendations and expertise of the rest of the client's care team, and setting clear boundaries regarding safety.

## Boundaries

Clear boundaries are essential for creating health and safety within the therapeutic rapport. When working with a trauma survivor, the YP may want to "rescue" them in one way or another. Yet a strength-based approach involves teaching clients how to care for themselves, rather than rescuing them (Courtois & Ford, 2016).

Establishing good boundaries starts in the first session when you educate clients about your policies and practices. Doing so lessens surprises or trust ruptures later in the therapeutic rapport. One of the first boundaries to set when working with minors is guardian consent. You must first obtain written consent from their guardian to treat clients who are minors. You may also meet with the guardian initially depending on the age of the client. Check your country's laws regarding age of majority and consent to treat. Other key team members may include a psychiatrist, school counselor, and other specialty therapists (like occupational or physical therapy). Be sure to obtain signed consent before speaking with a client's other team members. Teaching clients and their families about consent helps them understand their right to privacy. It also empowers them to make informed choices about who has access to their personal information.

Obtaining signed consent to speak to a client's other key providers also allows the YP to make another important boundary: not retraumatizing the client. It can be tempting for both the client and the YP to dive into the story of the client's trauma. However, sharing one's trauma story is something the client needs to do with their primary trauma therapist. The signed consent allows the YP to consult with this therapist to learn about a client's traumatic history. Repeatedly telling the story of their trauma is retraumatizing for a client, so it is important to guard against this happening.

Another boundary essential for safety is communicating your duty to report incidents of abuse and neglect. It is your ethical obligation to learn your country's laws around working with vulnerable clients. In the US, these laws are regulated by each state. In the State of Colorado, for instance, "a mandatory reporter is defined as a professional who is obligated by law to report known or suspected incidents of child abuse and/or neglect" (Colorado Department of Human Services, 2024, "What is a mandatory reporter?" section). In the UK, the Children Act 1989, which was updated in December 2023, lays out the statutory framework for safeguarding children (HM Government, 2023).

Being consistent in billing practices is another example of holding clear boundaries. It not only helps you value yourself, but also helps the client value their own therapy and healing. You can create a set of Client and YP Rights and Responsibilities to clarify boundaries and roles. Search the internet using the keywords "client rights and responsibilities" to find examples.

Establishing clear boundaries reduces the chance of burnout as you work with clients who have challenging histories and issues. It also helps you to track your own regulation needs as you hear challenging stories from clients. Having ensured you are well-regulated, let's explore how to help a client regulate their emotions and mood.

## Self-Regulation and Resources

*Self-regulation* is the ability to regulate one's affect and emotions, and it is an essential skill for clients to develop at the start of therapy. Ogden and Fisher (2015) say that self-regulation helps anyone (which here includes clients and YPs) to notice and change internal state through emotions and body sensations. This in turn helps clients learn how to stay within their own window of tolerance. Each client is unique, and we must take great care at the beginning of treatment to discover what yoga tool(s) truly help a client feel regulated. There is no formula—what works for one client may make another client feel uncomfortable and dysregulated.

Clients stabilize further when they're encouraged to use existing *resources* (Courtois & Ford, 2016; Rothschild, 2000). Rothschild (2000) categorizes resources into five classes: functional, physical, psychological, interpersonal, and spiritual (pp. 88–92). Functional resources are pragmatic like a safe place to live or a reliable car. Physical resources include physical strength and stamina. A client who embraces physical activity of any sort including but not limited to yoga should be encouraged to use these tools to further healing. Rothschild (2000) says that psychological resources encompass many traits such as intelligence, a sense of humor, and creativity. Interpersonal resources consist of one's social network, such as partner, friends, family, and pets. Spiritual resources include "belief in a higher power... adherence to religious practice, and communing with nature" (Rothschild, 2000, p. 91). Of these, yoga tools can be used to most easily cultivate physical, psychological, and possibly spiritual resources.

### Yoga Tools as a Physical Resource

Rothschild says physical resources "give many clients a greater feeling of confidence" (2000, p. 89). Any yoga asana and/or pranayama technique that helps a client feel regulated, present, and/or confident in their own body can be a physical resource. The Sa Ta Na Ma mantra (Figure 4.1; also referred to as a meditation in Kundalini Yoga) is a good starting point. Complete instructions are included in Appendix 8.

For physically inclined clients, standing poses like any of the three Warrior Poses or Tree Pose can increase body awareness as well as cultivate confidence. Figures 4.2–4.5 feature these four poses with variations, depending on a client's mobility and fitness. They are presented from least to most challenging, in terms of fitness and mobility.

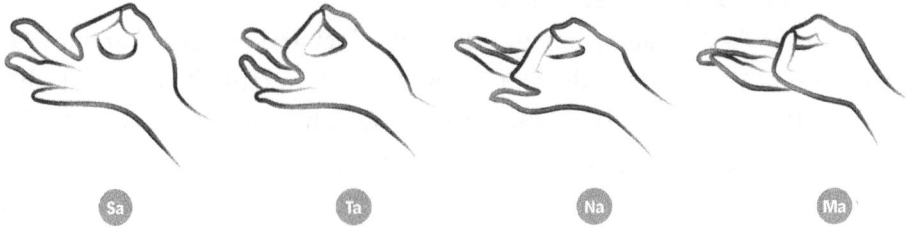

**Figure 4.1** Sa Ta Na Ma Mantra

*Illustrates the coordinating finger movements with the mantra Sa Ta Na Ma. This mantra is incredibly helpful for reducing anxiety for all three age groups covered in this book.*

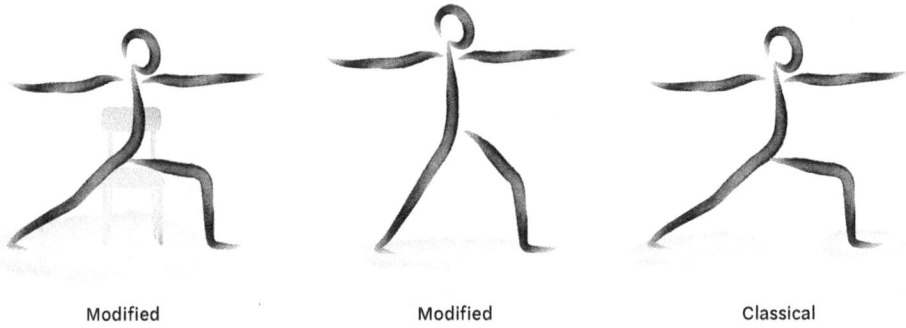

Modified                    Modified                    Classical

**Figure 4.2** Warrior II Pose Variations—Virabhadrasana II

*Depicts three variations of Warrior Pose II. Warrior II cultivates strength and stability in mind and body.*

Figure 4.2 features variations of Warrior II Pose. It is an accessible standing pose for many clients and can be a good place to start for building strength and balance.

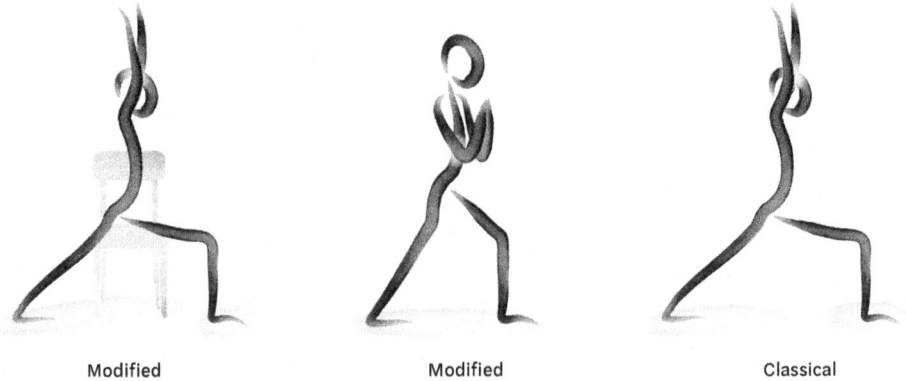

Modified                    Modified                    Classical

**Figure 4.3** Warrior I Pose Variations—Virabhadrasana I

*Depicts three variations of Warrior Pose I. Warrior I cultivates strength, openness, and energy in mind and body.*

Figure 4.3 illustrates variations of Warrior I Pose, which requires a bit more flexibility and mobility. While Warrior I Pose variations also take a bit more energy to do, they are also invigorating. We offer a variation with the hands folded in front of the chest, which lowers the amount of energy expended in the pose and can help protect the low back from too much lordosis—that is, too much inward curvature of the lumbar spine that can cause pinching and pain.

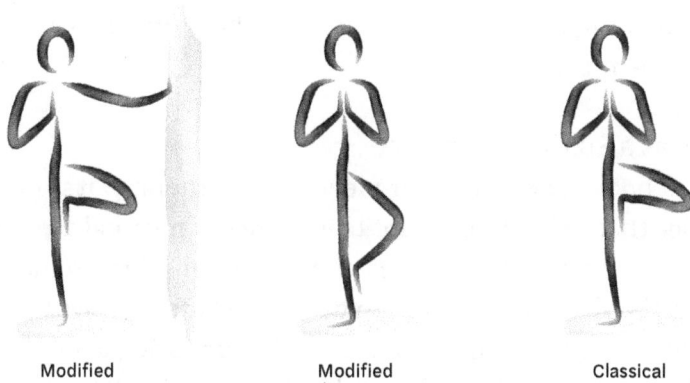

Modified　　　　　　Modified　　　　　　Classical

**Figure 4.4** Tree Pose Variations—Vrksasana
*Depicts three variations of Tree Pose. Tree Pose cultivates focus,
balance, and a sense of calm in mind and body.*

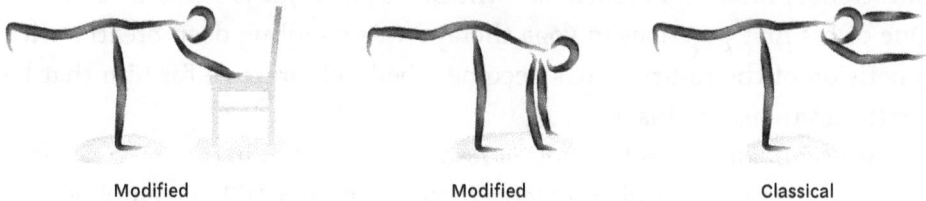

Modified　　　　　　Modified　　　　　　Classical

**Figure 4.5** Warrior III Pose Variations—Virabhadrasana III
*Depicts three variations of Warrior Pose III. Warrior III cultivates
strength, balance, and focus in mind and body.*

Figures 4.4 and 4.5 illustrate variations of the popular standing balances of Tree Pose and Warrior III, respectively. These poses build on the fitness of the first two warrior poses. They help clients focus through the challenge of balancing while also building confidence.

## Yoga Tools as a Psychological Resource

The *yamas*, *niyamas*, and *dharana* (concentration) practices are examples of yoga tools that can be employed in the service of bolstering clients' psychological resources. For instance, Devin practiced *ahimsa*, or nonviolence, toward themselves by taking study breaks from homework when they noticed spaciness. They also learned to practice *santosa*, or acceptance, rather than self-judgment when they felt panicky in class after a teacher assigned difficult homework. If you are not the client's primary therapist, be sure to coordinate with that provider to ensure that these practices align with the overall treatment plan.

## Yoga Tools as a Spiritual Resource

Though this book takes a secular view of yoga therapy, it's important to acknowledge that a client may want to explore the spiritual aspects of yoga. A client who wants to integrate this more spiritual side into the yoga therapy context should be encouraged to do so in whatever ways feels empowering and uplifting to them. To create good boundaries, a YP may want to separate the therapeutic from the spiritual by referring the client to a yoga teacher who can guide them in the spiritual aspects of their practice.

Clients who have an existing spiritual practice or religious faith can use *dharana* (such as visualization) and/or *pranayama* in conjunction with their devotional practices. For instance, Michelle's client Joe is a devout Catholic. One of his first practices in yoga therapy was coupling deep breaths with repetition of the rosary. It has become a bedrock practice for him that he continues to use to this day.

Rothschild describes three other resources essential in trauma treatment called *oases*, *anchors*, and *safe place* (2000, p. 92). In YTCT, we employ yoga tools to help clients create these three essential ingredients in CPTSD-informed treatment.

## Oases

An *oasis* is "an activity that demands concentration or attention" (Rothschild, 2000, p. 92). Mindlessly watching TV or scrolling on social media are not oases. Doing a challenging yoga pose (if that is within a client's ability and preference), or bringing all of one's attention to the present, are great oases. Five Senses Mindfulness Exercise is an easy and frequently used oasis by many therapists of all kinds.

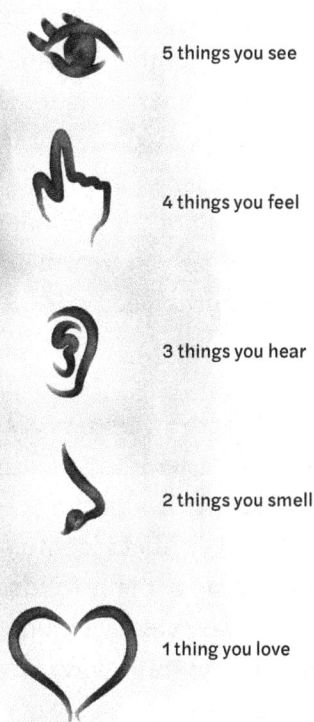

5 things you see

4 things you feel

3 things you hear

2 things you smell

1 thing you love

**Figure 4.6** Five Senses Mindfulness Exercise

*Illustrates the Five Senses Mindfulness Exercise—a commonly used practice in yoga therapy, psychotherapy, and mindfulness groups. It's great for all ages, especially children.*

## Anchors

An *anchor* is a "concrete, observable resource" (Rothschild, 2000, p. 93) already in the client's life. An anchor can be a person, a pet, a memory, or a place. It can also be a soothing activity like gardening or sewing: "A suitable anchor is one that gives the client a feeling (in body and emotion) of relief and well-being" (p. 93). Anchors are especially important in the treatment of all levels of trauma, because they are used in a process called "braking," which will be described shortly. Joe's practice of deep breathing while silently repeating the rosary is his anchor practice, as well as being a spiritual resource for him. The mantra mentioned previously, Sa Ta Na Ma, is a favorite anchor for many clients.

### Safe Place

Lastly, *safe place* is a very important resource for clients to learn as a form of self-regulation. A client's safe place is a physical location the client has been. Clients often pick places like a particular beach, mountain trail, vacation spot, or possibly family member's house. A YP can easily incorporate a client's safe place into other pranayama or visualization practices.

Rothschild (2000) says the safe place is a special kind of anchor in that it helps clients reduce stress when working directly with traumatic material. Though processing trauma is not formally done until Phase 2, the YP helps the client create a safe place early in treatment so they become familiar with it and can use it easily when the need arises.

## Stability

When helping clients cultivate awareness of their internal state, we need to proceed slowly. This is because **avoiding or numbing troublesome emotions, feelings, and body sensations is a protective adaptation for most (if not all) CPTSD survivors**. The inability to identify emotions is called *alexithymia* (Rothschild, 2000), and asking a client to identify feelings too soon can be triggering. Recall that calming yoga techniques like savasana caused Devin to dissociate. Even though the trauma was over, Devin continued to find it challenging—and even scary—to be aware of certain feelings and sensations.

### The Body as a Safe Space

For alexithymic clients, cultivating body awareness (also called *interoceptive awareness*) is indispensable (Rothschild, 2000). Clients build awareness of their internal state by identifying a neutral or *safe space* within the body. Different from the client's safe *place*, their safe *space* is a physical location in their body like the left pinky nail. It might also be a yoga pose like Child's Pose. If a client becomes triggered in their everyday life outside of session, they can then turn their attention to that safe space in the body to self-regulate (Rothschild, 2000).

To help Devin build interoceptive awareness, Michelle first introduced Devin to the idea of alexithymia. They were able to see that their severe dissociation was a way to stay away from body sensation. Michelle explained that the best way to do this was for Devin to share what body sensations or parts of the body felt "safe." She mentioned that for some people it is the tip of a finger, or even a fingernail.

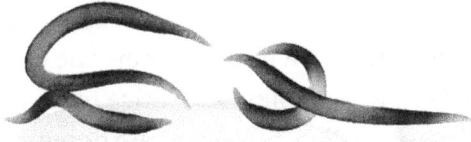

**Figure 4.7** Child's Pose—Balasana
*Depicts the classical version of Child's Pose, with arms outstretched.*

Devin said that observing transitory body sensations in short yoga vinyasas was calming. They felt safe knowing that whatever body sensation arose in one pose would soon transition to a new body sensation in the next pose. Noticing this transitory nature of body sensation allowed Devin the freedom to openly feel it, knowing it would not last for long. For instance, Devin could notice the side body stretch in Upward Salute Pose (hastasana) more fully, knowing they'd transition to another pose and set of body sensations soon. Devin added that they liked feeling the contractions in the arms and abdominal muscles in Plank Pose before transitioning to Cobra Pose (bhujangasana). In this way, they were using the body as a resource and anchor (Rothschild, 2000).

**Caution:** Rothschild (2000) warns that becoming aware of body sensation is contraindicated in two instances:

1. When a client's traumas were "so damaging to the bodily integrity that any attempt at sensing the body will overly accelerate contact to the trauma(s)."

2. When a client feels pressure to sense the body "correctly" (p. 106).

In these cases, it is best to stick to ensuring safety, strengthening the therapeutic rapport, and continuing to build other resources.

## Braking Versus Accelerating

Babette Rothschild (2000) likens trauma therapy to learning how to drive, where *braking* is the use of techniques that regulate the nervous system, whereas *accelerating* is the use of techniques to process the trauma (by intentionally eliciting the body sensations and feelings from the trauma). Most yoga therapy techniques can be used as either braking or accelerating interventions, depending how they are used and how the client relates to them. For instance, Child's Pose was a braking practice for Teresa (Chapter 2) who reported feeling calm and well-regulated while doing it.

The resources and yoga tools discussed thus far in this chapter have been examples of braking practices, since their intent was to induce feelings of calm and regulation for clients. Devin's "braking" practice was learning to notice neutral, present-moment body sensations during short vinyasas.

Accelerating practices are only offered to clients in Phases 2 and 3 of CPTSD treatment. "It is inadvisable for a therapist to accelerate trauma processes in clients or for a client to accelerate toward his own trauma, until each first knows how to *hit the brakes*—that is, to slow down and/or stop the trauma process" (Rothschild, 2000, p. 79). Accelerating interventions or practices widen a client's window of tolerance, but we don't work on them in Phase 1 when we're building safety and stability.

## Identifying and Labeling Feelings

As a client increases their body awareness, they can identify and label body sensations. Devin became more comfortable with labeling body sensations during yoga therapy sessions. For instance, while doing yoga vinyasa Devin developed the ability to label the contraction and/or stretch they felt in different muscle groups—the contraction in the arm muscles during Plank, or the stretch of the side body in hastasana. Over time, they also learned to label their feelings and emotions, also called *feelings identification*. Rather than dissociate, Devin could label feeling overwhelmed by schoolwork. And rather than withdraw, Devin learned it was okay to share with Michelle if they felt frustrated or confused by an instruction she gave. **As discussed previously, when an individual has unresolved and untreated CPTSD, their reaction to a trauma trigger is automatic. Learning to identify feelings helps slow this process down.** It is also the first step to increasing emotional awareness, which is "the ability to recognise and make sense of not just your own emotions, but also those of others" (Darcy, 2023, "What is emotional awareness?" section, para. 1).

Clients will often learn the skill of feelings identification with their primary therapist (if this is not you). As YPs, we can also encourage feelings identification. How we ask clients about their feelings depends on their age. Children 5–12 years old respond best to a graphic chart that features pictures rather than words. Amy Wheeler's Mental/Emotional State Assessment feelings chart for children shown in Figure 4.8 is an excellent example of this.[1]

# How do you feel?

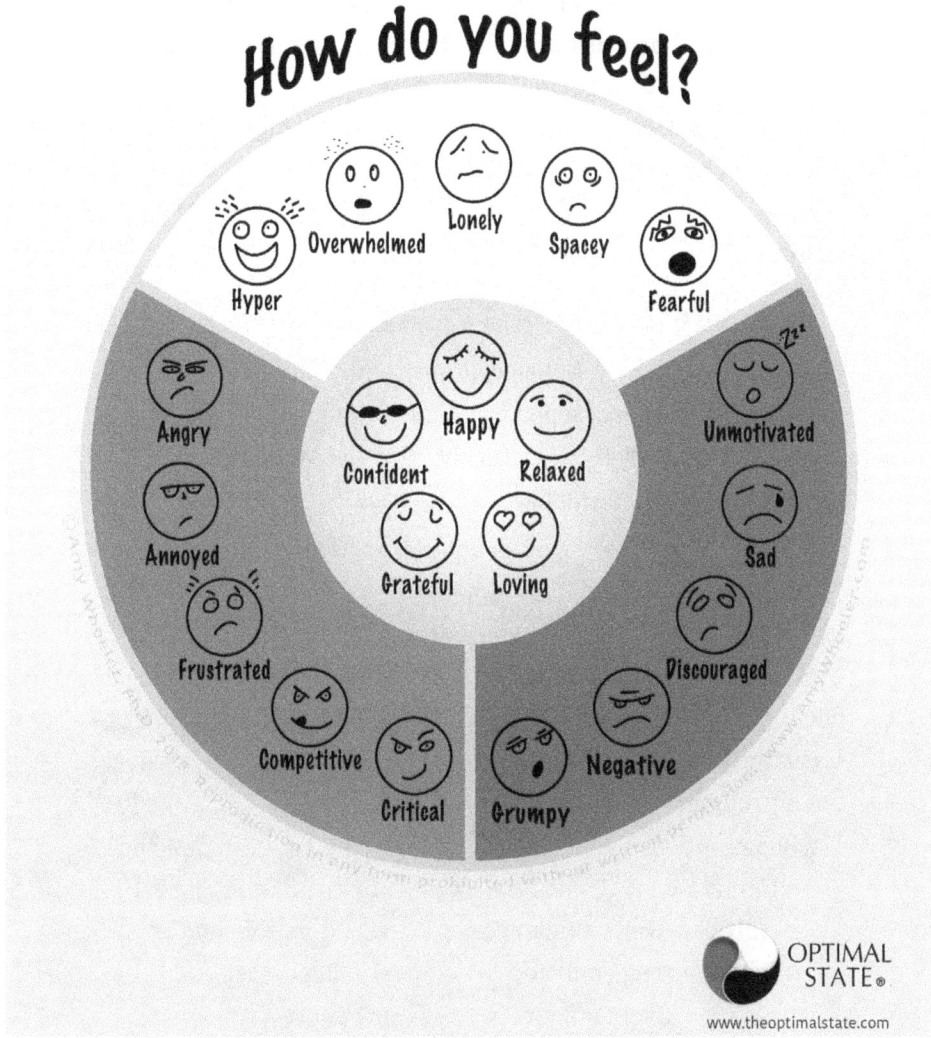

**Figure 4.8** Amy Wheeler's Mental/Emotional State Assessment Feelings Chart for a Child.
Source: Amy Wheeler

Adolescents aged 13–18 years old respond best to verbal interaction about their internal state. Yet they don't often respond well to "How are you doing?" For adolescents, it's best to frame the question as a three-part answer such

---

1   These charts have been published on Amy Wheeler's mental health mobile app since 2018. They have been used in training programs since 2015.

as the Rose-Bud-Thorn exercise. The University of Colorado Boulder offers a helpful description of how to set up this exercise with children or adolescents at www.colorado.edu/researchinnovation/rose-bud-thorn. Adolescents are asked to share something in their week that was good (the "rose"), something in their week that was hard (the "thorn"), and something that they are excited about or are working on (the "bud").

Lastly, Wheeler's Mental/Emotional State Assessment Feelings Chart for adults shown in Figure 4.9 is an excellent tool to use with adult clients. The advantage to Wheeler's feelings charts is that they integrate the gunas, a key component of the YTCT presented in this book.

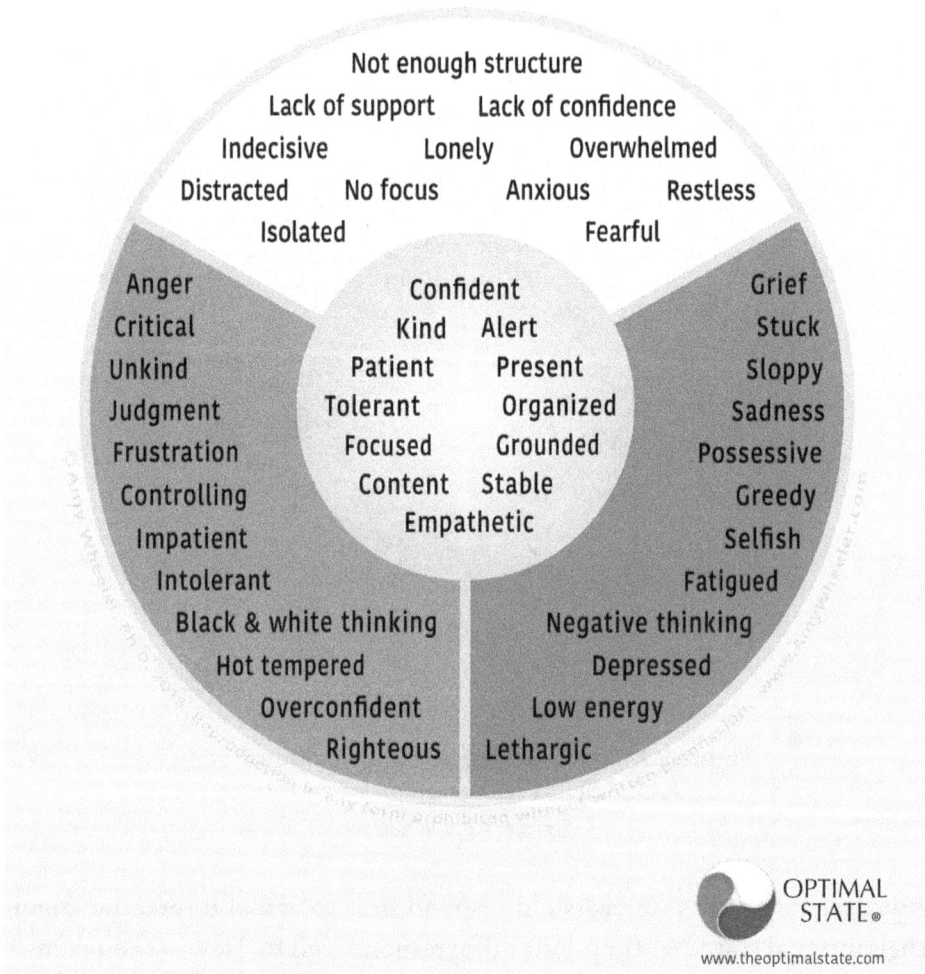

**Figure 4.9** Amy Wheeler's Mental/Emotional State Assessment Feelings Chart for an Adult.
Source: Amy Wheeler

Chapters 8–10 offer developmentally appropriate details to help clients identify and label feelings for each of the three age groups. In addition, copies of Wheeler's two feelings charts listed above can be found in Appendices 2 and 3. Having explored how to help a client identify and label their own feelings, let's turn again to the interaction between YP and client with regards to how we engage.

## Engagement
### Sequence of Engagement
When it comes to engaging with clients, we need to consider our *own* state before the client even walks through the door. Bruce Perry developed the Sequence of Engagement (2020a) to describe what happens between a caregiver and client when they first interact. He emphasizes that we as providers need to be fully regulated ourselves before we interact with clients. "If you're regulated, you have a chance at helping the other person be regulated, of connecting with them and then communicating with them" (Perry, 2020a, 5:17–5:25).

As a neuroscientist and a child psychiatrist, Perry understands more than most the significance that brain processing has on our ability to communicate effectively with others, most especially clients who suffer from CPTSD. The Sequence of Engagement illustrates that many steps occur between something we say and how the message is received. Watch Dr. Perry's video on the topic at www.youtube.com/watch?v=LNuxy7FxEVk

Perry offers a helpful mnemonic device that sums up this complex process: Regulate, Relate, Reason. Essentially what this means is that we as providers need to *regulate* ourselves before we can effectively *relate* (interact) with clients (and colleagues) and then be able to *reason* (effectively communicate) with them.

Even if your nervous system is well-regulated, your client's may not be. How do you respond to that? Let's consider 16-year-old Devin again. Devin appeared to be on the verge of tears when they came to session. Unbeknownst to Michelle, they'd just had a fight with their mom. Michelle asked, "How are you?"

"Fine," Devin said blankly, staring into space. They looked away and rolled their eyes.

Michelle noticed her own heart beating faster and wondered what caused Devin to shut down. But she also recognized that it probably took a lot for Devin to even answer her question (or possibly to show up to session).

The fact that they responded to her question meant they hadn't completely dissociated or disconnected. This was progress. To calm her own nervous system, Michelle took a deep breath. She noticed that Devin did the same, so she continued to breathe deeply and said quietly, "Hey, I'm just going to take some deep breaths. I'll check in with you in a few minutes." Devin nodded, still looking down. They practiced together in silence for a while, then Michelle asked, "What would you like to do right now?" Devin made eye contact for the first time and said, "Can we do Sa Ta Na Ma?"

This scenario illustrates the use of the Sequence of Engagement. When Michelle noticed Devin's frozen stance, she knew this was a sign of dysregulation. She also knew that behind their frozen exterior, Devin was probably reading her nonverbal body language with hypervigilance and began to constrict by shutting down. To effectively relate with them, Michelle needed to regulate her own nervous system, so she took deep breaths. Whether consciously or not, Devin started to do the same. Michelle saw this and continued. Once both seemed more regulated, Michelle asked what they needed, and Devin was able to ask for a yoga tool they knew worked for them.

## Co-Regulation

Breathing together in this way is an example of *co-regulation*, where two individuals' interactions and behaviors are continuously influenced and modified by each other (Bornstein & Esposito, 2023). Co-regulation can include a calming presence, soothing tone of voice, verbal reassurance and validation, modeling of regulating behaviors (like deep breathing), and providing an environment that offers emotional and physical safety (Complex Trauma Resources, 2024). Notice how most of these behaviors are nonverbal in nature.

## Nonverbal Communication

Perry (2020a) argues that nonverbal communication is essential to "getting the meaning and intentionality of communication across" (7:07). In 1972, Albert Mehrabian wrote *Nonverbal Communication* that showed 55% of human communication occurs through body language and facial expressions and 38% occurs through tone of voice. That means a mere 7% of communication is verbal (Mehrabian, 1972). While the words we say do matter, they don't matter nearly as much as our nonverbals. Due to its mind–body nature, yoga therapy is uniquely suited for cultivating co-regulation and effective communication with clients of all ages. And it is especially effective for children and adolescents, whose language skills and brain development are still in process.

## Body Awareness

Nonverbal communication is related to another vital aspect of how we engage with clients: *body awareness*. Babette Rothschild (2000) says that "body awareness implies the precise, subjective consciousness of body sensations arising from stimuli that originate both outside of and inside the body" (p. 101). **Rothschild also notes that cultivating body awareness has its roots in yoga and meditation.**

First and foremost, you the YP must be aware of your own internal state before meeting with a client. Let's take a closer look at how a practice like Mindful Transition cultivates body awareness. In Mindful Transition, you start by taking deep breaths and noticing current body sensations. This is called *interoception*, sensing stimuli from inside the body (such as tension, hunger, the flow of breathing). At the same time, you allow yourself to observe stimuli from outside the body (sounds, smells, the kinesthetic feel of whatever you're sitting on). This is *exteroception*—sensing stimuli from outside the body with your five senses.

Increasing your own body awareness through a practice like Mindful Transition allows you to be more present and grounded (regulated). This in turn allows you to observe clients' nonverbal communication, as well as teach them how to practice body awareness for themselves. Rothschild (2000, p. 102) offers an invaluable list of words and phrases that help clients identify body sensations. Here is a sample of that list:

> Breathing: speed and depth; position of a body part in space; pulse rate, heartbeat; pain, burning; vibration, shaking; tense/relaxed; big/small; hot/cold; restless/calm; movement/still; heavy/light; empty/full; expansion/contraction; soft/hard; tight/loose.

## Collaboration

As YPs our goal is to collaborate as well as co-regulate with our clients. Schwartz (2021) emphasizes the importance of collaborating with clients to empower them in their treatment. Engagement in Phase 1 of CPTSD-informed yoga therapy also includes familiarizing clients with the window of tolerance to ensure we match yoga interventions to a client's current window of tolerance. This window of tolerance will change (hopefully widening) over the course of treatment. It is important to check in with clients about their current window at each phase of treatment.

## Achieving Phase 1 Goals

As we have seen, the goal of Phase 1 is to help the client cultivate safety and stability in their life, relationships, and within themselves. How is this accomplished? As Babette Rothschild (2000) puts it, the client learns to put on the brakes—that is, stay away from traumatic content and sensations. The client learns to use the window of tolerance and yoga tools to:

- Increase interoception (body awareness)
- Help identify and label feelings

With its body-based and holistic approach, yoga therapy helps the client integrate what they have learned in Phase 1 and prepares them for Phase 2. With time and practice both in yoga therapy sessions and on their own, the client learns to use all these tools to become aware of when they're moving outside the therapeutic window. Once the client can regularly use yoga tools to intentionally re-regulate when they *do* go outside the window, they are ready for Phase 2.

## Phase 2: Trauma Processing

To provide Phase 2 treatment to a client, the YP must have the skills, training, and expertise to offer formal trauma therapy, also called trauma-focused care. Though trauma-focused care is beyond the scope of this book, we offer a detailed description of Phase 2, and how yoga therapy can be effectively incorporated into this stage of a client's healing process. If this phase and level of care is beyond your scope of practice, you would work with the primary trauma therapist to coordinate and integrate care.

Phase 2 can be seen as a form of *exposure therapy*, a psychotherapeutic intervention developed by Edna Foa (Treleaven, 2018) and commonly used to treat general anxiety. Recall the snake scare in Chapter 2: if one developed a fear of snakes after this incident, exposure therapy could help "expose" the individual little by little to their fear until it was extinguished or manageable enough to take a walk in the woods again. When used as a treatment for general anxiety, it is considered best practice to expose the individual to their fear as soon as possible.

Exposure therapy is also used to treat PTSD. However, in the treatment of PTSD, the client first needs to develop effective coping and calming skills before facing their fears. Phase 2 of trauma treatment at any level (i.e., for both PTSD and CPTSD) is a form of exposure therapy in that the client begins to face rather than protect against traumatic material. For over 25 years, trauma experts have recognized that the body holds the key to healing trauma (Courtois & Ford, 2016; Levine, 1997; Ogden & Fisher, 2015; Rothschild, 2000; Schwartz, 2021; van der Kolk, 2014). Yet Rothschild (2000) notes that intentionally becoming aware of body sensations associated with trauma is "one of the great challenges of trauma therapy" (p. 116).

Rothschild (2000) refers to this phase of treatment as using the "body as diary" (p. 116). As we have seen, the "memory" of trauma is stored in the body as sensations. When a trauma is triggered, the individual re-experiences trauma as those sensations arise in the here and now. This is why it is so important to move slowly and with intentionality at this phase of work. Clients need to feel in control of the process. To do so, a client must be able to self-regulate, so that they can re-examine past traumas from the lens of the learning brain (Ford, 2020).

**For these reasons, yoga therapy is the perfect complement to complex trauma treatment: it offers a gentle, mindful approach to body-based work that empowers clients to increase somatic awareness with intention and at their own pace.** Here, the "pace" and timing specifically refer to the use of exposure therapy at this phase of treatment. By working closely with the primary therapist, the YP can help support and augment the client's ability to tolerate the distressing content as they work through traumatic memories and re-experiencing in their primary trauma therapy. For instance, when at CHCO (Children's Hospital Colorado), Michelle worked with a client who suffered from stomach migraines that were exacerbated by stress. This patient and her family were seen by a family therapist (also at CHCO) for traumas the whole family had endured.

Michelle and this therapist recognized together that the patient was holding a lot of family pain and stress that seemed to lead to an increase in her stomach migraines. In yoga therapy sessions, the patient learned to use breathing techniques to increase her interoceptive awareness. Through deep breathing, the patient became aware of how family traumas impacted her. She'd tried to "protect" her family from the damaging effects of this by stuffing those feelings down. She reported feeling a mix of sadness, anger, and confusion. Michelle encouraged her to talk about these difficult feelings in family sessions, where the family therapist was able to support the patient's experience and help her family understand how brave it was for her to share these painful experiences. After several months of family and yoga therapy, the patient reported a decrease in stomach migraines, as well as an increase in her self-esteem and confidence.

## Review Client's Progress

To proceed smoothly and safely into Phase 2, consider the checklist below to determine a client's readiness. The client, their primary therapist, and you agree that the client demonstrates:

- Safe, trusting rapport with you their YP and with the primary therapist

- An increase in emotional regulation skills—they can use their "brakes" by using their various resources (such as anchors, oases, safe place, and safe space)

- The ability to identify body sensations and feelings more readily

- Self-compassion—the client asks for help and uses self-compassion when struggling

On the one hand, Phase 2 should not proceed if a client does not have a primary trauma therapist who has been actively working with the client on Phase 1 first. On the other hand, Phase 2 trauma therapy can be much more effective for a client when yoga therapy is integrated into the overall treatment plan, because of the powerful body-based tools that it has to offer.

The *trauma narrative* is one of the key interventions the primary trauma therapist introduces to the client in Phase 2. "The trauma narrative is a psychological technique used to help survivors of trauma make sense of their experiences, while also acting as a form of exposure to painful memories" (Therapistaid, 2024, "Trauma narratives" section). This technique is considered a form of exposure therapy and is a psychotherapeutic skill that needs to be conducted by a trained, experienced trauma therapist. While it can be a very effective tool on its own, Michelle has found that the trauma narrative is more healing when it is paired with yoga therapy.

The trauma narrative helps the client take control of their story by telling it in their own words and from their own perspective. This is vital to a client feeling a sense of agency and restored empowerment. In addition, the trauma narrative helps the client recognize that their trauma has a beginning, middle, and end. (Recall that one of the worst parts of trauma is that it feels never-ending.)

But the trauma narrative also exposes the client to the bodily triggers and sensations that were present during the trauma. Including yoga therapy in trauma treatment at this phase can greatly help the client build awareness and tolerance of the aversive body sensations that arise while they are sharing and processing their trauma narrative without becoming flooded. When the YP and the primary trauma therapist work collaboratively during Phase 2 of a client's trauma treatment, they help the client further integrate and heal from the trauma.

## Using Yoga Tools to Process Trauma

The goal of Phase 2 is to help the client cultivate a sense of hope, empowerment, and agency (Courtois & Ford, 2016). To that end, the YP offers the client yoga tools that help them widen their window of tolerance. This is an exciting and challenging time for both the client and the YP. Each client is different and what works well with one client may not work at all with another.

Before we explore general principles for how to tailor yoga tools for Phase 2 with a client, let's consider our adolescent case study. When Devin was ready for Phase 2, they learned to use the awareness of moment-to-moment body sensations that they'd cultivated during active yoga practice into less-active and more restorative yoga poses. Recall that they increased their body awareness in short yoga vinyasas but felt triggered by calming poses like savasana. They used to feel that the "floaty" sensation they felt after yoga was too much like dissociation. But over time and with practice, they said they were able to slow things down and notice that the sensation after yoga was a "feeling of peace and being present," *not* dissociation.

"It's like when there's noise and finally there's silence. That's what it feels like after yoga. Also, I can feel like a human being who deserves respect." Devin's sentiment that they now felt like a person—a human who deserves respect—is the hallmark of someone who has regained a sense of hope and empowerment. Other clients say things like, "I see my worth now." These powerful statements express the tremendous courage and work it takes to transform the inner wounds of CPTSD that shatter one's sense of self, to an empowered sense of self-worth and humanity.

While there is no exact formula, the rule of thumb at this phase of treatment is to start where the client is. Devin needed to start with more active yoga, because stillness caused dissociation. It took nearly two years of regular yoga therapy sessions and practice on their own to move into Phase 2, where they could tolerate a slower pace and do savasana at the end of practice.

Other clients who feel depressed and "stuck" may prefer a slower start to yoga therapy. A practice like Sa Ta Na Ma mentioned at the beginning of this chapter is best for these clients.

## Phase 3: Integration of Skills and Knowledge

The goal of Phase 2 is to shift from victimhood and powerlessness to a sense of hope, empowerment, and agency (Courtois & Ford, 2016). Phase 3 is a con-solidation of all the skills learned in Phases 1 and 2. The client can apply "the skills, knowledge, and increased self-worth and self-confidence acquired in the first two phases to all the facets of current (and future) daily life" (Cour-tois & Ford, 2016, p. 121). To ensure a smooth, safe transition from Phase 2 to 3 we follow a similar checklist used in the last phase transition. Like Phase 2, Phase 3 requires a trauma-focused level of care, since a client cannot inte-grate skills and knowledge until they have processed the trauma(s).

### Review Client's Progress

Use the checklist below to determine a client's readiness. The client, their primary therapist, and you the YP agree that the client demonstrates:

- Continued safe, trusting rapport with you their YP and with the pri-mary therapist

- Consistent use of self- and emotional regulation skills

- Increased self-compassion—the client both asks for help and uses self-compassion when struggling

- Increased sense of confidence and agency

### Relationships and Lifestyle

One of the hallmarks of Phase 3 is that clients gain what is known as "earned secure" attachment (Courtois & Ford, 2016, p. 121). Through healthy interac-tions with their primary therapist and you their YP, the client's attachment style changes. They may let go of relationships that aren't serving them. They seek out and establish relationships that are more supportive, reciprocal, and nurturing. Most importantly, clients at this phase show a more positive relationship to themselves—their bodies and health (mental/emotional as well as physical). If a client has a spiritual or religious practice, they often talk about how they use these practices as part of their continued wellness at this stage.

## Self-Care Practice: Healthy Boundary

Reading about the many ways in which CPTSD survivors suffer and experience disruption in their lives can be triggering. It's important to take time to practice self-care to process and let go of the material you just read. The first step in good self-care is healthy boundaries, so let's start there.

While you might think that you want to feel everything your client is telling you—or that you feel from them—this is not a sustainable way to practice. In fact, this is a formula for burnout. Instead, it is best to visualize an invisible boundary between you and clients. In addition, as you listen to your client's words, listen only with your ears. For those of us who are visual, take care not to visualize what your client tells you. Visualizing makes the experience more real, and harder to separate from. This is a technique Michelle's supervisor taught her when she interned at a rape crisis center, and it made a huge difference for her.

Incorporate your boundary visualization into Mindful Transition if you like. To do this, start as usual by noticing your internal state. How do you feel after reading this chapter? What are your thoughts, feelings, body sensations, and state of mind? Take some deep breaths. From the body sensations you've noticed, what kind of wall would serve to protect and nurture you? Perhaps all it takes is a membrane as thin as a soap bubble. Imagine this membrane that supports you to be present with your client's experience without taking on their burden.

## Chapter Summary

- A phase-based approach is the best course of treatment for those who suffer from both PTSD and CPTSD.

- The goal of Phase 1 is to help the client cultivate safety and stability in their life, relationships, and within themselves.

- An individual's reaction to a trauma trigger is automatic and out of their control before they start treatment. Identifying body sensation (interoception), and then feelings, helps slow this process down.

- The client's avoidance or numbing of troublesome emotions, feelings, and body sensations is a protective adaptation for most (if not all) CPTSD survivors. As such, increasing awareness means letting go of these adaptations, which takes time and patience on the part of the client as well as the YP.

- Yoga therapy is the perfect complement to complex trauma treatment: it offers a gentle, mindful approach to body-based work that empowers clients to increase somatic awareness with intention and at their own pace.

- The goal of Phase 2 is to shift from victimhood and powerlessness to a sense of hope, empowerment, and agency.

- Phase 3 is a consolidation of all the skills learned in Phases 1 and 2, and therefore is an integration of skills and knowledge.

# The Fundamental Movements and Yoga Tools

## Integration
### Fundamental Movements: The Origin Story

In this CPTSD-informed yoga therapy model, yoga tools are applied using the panchamaya kosha, the gunas, and the *six fundamental movements* (Frank, 2024, para. 4). Gestalt and somatic psychotherapist Ruella Frank introduced this concept in her book *Body of Awareness: A Somatic and Developmental Approach to Psychotherapy* (2001). The fundamental movements (FM) are yield, push, reach, grasp, pull, and release (Frank, 2013). They represent what Frank calls "a movement vocabulary that develops in the first year of life and continues to be essential to all our interactions throughout life" (2013, 0:10–0:19). As babies, our developing movements inform our relationships—with ourselves, others, and the environment around us. In this way, the movements articulated in the FM are closely associated with one's attachment style.

Also known as *fundamental actions* (Aposhyan, 2007), *satisfaction cycle* (Schwartz, 2018), and *developmental actions/movements* (Frank, 2001), the original inspiration for the FM came from Bonnie Bainbridge Cohen (Frank, 2001, 2024). Creator of Body-Mind Centering™ (2024), Bainbridge Cohen conceived of a set of *developmental movement patterns* that is the basis of Frank's fundamental movements. Bainbridge Cohen's more than 50 years of research and work has inspired those in the fields of "movement, dance, yoga, bodywork, physical and occupational therapy, psychotherapy, child development, education, voice, music, art, meditation, athletics, and other body–mind disciplines" (Bainbridge Cohen, 2024, para. 2).

We focus on Frank's conceptualization of movement because the FM "demonstrate how movement plays a critical role in a developing self-awareness for the infant and in maintaining a healthy self throughout life" (Frank,

2001, p. 11). Frank (2001) notes that the movements learned in infancy teach the child what is "me and not me" (p. 14). Frank goes on to explain that these patterns echo into adult experience. This emphasis on the relational aspect of movement works well with CPTSD-informed yoga therapy, because at its core, complex trauma is relational trauma. Understanding the six fundamental movements can strengthen a YP's attunement to clients by increasing awareness of nonverbal body cues that arise during sessions (Frank, 2001).

## Integration of Fundamental Movements into Yoga Therapy

This chapter is divided into five sections—one for each FM (except for grasp and pull, which are presented in the same section, because they frequently occur together in physical, emotional, and psychological movement). In each section we define the movement, yoga tools that cultivate its qualities, and how to use yoga tools therapeutically, especially for the treatment of CPTSD symptoms. Before delving into a description of each movement, let's consider the FM's relevance to CPTSD-informed yoga therapy.

As Australian trauma therapist Monique Pangari explains, "Movement patterns that have not been adequately embodied can create challenges in being able to fully relax, learn, process our emotions, [and] express and ask for our needs to be met, all of which can have a huge impact on our relationships, communication and learning" (Pangari, 2022, para. 3). **Integrating the fundamental movements into yoga therapy allows the client to not only become aware of the traumas held in the body, but also learn new movement patterns.**

When a child is nurtured in a safe, healthy environment with the rhythm of routine, they naturally learn the FM. Much like the three gunas that are constantly "in dynamic interaction" (Frawley, 1999, p. 28), the child organically moves from one FM to the next (Frank, 2013). Such dynamic flow is the healthy state of a flexible, responsive nervous system.

Imagine a toddler, peacefully resting in a parent's lap. The toddler is *yielding*—their body leans into and receives the support of the parent. Suddenly, the child spots a colorful toy nearby. In this case, the child may *reach* with their eyes before they *push* against the parent to be let down. A loving parent will make sure the child exits their lap safely. Once on their own, the child can then *reach* with their arm and hand to *grasp* and *pull* the toy toward them. The child will enjoy making this dazzling new object its own by playing with it for a time. And then finally when the child has satisfied their curiosity and tired of the toy, they will *release* it. This dynamic flow of the child's movements, and the safe and loving interactions with the parent, are all part of the dance of the fundamental movements (Frank, 2001).

However, when a child is raised in a chaotic, unpredictable, and/or unsafe environment, the FMs are disrupted. **These disruptions show up in an individual's patterns of relating in their life as hyper-arousal (a *rajasic* state of too much mobilization—a chaotic environment) and/or hypo-arousal (a *tamasic* state of collapse or numbing—a neglectful environment).** When the stressors are pervasive, chronic, and acute, the child develops rigid and fixed ways of being and relating to themselves and the world that mirror disturbances in their FM. Let's consider the following examples (the FM are bolded and the gunas are italicized).

A baby who doesn't receive enough "tummy time" (National Institute of Health, n.d.) may become anxious and grow up to be an adult who can't relax. This is someone who has a *rajasic* relationship to **yield**. A child who witnesses his older brother being beaten when he stands up to an abusive parent may learn to become passive. The child may become an adult who finds it difficult to create boundaries or ask for what he needs. He has a *tamasic* relationship to **push**. A baby born into a South Asian brothel will learn that she and all the adult women around her aren't afforded the opportunities of others. She may assume she can't or shouldn't bother to **reach** for her dreams (a *tamasic* state of learned helplessness). Similarly, an African American boy with a sharp intellect and talent for AI may find that his dream of becoming a computer engineer is out of his **grasp** due to systemic racism. Due to societal constraints, he may feel forced into a *tamasic* relationship to grasping what should be in reach for him. And lastly, a child who is abandoned by a parent early on may learn that if she doesn't take what she wants, she won't get anything. She may develop a *rajasic* relationship with **pull**, and take what isn't hers, perhaps by overtly stealing or more subtly by taking credit for others' work.

## Application of Fundamental Movements in Yoga Therapy

In the YTCT model, the FM are integrated into yoga therapy treatment in the following ways.

### Assessment and Treatment Planning

At the beginning of treatment, the YP collaborates with the client to assess and determine their treatment plan based on information gathered from the panchamaya kosha, gunas, and FM (Chapter 7 lays out the model in its entirety). Examining a client's functioning in each of the five koshas helps the YP determine the target kosha(s) for treatment goals. Assessing how the gunas are currently influencing the client's FM helps the YP determine the objectives of those goals.

## Treatment Sessions

During yoga therapy treatment, the YP uses the fundamental movements in one of a few ways. First, the YP employs yoga tools to remedy one or several FMs where the client seems stuck. For instance, recall that Teresa (Chapter 2) had difficulty relaxing. She said she felt suffocated and wanted to scream when doing savasana in a yoga class. In the YTCT model, we would say her hypervigilant reaction to savasana demonstrated a *rajasic* relationship to the FM of yield. To remedy this, Michelle taught Teresa the Wave Vinyasa (Chapter 2), in which she repeated a moving sequence—a *rajasic* action— of yoga poses that included brief holds of Child's Pose (a yoga posture with yield qualities). After several rounds, Teresa could stay in the yielding posture of Child's Pose for a few more seconds with each round.

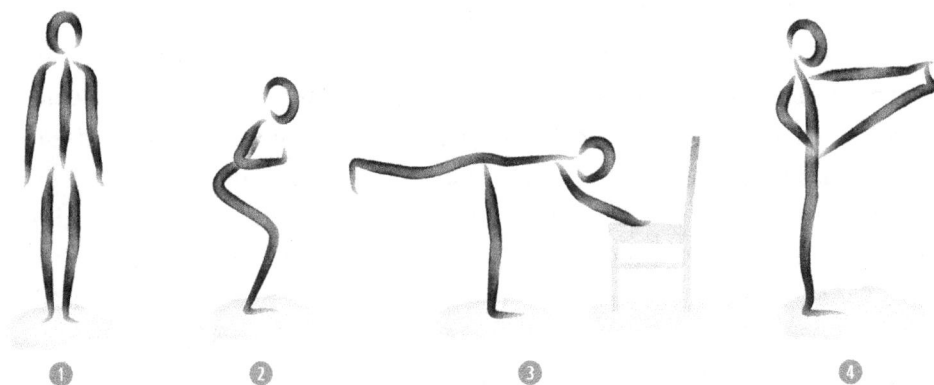

**Figure 5.1** Rajasic Vinyasa
*Depicts a challenging sequence of yoga poses that energizes and cultivates focus.*

Conversely, the YP may use a yoga sequence that mimics the entire fundamental movements to help a client feel a sense of embodied accomplishment and satisfaction if they are stuck in old patterns. For example, later in treatment Teresa complained of feeling stuck in old patterns of relating to her ex-husband. Talking through these old patterns didn't help her, because as she put it, she tended to "get stuck in my head." Feeling stuck is a *tamasic* feeling, so Michelle suggested they try a new vinyasa to help her feel strong, powerful, and capable. This time, Michelle created a standing yoga vinyasa. (Standing poses and vinyasas are more *rajasic* in nature.)

## The Fundamental Movements and Yoga Tools

Now let's consider how the fundamental movements and the eight limbs of yoga work together. For each FM we offer examples from many (sometimes all) of the eight limbs that exemplify that FM. In addition, the gunas (sattva, rajas, and tamas) are integrated into the description of each movement in the following way: we consider the healthy expression of each movement as *sattvic* (balanced, harmonious) and give examples of yoga tools that cultivate this healthy expression. Then two expressions of disruption for each movement are considered: its *rajasic* (hypervigilant, hypermobile) expression and its *tamasic* (collapsed, dissociated, disconnected, muted) expression.

### Fundamental Movements as Integrative Framework

The FM also provide an integrative framework in which to consider the seven limbs of yoga other than asana. For instance, we list *ahimsa* (nonviolence) under the first FM of *yield*. In essence, ahimsa in the therapeutic context means safety. A child who can yield into the arms of the caregiver feels safe. Likewise, a client who can find safety in various yoga poses and practices is yielding. For this to happen, the YP must provide a safe space. In this sense, safety (Phase 1 of CPTSD-informed treatment), ahimsa (which falls within the yogic limb of the yamas), and yield (the first developmental movement) are synonyms.

For each movement, we list possible yoga tools from the limbs of yoga that embody the qualities of that movement. Each list is illustrative, not exhaustive. Use the lists as springboards for your own ideas. With regards to the yoga asanas, many (if not most) asanas embody several of the FM at once. So, a pose listed under one FM might easily be listed under a different one. For instance, Child's Pose is usually performed with the arms outstretched on the floor. As such, we have included it in the list of asanas in the *Reach* section. However, we have also included Child's Pose in the *Yield* section with the hands stacked under the head.

### Fundamental Movements Within Yoga Asana

With regards to asanas, we have purposefully included a wide range of asanas that suit different fitness levels. We offer modifications with props like a chair for Simple Sitting Pose (sukhasana) and with a strap for Seated Head-to-Knee Pose (janu sirsasana), because these are such commonly used poses. This book assumes that the reader is well-versed in anatomy and physiology for yoga asana. If we present a pose that is not already in your teaching repertoire, please disregard it.

We do not address the use of partner poses in this first book. While partner poses can be incredibly healing when used at the right phase of treatment (most likely Phases 2 and 3), they can be problematic in Phase 1 because they involve touching and proximity. This is triggering for most clients early in—and sometimes throughout—treatment.

## Accessibility

Finally, yoga tools presented in this chapter tend to be good for all three age groups. In some cases, you will see two or more frames for an asana—the first frame(s) show modifications and the second or last frame shows the classical pose. Offer instruction and modification that are appropriate for each client, given their mobility, flexibility, and strength. Using a standardized range of motion assessment during the intake session is a great way to ensure this.

Another vital consideration is how long the YP invites the client to stay in a particular pose. The general rule is the younger the client, the less time they should spend in a pose. For instance, whereas a physically fit adult can hold Downward Facing Dog Pose (adho mukha svanasana) for 10–20 seconds, an 8-year-old should hold this pose for no longer than 5 seconds.

Yoga therapy is not a one-size-fits-all process. Consider the unique needs of each client and how best to help them heal the disruptions in their movement and relating patterns. Use the following lists as reference for possible starting points, but not prescriptively.

## Sattvic Yield: Relaxed Alertness

When securely attached, an infant experiences a sense of safety, trust, and connection in the arms of the caregiver; this is **yield**, the first movement of the fundamental movements that starts in the womb when a fetus is held within the mother's body (May, 2022). A healthy, **sattvic** expression of yield is a state of relaxed alertness. To yield, we must fully "surrender (our) weight into gravity" (Schwartz, 2018, "Yield" section). The breathing is deep, perhaps with an extended exhale; and while relaxed, yielding also has a quality of alertness. May (2022) notes that there is gentle muscle tone, especially at the places of contact with the caregiver.

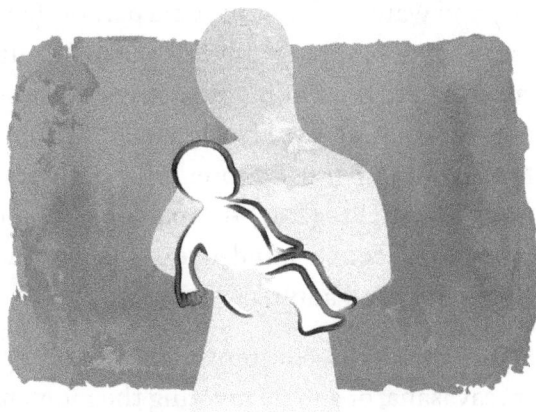

**Figure 5.2** Sattvic Yield
*Depicts the relaxed alertness of the first fundamental movement yield,
such as when a baby relaxes into the arms of a loving caregiver.*

In the therapeutic relationship, yielding shows up as trust and connection between client and YP when the client feels safe. Yet survivors of CPTSD often find this difficult. **As such, many survivors need to spend a longer time in Phase 1 of treatment.** Keep in mind that some clients may remain in Phase 1 for the duration of treatment, where they learn to trust themselves and increase body awareness while building a safe, stable rapport with you the YP.

## Yoga Tools for Sattvic Yield

**Yama:** Two yamas are particularly relevant to the FM of yield: ahimsa and aparigraha.

- *Ahimsa:* We can only yield when we feel safe. Thus *ahimsa*, or non-violence, can be seen as a form of yielding in that the act of not engaging in harm creates safety. Yoga practices that cultivate compassion and self-compassion help create this quality of security. Age-appropriate poems, songs, and chants can help little ones aged 5–12 years old develop self-compassion. Gail Silver's article "Metta (Loving-Kindness) Meditations for Kids" (2018) is a great resource for such practices. For other adolescents or adult clients, any guided meditation that fosters compassion and loving kindness also works.

- *Aparigraha*: This is the yama of nonattachment or letting go. When a client is ready and wants to let go of some part of their "story" through yoga practices, they are tapping into this yama. Mindfulness practices that bring attention to present moment sensation are great strategies to help clients let go. Both the Five Senses Mindfulness Practice and the Sa Ta Na Ma mantra (see Chapter 4 for both practices) are great examples. Jack Kornfield's (2017) *A Mind Like Sky* audio meditation (https://jackkornfield.com/a-mind-like-sky) is another great resource for older adolescents and adults.

**Niyama:** The practice of *santosa* (contentment and acceptance) through guided meditation, savasana, or simply savoring the moment are other ways to offer clients a chance to yield.

### Five Senses Game (for 5–12-year-olds)

Michelle developed a *Five Senses Game* for primary school children that helps them savor and experience each of their five senses in an interactive way. With one child, this game will take 20–30 minutes. With a group of children, allow 45–60 minutes. Be sure to plan this game in advance by finding out if the child/children are allergic to, or find aversive, any foods or scents.

*Sight*: Play "I spy with my little eye" with the child or group. If you are unfamiliar with this children's game, here is a cute YouTube video from Kalm Kids (2024) that you can watch and use with children: www.youtube.com/watch?v=HMp2Aj7Z9uc

*Sound*: Use a singing bowl or bells to bring the child/children's attention to sound. Alternatively, do a short meditation on sound during which you bring the children's attention to various sounds around them, especially pleasant and/or neutral sounds.

*Exception: Sound can be a trigger for many survivors of CPTSD. Be sure to find out if the child/children have any sound triggers before playing this part of the game. If a client does become triggered during a session, end the triggering practice right away and help the client use one of the anchors or oases (Chapter 4) to re-regulate.*

*Touch*: The child/children are offered an object (stuffy or another toy) that they can't see. If comfortable, the child/children can close their eyes, and the YP places the object in their hands. If not, the child/children keep their eyes open, and the YP places the object on the floor behind them within hand's reach, allowing the child to reach for and explore the object behind their back. Children are asked to guess the color(s) and what the object itself is before looking at it.

*Smell*: Ensuring that the scent to be used is neither an allergen nor offensive to the child/children, the YP passes around vials of essential oils or other pleasant scents. This exercise brings up many memories that children like to share. Be sure to allow time for sharing.

*Taste*: Mindful eating—This exercise comes directly from Marsha Linehan's Dialectical Behavioral protocol, an evidence-based therapy treatment Michelle was formally trained in and practiced at CHCO. Contact parents ahead of time to determine what, if any, allergies each child has. Foods like grapes or fruit gummies in individually wrapped bags are good options. Once again, the child/children can close their eyes or leave them open. Instruct the child/ group to eat the food item very slowly, encouraging pauses when the food is in the child's hand, after they have put the food in their mouth but have not chewed yet, and after one chew. Once chewing, suggest the child/group chew as slowly as possible, noticing how a familiar food may taste different simply from eating it mindfully.

*Exception: The taste exercise in this game may not be appropriate or possible in some settings. In this case, replace this part of the game with a "What I love" section where the child/children are asked to think about something or someone they love and share.*

## Asana:

**Caution:** those with sexual trauma may have difficulty with most or all supine poses, especially those over a bolster. Be sure to check with the client about their comfort level and feelings of safety, and observe their body language, before and while using these poses. This is a good moment to practice Look-Feel-Sound (see Chapter 7) to be mindful of nonverbal communication.

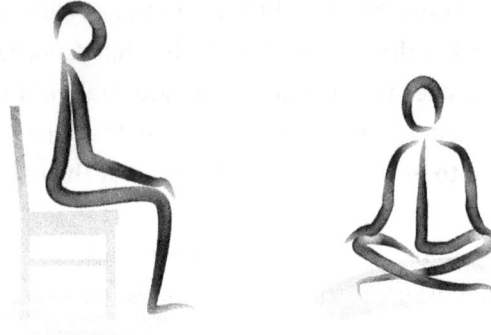

Modified                                    Classical

**Figure 5.3** Simple Seated Pose—Sukhasana

*Depicts two variations of Simple Seated Pose, which encourages relaxed alertness when seated.*

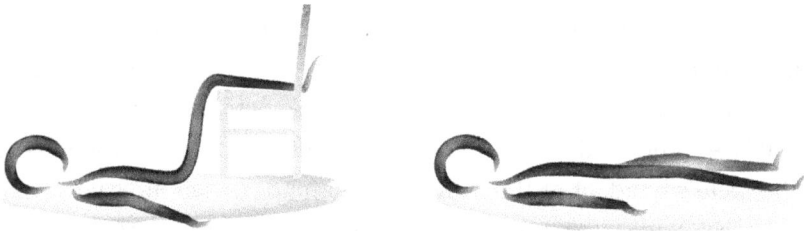

Modified                                    Classical

**Figure 5.4** Relaxation Pose—Savasana

*Depicts two variations of Relaxation Pose, which encourages
relaxed alertness when lying down.*

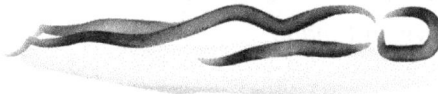

**Figure 5.5** Lying on Belly

*Depicts Lying on Belly Pose—this may not be possible for clients with neck, shoulder,
or back issues. Be sure to do a range of motion assessment before recommending it.*

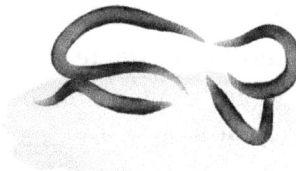

**Figure 5.6** Child's Pose with Hands Under Head—Balasana

*Depicts another variation of Child's Pose with the hands under the head. This
is a good variation for clients with neck, shoulder, or back issues.*

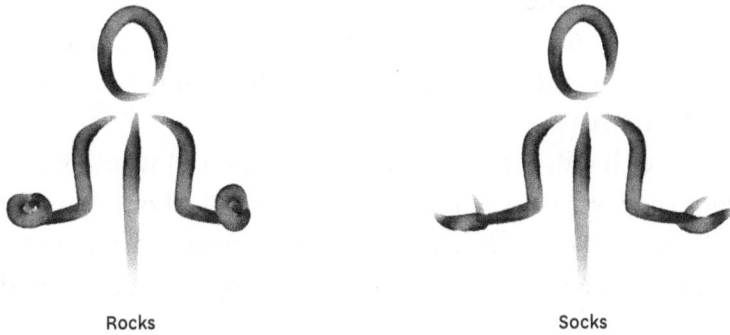

Rocks                                                        Socks

**Figure 5.7** Rocks and Socks

*Depicts the practice Rocks and Socks: inhale and ball up the hands (rocks), exhale and release the hands (socks). Repeat 3–5 times. Good for all ages, especially children.*

**Pranayama:** Any breathing practice that increases the exhale and/or awareness of exhale such as counting breaths with extended exhale.

*Exception: Bear in mind that some clients may be triggered by breathing practices, just like Devin (Chapter 4), or they may be too young for formal breathing practice (Chapter 2). Be sure to collaborate with the client and their care team to avoid any practices, including breathing, that are not appropriate or are triggering for them.*

**Dharana:** Any concentration practice that allows the client's mind and body to relax and settle into the present moment helps cultivate yield. For instance, a body scan such as Yoga Nidra can be helpful.

**Dhyana:** Guided meditations that help clients feel relaxed and a sense of belonging can cultivate yield. Using a client's established Safe Place (Chapter 4) is a great example.

Difficulties with yield occur when an individual either did not receive the consistent, nurturing care from caregivers, or safety and connection were ruptured through interpersonal traumas. Clients may relate to yield in a hypervigilant, constricted way, or may dissociate rather than yield.

## Rajasic Yield

*Rajasic yield* means that a client is experiencing hypervigilance and/or constriction. Recall Teresa from Chapter 2: she was a high achiever who had difficulty relaxing. Poses like Relaxation Pose made her feel panicky (a form of hypervigilance), whereas Chataranga felt more comfortable. This is an example of a client who possesses too much mobilization in the sympathetic nervous system. For her, doing the Wave Vinyasa (Chapter 2) helped her slow her movements down until she could spend increasing amounts of time in Child's Pose.

On the other hand, sometimes Devin (Chapter 4) would stare off into space. Once they were out of this state, they'd talk about racing thoughts going through their head. This was a sign they were in a state of constriction. Using movement such as vinyasa often helped them shake this feeling state.

## Tamasic Yield

*Tamasic yield* means a client is in a collapsed state. This collapsed yield can show up for a client through hypo-arousal, and possibly some level of dissociation. Like Teresa, Devin (Chapter 4) also didn't like savasana. But whereas Teresa felt panicky in it, Devin tended to dissociate, or mentally collapse. The state of collapse that occurs when someone dissociates can mimic yield (Bainbridge Cohen, 2023; Schwartz, 2021). Thus, it is very important to differentiate. "When I collapse... I have lost the sense of self in relation to gravity" (Bainbridge Cohen, 2023, 0:27–1:07).

To help Devin relate to *yield* in a sattvic (or balanced) way, Michelle the YP helped them identify what body sensations felt safe. Devin noticed that they felt safe increasing their awareness of body sensations in short, active vinyasas (review Chapter 4). This process is known as *pre-yield*—where the individual builds interoceptive awareness to relate healthfully to yield. Once Devin felt safe noticing transitory body sensations, they were able to slow down both their movements and their mind until they themselves recognized that the "floaty" feeling after yoga was not dissociation but relaxation. This new awareness showed their increased ability to *yield* rather than *collapse.*

As the examples of Teresa and Devin show, clients usually need a repertoire of poses in the form of short vinyasas or tailored sequences to heal the unique disruptions in their FM.

## Sattvic Push: Boundaries and Independence

Each of the FM relies on the previous one (Schwartz, 2021). When we feel safe enough to yield into gravity, we can then push against our connection to the earth. The pushing action is what allows a baby to push with arms, legs, belly, and head to eventually crawl (Frank, 2013; May, 2022; Schwartz, 2018). Center for Somatic Studies Founder Dr. Ruella Frank (2013) calls the pushing action a "separating from while including the other" (1:30–1:33). Because this movement is what allows babies to be more independent, it is considered the movement that creates boundaries. When I extend my arm out with a flat palm, I am saying "no."

In addition, push is associated with strength, because we must engage our core to push (May, 2022). Right now, try pressing your palms against each other. Notice as you push your hands your core engages. Lastly, May (2022) says that push is associated with assertiveness and self-esteem, because it helps us align our posture.

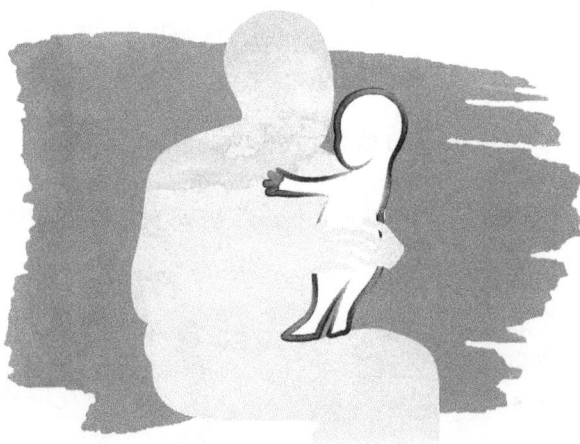

**Figure 5.8** Sattvic Push

*Depicts the second fundamental movement push, illustrated by a baby pushing with hands and legs against the caregiver. This movement facilitates independence and boundaries.*

## Yoga Tools for Sattvic Push

**Yama:** Clients can use the yama of *brahmacharya* (self-control, moderation) to create better boundaries with others by not giving their time and energy to those who don't support or nurture them.

**Niyama:** The niyamas of both *tapas* (perseverance) and *svadhyaya* (self-reflection and introspection) can be very useful in helping a client cultivate strength and a sense of self.

**Asana:**

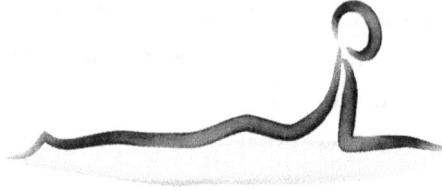

**Figure 5.9** Sphinx Pose—Salabhasana Prep
*Depicts Sphinx Pose, which encourages a supported form of pushing into the floor.*

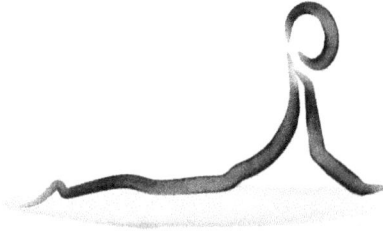

**Figure 5.10** Cobra Pose—Bhujangasana
*Depicts Cobra Pose, an active but still supportive form of push. Be sure to do a range of motion assessment to ensure a client does not have back or shoulder issues.*

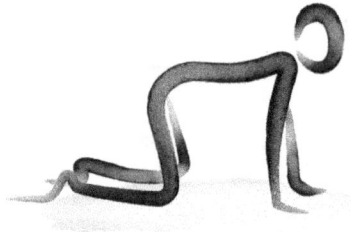

**Figure 5.11** Table Pose—Bharmanasana
*Depicts Table Pose, which encourages push with both arms and legs.*

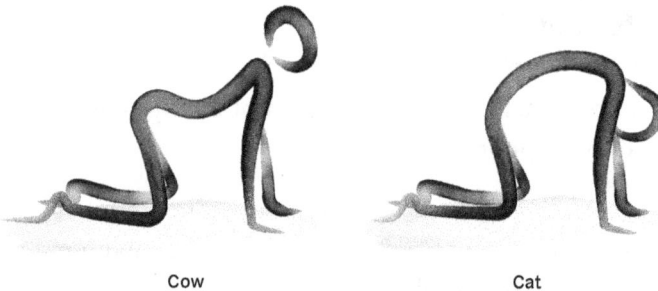

Cow                    Cat

**Figure 5.12** Cat-Cow Pose
*Depicts Cat-Cow Pose, which massages the spine while also encouraging push with arms and legs.*

Modified　　　　　　　　　　Classical

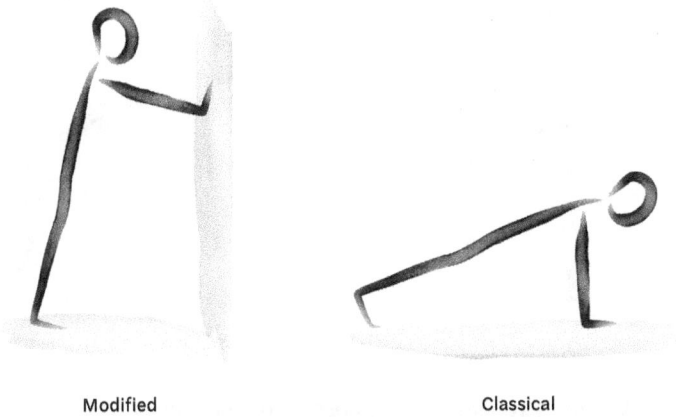

**Figure 5.13** Plank Pose—Phalakasana

*Depicts two variations of Plank Pose. The first variation is great if a client has shoulder/
neck issues. The second variation is more challenging, requiring upper body strength.*

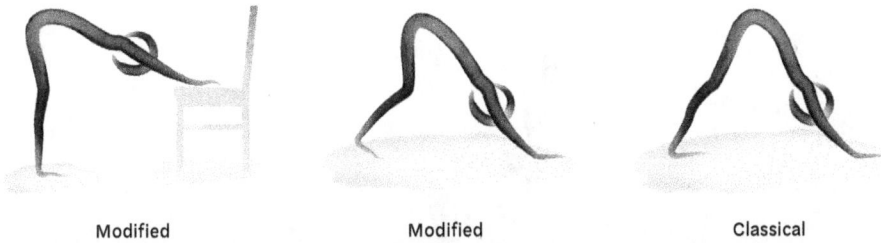

Modified　　　　　　　　Modified　　　　　　　　Classical

**Figure 5.14** Downward Facing Dog Pose—Adho Mukha Svanasana

*Depicts three variations of Downward Facing Dog Pose. This pose is great for lengthening
the back, and engaging many muscle groups and FMs at the same time.*

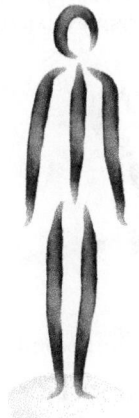

**Figure 5.15** Mountain Pose—Tadasana

*Depicts Mountain Pose, the quintessential yoga pose that also emphasizes the FMs
of push through the legs, as well as yield through connection with gravity.*

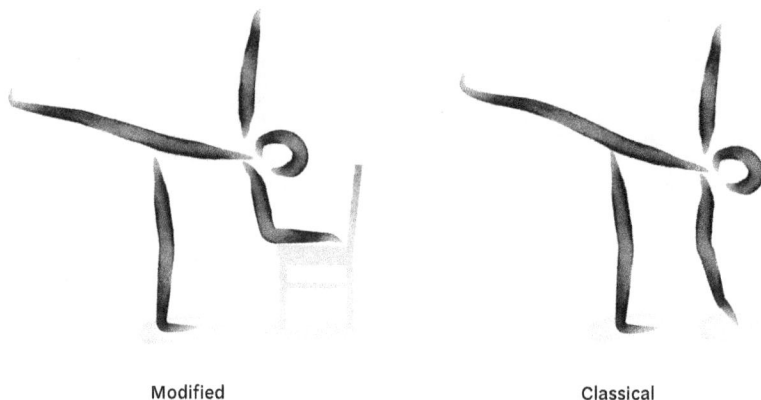

Modified                                    Classical

**Figure 5.16** Half-Moon Pose—Ardha Chandrasana

*Depicts two variations of Half Moon Pose, which emphasizes push through one side of the body in both the arm and leg.*

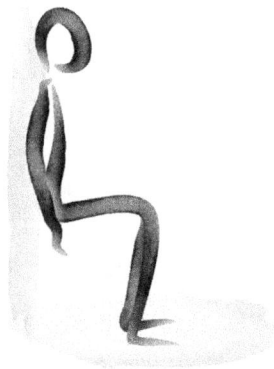

**Figure 5.17** Wall Sit

*Depicts a wall sit—a very intense and energizing form of push. This pose is great for clients who prefer intensity to decrease anxiety and increase emotion regulation.*

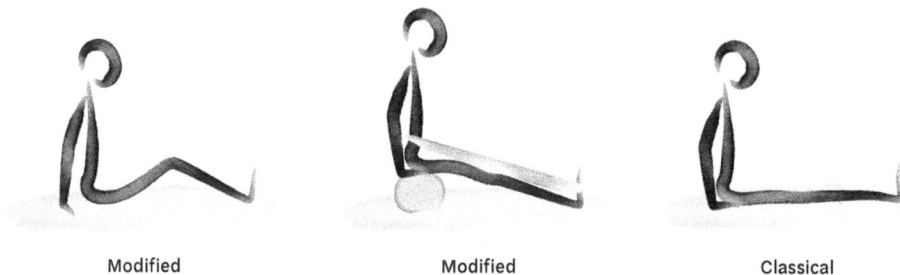

Modified                    Modified                    Classical

**Figure 5.18** Stick Pose—Dandasana

*Depicts three variations of Stick Pose, depending on a client's flexibility. Notice the push primarily through the arms but also through the legs.*

**Pranayama:**

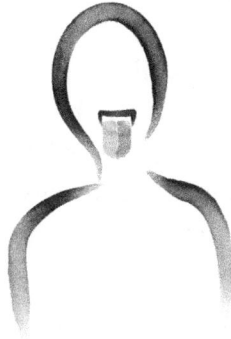

**Figure 5.19** Lion's Breath—Simha Pranayama

*Depicts Lion's Breath, where one exhales with a loud "aaahhh!" This breathing technique cultivates push by emphasizing the exhale. It helps release tension, and is fun for all ages.*

**Dharana:** Concentration or visualization practices that focus on creating boundaries are useful. For example, try using the Sa Ta Na Ma mantra (Chapter 4) against a wall or other surface to help clients feel the FM of push while they recite it.

**Dhyana:** Try using a guided meditation that helps a client create boundaries, such as visualizing a protective barrier between themselves and others.

Disruptions in the push can occur when a child is not allowed to create healthy boundaries. If parents were aggressive or overbearing, a child may become overly accommodating. Conversely, a child may adopt the aggressive stance of a caregiver as a defense. Also, if a child experiences chronic neglect from a parent, they may not have had the opportunity to explore this movement fully.

## Rajasic Push

Somatic psychologist Jennifer May (2022) points out that because the fundamental movements are constantly in relationship, when there is an excess of one movement, there is a deficit of another. For instance, someone who exhibits an over-abundance of push also shows a deficit of yield. This can be seen in clients who complain that they push others away. A client may "feel protected but not connected" (May, 2022, 1:26). The tendency to disconnect and isolate by pushing others away is a form of hypervigilance and rajasic push. For example, one of Michelle's clients who desperately wanted to have a fulfilling romantic relationship kept pushing her partners away. This client benefitted from doing Viloma Breathing (mentioned in the above yield section), which helped her increase her ability to yield and decrease her desire to push others away.

Another way a client may exhibit a rajasic push is through constriction. Recall that *constriction* (Chapter 3) is when the nervous system narrows one's focus and effort to ensure the best possible chance of survival (Levine, 1997). If a client becomes hyperfocused during a session—perhaps on something they felt they did wrong in a pose, or something you the YP said to them—they may likely be exhibiting constriction. As with many triggers, the best thing the YP can do is stop whatever technique they may be practicing and/or gently ask what they notice in their body at that moment. This not only distracts the client from whatever may have triggered them; it also allows the client to use their body sensation to yield into the present moment.

## Tamasic Push

When an individual was or is not allowed to exercise boundaries with others in their life, they may exhibit not enough push and too much yield (May, 2022). This can be seen in clients who don't know how to say no or make decisions. Such a client may seem very agreeable at first, until it becomes apparent that they want you the YP to make all the decisions.

When this is the case, the YP can do two things: first somatically with yoga asana, and then with the therapeutic interaction. Somatically, the YP can suggest that the client practice Mountain Pose with legs slightly bent to feel their weight supported by gravity. Once the connection to the floor and gravity is established, the YP invites the client to push firmly against it by straightening and bending the legs a few times.

When and if the client remarks on their own that they can feel the floor, feel their center or core, or in any other way indicates that this pushing Mountain Pose practice was pleasant, the YP knows the client is ready for the next step. In this second step, the YP gently brings the client's attention to their tendency to defer decisions to others—many times, clients are already aware they do this. The YP can then invite the client to make a choice between two poses or practices they like. Even if the client is unable to do this, the YP acknowledges the client's bravery in noticing their tamasic push and reassures them that this awareness is progress in and of itself.

## Sattvic Reach: Curiosity

Babies show curiosity by reaching (Frank, 2013). They reach for both objects and people. Frank (2013) says the reach gesture is expressed in the eyes, mouth, and limbs, and excitement about reaching out is influenced by who or what is reached for. Reach is associated with satisfying needs, as well as power, ownership, and "healthy entitlement" (May, 2022, 6:27). When a child is chronically neglected, they are not given the opportunity to develop this fundamental movement.

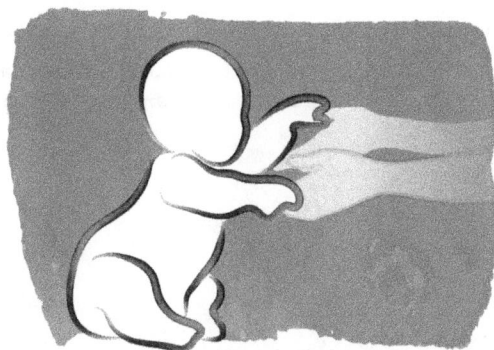

**Figure 5.20** Sattvic Reach

*Depicts the third fundamental movement of reach, as illustrated by a baby reaching for its caregiver. This movement evokes curiosity and wish to connect with the outside world.*

## Yoga Tools for Sattvic Reach

**Niyama:** Reaching takes energy, and so the niyama of tapas (perseverance) applies as much to this FM as it does to the last. The YP can help a client cultivate tapas by noticing the activity of muscles and movement within their yoga therapy session, as well as throughout their day outside of therapy.

**Asana:** Almost all standing (and standing balance) poses have some degree of reach in them. Since we have featured many of these already in other FM sections, we will highlight others we have not listed yet.

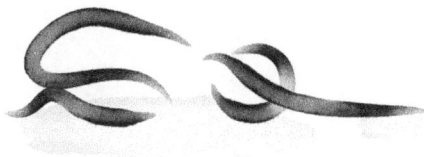

**Figure 5.21** Child's Pose—Balasana

*Depicts the classical version of Child's Pose. With the arms outstretched, this pose offers a supportive form of reach.*

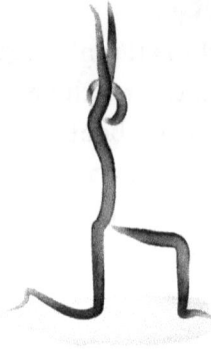

**Figure 5.22** Dragon Pose—Uttan Pristhasana

*Depicts Dragon Pose, which encourages a reach with the arms. Try combining with Lion's Breath with child clients: inhale arms up, and exhale sweep arms down as you exhale "aaahhh!"*

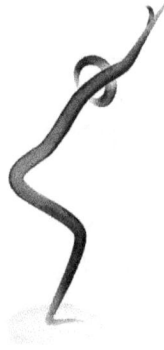

**Figure 5.23** Chair Pose—Utkatasana

*Depicts Chair Pose, an energizing, active form of reach. Be sure to do a range of motion assessment before introducing a client to this pose.*

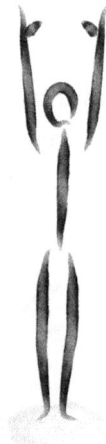

**Figure 5.24** Upward Salute—Urdhva Hastasana

*Depicts Upward Salute Pose, which combines the push of the legs in Mountain Pose with a reach of the arms. This pose helps cultivate a sense of grounding as well as upliftment.*

Modified        Classical

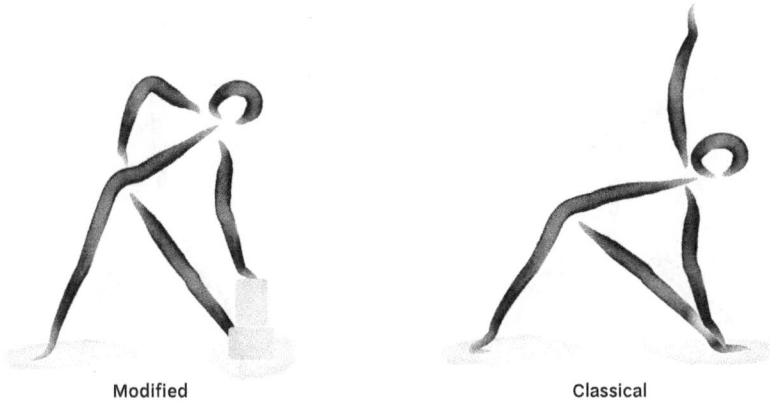

**Figure 5.25** Triangle Pose—Utthita Trikonasana

*Depicts two variations of Triangle Pose, depending on a client's flexibility. Standing poses by nature have a push and reach quality in the legs. Triangle adds a reach of the arm(s).*

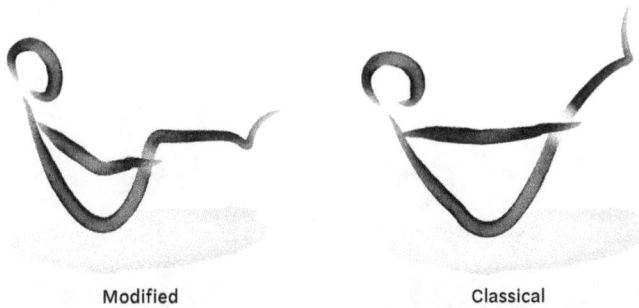

Modified        Classical

**Figure 5.26** Boat Pose—Navasana

*Depicts two variations of Boat Pose. Clients with low back issues will be safer in the first variation. This pose offers a very active reach through the legs.*

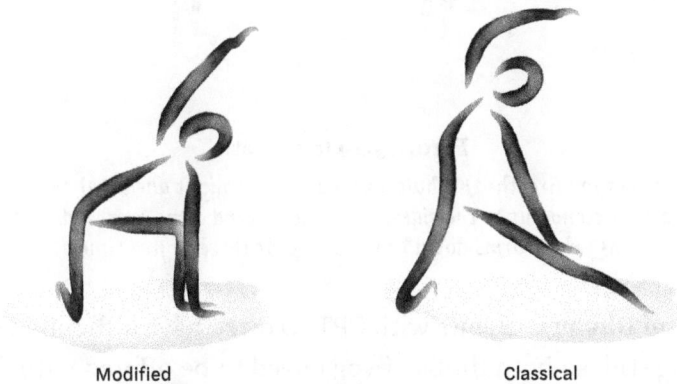

Modified        Classical

**Figure 5.27** Gate Pose—Parighasana

*Depicts two variations of Gate Pose. Like Triangle Pose, it offers the action of reach through the side body. Clients with herniated discs should avoid this pose.*

Modified                                    Classical

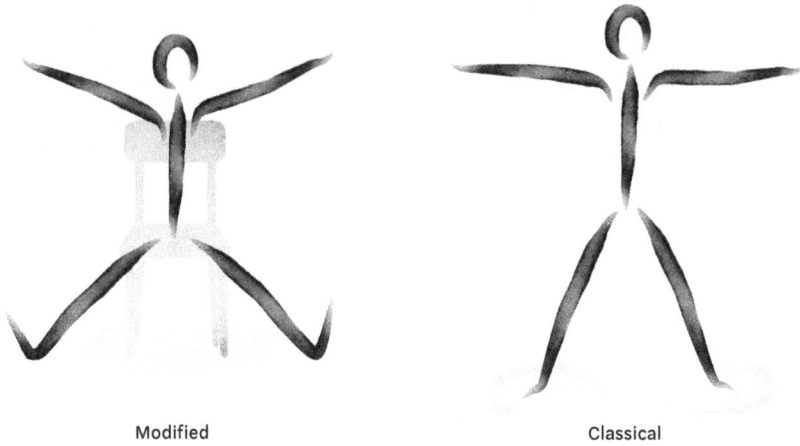

**Figure 5.28** Five-Pointed Star Pose—Utthita Tadasana

*Depicts two variations of Five-Pointed Star, in which all limbs and the head reach. This pose encourages the client to expand the space they embody—to literally take up space.*

**Pranayama:**

①                    ②                    ③                    ④

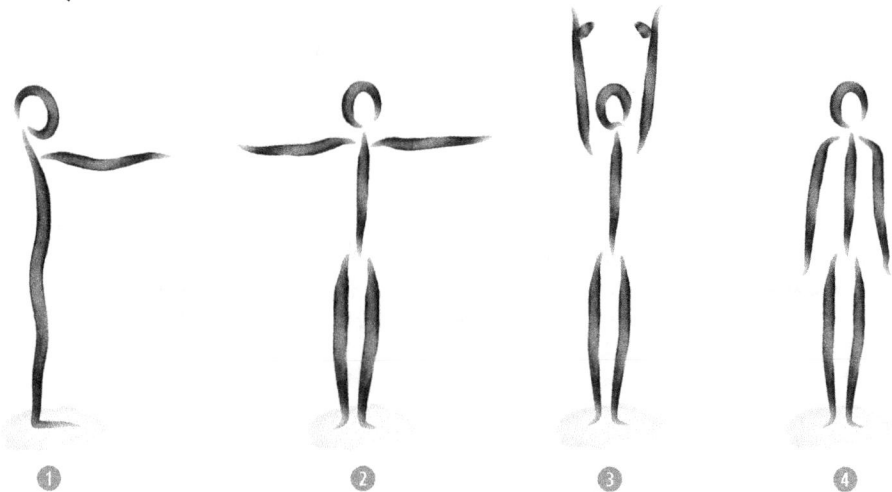

**Figure 5.29** Joy Breath

*Depicts Joy Breath: 1) inhale, extend arms straight ahead; 2) exhale, arms extend out to the sides; 3) inhale, extend arms overhead; and 4) exhale arms down to sides. Repeat three to five times.*

**Dharana and Dhyana:** Clients with CPTSD often have difficulty with focusing or being still, so both limbs of yoga need to be offered with fine-tuned attention to how the client responds to them. Proceed at the client's pace so that they don't become frustrated or triggered. See the next section for guidance on how to help a client re-regulate if they find a yoga tool frustrating.

## Rajasic Reach

A client who says they feel desperate or frantic may struggle with overreach. If their reach is too intense, it can come off as needy or demanding (May, 2022). If a client says they feel like they wear their friends or partners out, their reach may be too strong. An overly strong reach is also associated with reaching out for that which is not ours. On the other hand, if a client says they tend to over-extend themselves, this may be a sign they reach without receiving. They continue to reach but come up empty-handed.

Joe (Chapters 2 and 3) often felt like he tried too hard in relationships without getting a lot of support in return. One of his favorite practices was to do X-Ray Pose over a bolster. He said he felt like all the tension drained out of him like water out of a CamelBak water bag. By allowing himself to yield to the support of the bolster, he could reach in more productive, fulfilling ways in his life.

Any time a client shows signs of straining during a yoga therapy session, they are demonstrating a rajasic reach. Many clients (not just those with CPTSD) may at first work too hard in calming/focusing practices such as pranayama, dharana, and dhyana. Struggling in this way is a form of rajasic reach. One way to avert this struggle and frustration is to offer the technique at a faster pace than usual. For instance, the Sa Ta Na Ma mantra can be taught at a fast pace, and then the speed gradually decreased over the course of the recitation. Starting at a faster, more rajasic pace is often calming for a client who is feeling anxious. As you continue to repeat the mantra together, you gradually slow the speed down until there is lots of space between the syllables. The YP should observe the client's facial expressions, body posture, and movements to determine when they are ready to slow the mantra down further. If a client naturally closes their eyes during the technique, this is a positive sign that they are feeling calmer.

If instead you notice the client fidgeting, opening their eyes, and appearing tense and distracted, gently instruct the client to stop the technique and relax. If the client exhibits more rajasic behavior like this, suggest a walk or some simple yoga activity that meets their energy. Sometimes a rajasic reach can flip suddenly into a tamasic stance. For instance, if after appearing strained the client exhibits a far-away stare and/or collapsed posture, you will still want to help the client move but more slowly. Using a technique like 5-4-3-2-1 can help a client reconnect with present moment sensation and experience.

## Tamasic Reach

Hesitation or lack of reaching may indicate that an individual doesn't feel deserving (May, 2022). The person may feel like they are a burden, or fear being rejected or invalidated. While a weak reach may be related to a client's home life, it can also occur due to bullying. If a client experienced chronic bullying, they may feel hesitant to reach out for what they need.

# Sattvic Grasp/Pull: Connecting to the World

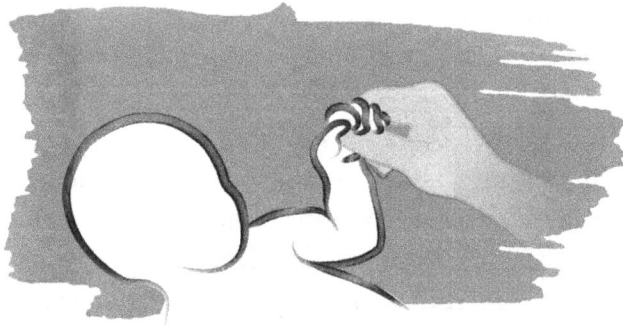

**Figure 5.30** Sattvic Grasp/Pull
*Depicts the fourth and fifth fundamental movements of grasp and pull. The baby learns to grasp and pull people and objects toward it to connect with the world around it.*

Grasp and pull are often discussed together, given how intertwined these two movements are. Frank (2013) points out that when a baby reaches for something, grasping soon appears. Pulling is how the baby finally connects with the thing or person they grasped for. "From the act of grasping and pulling comes the experience of 'me and you,' and the degree to which 'me and you' becomes 'we'" (Frank, 2013, 3:50–3:58).

Again, neglect can cause disruption in the grasp/reach movements. In addition, if an overprotective caregiver withholds too many things from a child, they will have difficulty with this (May, 2022): "On a broader cultural sense... there's things out of reach for certain groups in society, whether it's people of color, LGBT, women, (or the) elderly" (3:57–4:14).

Because grasp/pull issues can develop because of societal injustice and exclusion, it is important to pay attention to what a client can change in their life. For instance, if a client feels like their career has stymied due to systemic racism, no amount of yoga postures using straps will alleviate their pain. If a client brings these painful societal realities up in yoga therapy, consult with the individual trauma therapist. In collaboration with both the provider and the client, the YP may find creative ways to help the client feel the satisfaction of grasp/pull as they learn to do it in their primary therapy setting.

## Yoga Tools for Sattvic Grasp/Pull

**Niyama:** *Svadhyaya* (self-reflection) can be a particularly powerful practice at this stage. Clients often can't see how far they've come. This is one of the most powerful aspects of therapy—we the care team can often see a client's progress before they do. They've been so busy struggling and judging themselves, they may not notice how far they've come. Once a client has developed the ability to move smoothly and easefully through the fundamental movements to this point (where they can grasp and pull toward them what they couldn't before), they may need help noticing the change. Self-reflection practices help clients notice and appreciate their progress and positive change.

**Asana:** Many twists and any pose using a strap or a bind (i.e., clasping one hand with the other) embody the FM of grasp/pull. (Recall that straps and other yoga props that may be used to harm oneself should be kept in a secured, locked place if a client is actively suicidal.) Here is a selection of poses that especially highlight this dual movement.

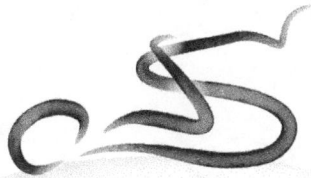

**Figure 5.31** Knees-to-Chest Pose—Apanasana
*Depicts Knees-to-Chest Pose—a supported form of grasp/pull that adds the fundamental movement of yield.*

Modified          Modified          Classical

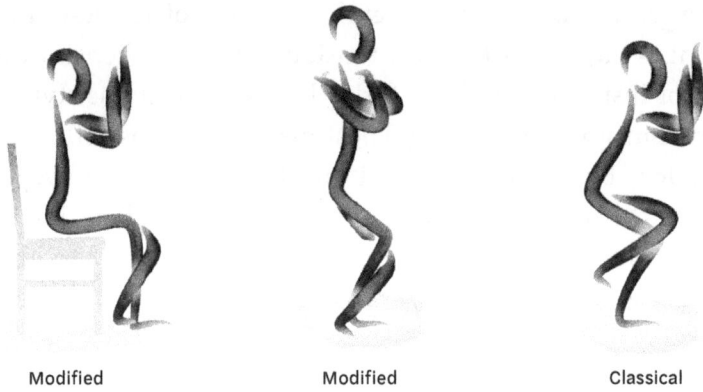

**Figure 5.32** Eagle Pose—Garudasana

*Depicts three variations of Eagle Pose, which embodies grasp/pull while holding it, and then reach when coming out of it. Great for clients who struggle with all three FMs, and many do.*

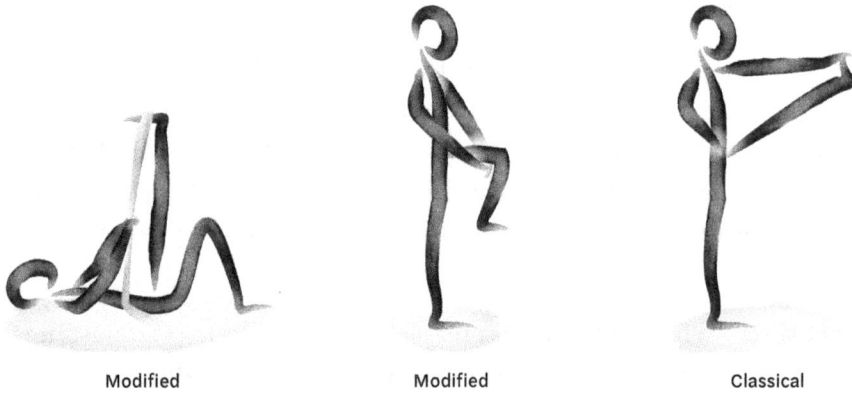

Modified          Modified          Classical

**Figure 5.33** Extended Hand-to-Big-Toe Pose—Utthita Hasta Padangusthasana

*Depicts three variations of Extended Hand-to-Big-Toe Pose. Variation 1 adds the support of the floor, making it a lovely combination of five of the six FMs.*

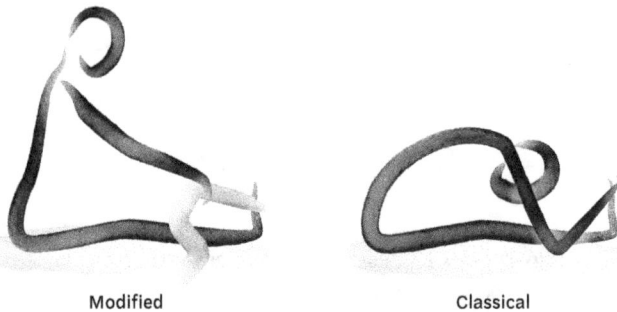

Modified          Classical

**Figure 5.34** Seated Forward Fold Pose—Paschimottanasana

*Depicts two variations of Seated Forward Fold, depending on a client's flexibility. This pose creates a holistic grasp/pull, where the upper body reaches toward the lower body.*

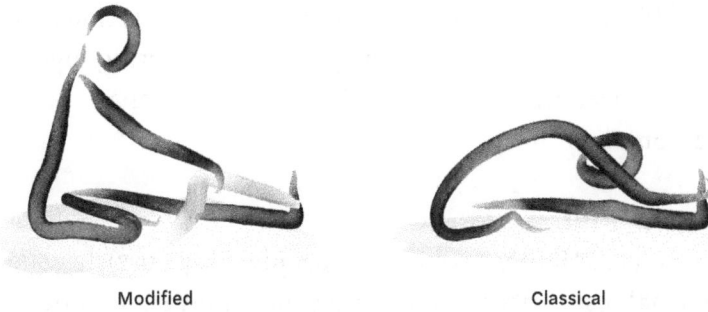

Modified                                Classical

**Figure 5.35** Seated Head-to-Knee Pose—Janu Sirsasana

*Depicts two variations of Seated Head-to-Knee Pose. Crossing the body adds a twist that creates an integrating effect for mind and body.*

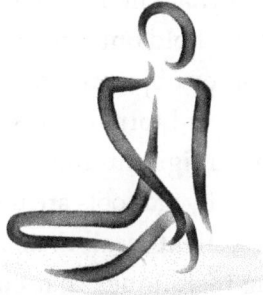

**Figure 5.36** Simple Seated Twist Pose—Parivrtta Sukhasana

*Depicts Simple Seated Twist Pose. Adding a twist to the grasp/pull quality of the pose not only helps release spinal tension but also creates integration, an important quality to cultivate for those suffering from any level of trauma.*

**Pranayama:**

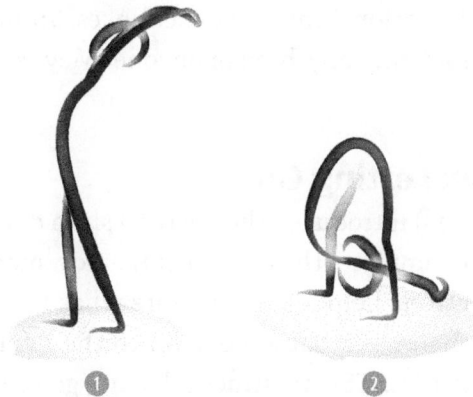

①                                ②

**Figure 5.37** Elephant Breath

*Depicts Elephant Breath: 1) inhale, clasp hands overhead, and 2) exhale, sweeping arms down, and possibly between legs. This energizing breathing technique is fun for all ages, especially children.*

**Dharana and Dhyana:** Any visualization or guided meditation practice that helps a client set an intention and imagine it manifesting highlights this FM. The YP can teach the client Yoga Nidra with an emphasis on intention-setting to accomplish this.

## Rajasic Grasp/Pull

One can hold on too tightly to objects or people (May, 2022). If a client experienced financial insecurity as a child, they may show signs of poverty mentality (fear of being poor) even if they're objectively wealthy. A client may instead cling to a loved one for fear of abandonment or rejection. These are forms of hypervigilance.

May (2022) aptly points out that clients sometimes hold onto a tendency or behavioral pattern. "If I don't hold onto my depression, who am I?" When a client zeroes in on a person or object as though that person/object will save them—this is the constricted form of grasp/hold.

When clients exhibit hypervigilant and/or constricted expressions of rajasic grasp/pull, a few types of yoga tools are useful. Practices that emphasize the FM of push can help a client recall their own strength. And practices like meditations or focusing techniques that cultivate witness consciousness can help clients let go of their "storylines" and see a bigger picture that allows them to let go of unhealthy attachments.

## Tamasic Grasp/Pull

Having difficulty holding onto either people or possessions can be a common issue for survivors of CPTSD. When interpersonal traumas disrupt and rupture meaningful relationships and experiences, an individual may distrust the ability to hold onto anything or anyone (May, 2022; Schwartz, 2021).

# Sattvic Release: Letting Go

Ruella Frank (2001, 2013) introduced the idea of a sixth developmental movement—*release*—that completes the fundamental movements. Frank explains that the first five actions help a baby explore what they desire. The sixth action of releasing helps the baby move on to the next thing. This is an important milestone in CPTSD treatment: letting go of what *was*, to move on to what *is*.

As we have seen, survivors of CPTSD cannot simply "let go," because the traumas are locked in their bodies and nervous systems. "Letting go of what *was*" means first working through the allostatic load in their cells and nervous system to find homeostasis. "Moving on to what *is*" means learning new movement patterns that restore (or create for the first time) equilibrium in a client's body, mind, and life. CPTSD-informed yoga therapy tailors treatment plans and practice to the client's needs, allowing them to find this balance.

One of the best yoga tools to foster this final fundamental movement is *isvarapranidhana*, devotional practices that cultivate trust in the process of life. Such yoga tools can help a client build trust in themselves and life, which allows them to let go to feel satisfied and fulfilled. If a client already has a religious or spiritual practice, encourage them to integrate their spiritual rituals with yoga tools. For instance, Joe (Chapter 3) used his religious practices with deep breathing to cultivate devotion. A regular meditation practice also helps cultivate trust in oneself and life and can lead to profound insights into the nature of pain and suffering in life.

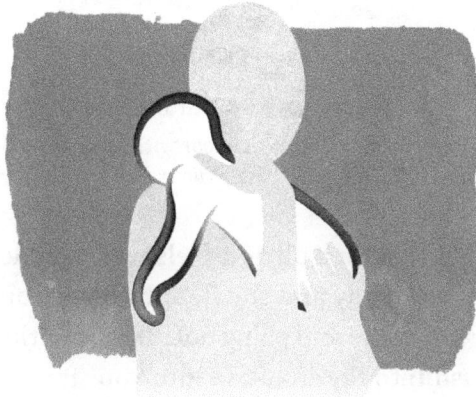

**Figure 5.38** Sattvic Release

*Depicts the sixth and final fundamental movement of release, illustrated here as a baby relaxing against the caregiver. Release is the action of yielding after the cycle of FMs are complete. Clients with CPTSD may have little experience with this fundamental movement. Releasing (or at the very least reducing) the effects of trauma locked within a client's body and mind is one of the goals of CPTSD-informed treatment.*

## Self-Care Practice: Fundamental Movements Vinyasa

The best way to learn the movements of the FM and how they relate to yoga therapy is to practice them together in an integrated way. Below we offer you a yoga vinyasa in which each yoga asana represents a movement in the fundamental movements. We have purposefully pared the asanas down to their most elemental movement to mimic the fundamental movements of an infant. Once you develop an understanding of how the two relate, we invite you to experiment with other yoga poses to create your own FM yoga vinyasa.

Before practicing the sequence below, take note of your state. How do you feel right now?

Now, we invite you to roll out your yoga mat and lie on it in a comfortable position. We have chosen to show Lying on Belly in our sequence, because it most closely resembles what infants do when they first learn to yield. However, it is important to take whatever position is most comfortable for *you*. So, choose a pose that feels most relaxing and supportive to you.

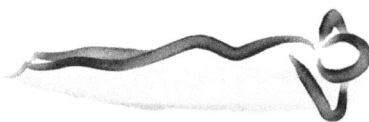

**Figure 5.39** Round 1: Yield

*Depicts Round 1: Yield—lie face-down on the floor with hands below forehead to support the neck. Feel free to do a different yield pose of your choice if you have neck/back issues.*

Linger in the yield position for a bit, if it feels comfortable. Notice the points of contact between your body and the floor beneath you. We invite you to notice your breath, coming in and going out. Then—without moving—bring the intention to push into Sphinx Pose into your mind. Notice what happens in your body. Do you feel a tightening in the abdominal muscles? A tensing in the arms or legs?

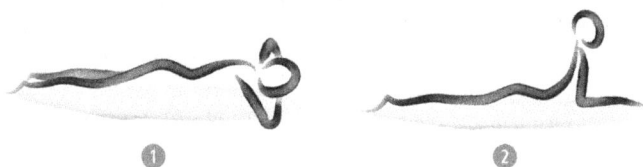

**Figure 5.40** Round 2: Yield-Push

*Depicts Round 2: Yield-Push—1) come back to Lying on Belly and then 2) push body to Sphinx Pose, noticing the muscle movements and body sensations that arise to make this transition.*

When you're ready, move mindfully into Sphinx Pose. Notice what thoughts, feelings, and states of mind arise as you transition from relaxed alertness into the more active movement of pushing the elbows into the floor. Notice your abdominal, back, and leg muscles. Take a few deep, even breaths here and relish the sensations.

Once again, come back to your original yield position. How does it feel different after the activity and stretch of Sphinx Pose? Take a deep breath in and a long slow breath out and note those differences. Then as you're ready, move back into Sphinx. How does it feel different the second time around?

Now, prepare to move from Sphinx to Child's Pose. This is a big transition. Many muscle groups must coordinate to make this shift. As you move, notice what muscles engage. Notice not only that the arms push and reach forward, but also that the hips reach back. Take some deep breaths here, and notice the stretch in the back, the different impact gravity has on the body in this position. Make whatever adjustments help you feel more relaxed and supported in this pose.

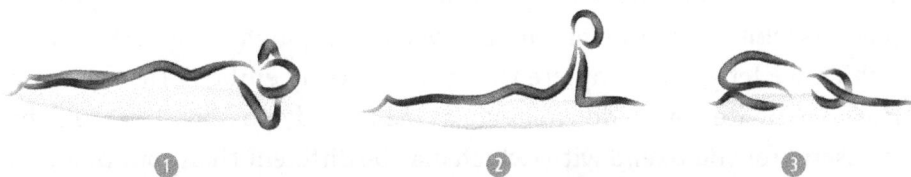

**Figure 5.41** Round 3: Yield-Push-Reach

*Depicts Round 3: Yield-Push-Reach—1) once again lie on the belly; 2) push into Sphinx; and 3) reach back into Child's Pose. How does each movement feel different on round 3?*

Come back to your yield position. How does this round feel different? As you move from Sphinx to Child's Pose, notice differences there. Pause for a moment in Child's Pose. Then mindfully move from Child's Pose into Table. Just as an infant must make many attempts to come to all fours, notice how this transitional movement from Child's Pose to Table Pose is significant— again, many muscle groups must engage to allow this action.

Now, when you're ready, mindfully reach your right arm out, as if for an object or person. Imagine grasping onto it and pulling it toward you. Focus on thoughts, feelings, and body sensations as you do so. How does it feel to reach, grasp, and pull? Try this action with your left arm. Is there a difference between the sides?

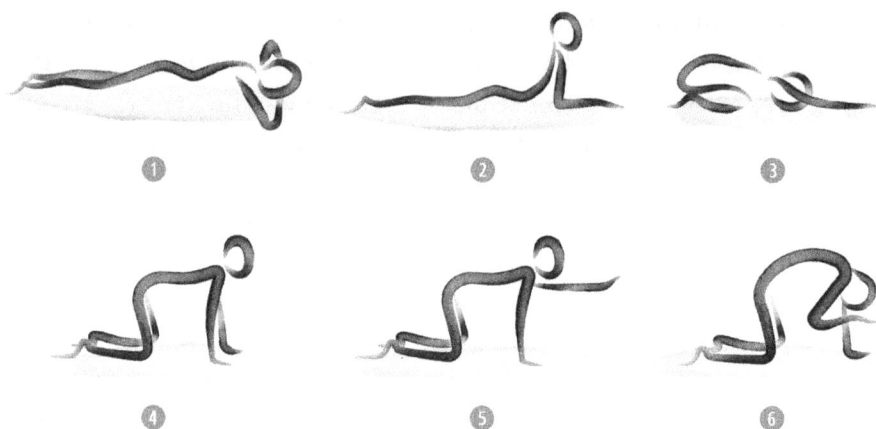

**Figure 5.42** Round 4: Yield-Push-Reach-Grasp/Pull

*Depicts Round 4: Yield-Push-Reach-Grasp/Pull—Repeat the last round, then transition to Table Pose. Envision an object you want to reach for as you extend your arm, then imagine pulling that object toward you as you bend your extended arm into your body.*

In the final, fifth round, you will move through the entire sequence all the way back to your original yield position. Moving back to this first position represents *release*—the fundamental movement highlighted by Ruella Frank, in which we let go to complete the cycle. To truly embody the feeling of release, we invite you to do whatever asana or body position feels relaxing and easeful for you to end with (which may be different than your first position). For instance, would you prefer to rest on your back, or in Child's Pose, or curled up on your side? As you move into this final movement, notice again the shift of thoughts, feelings, and body sensations that accompany release.

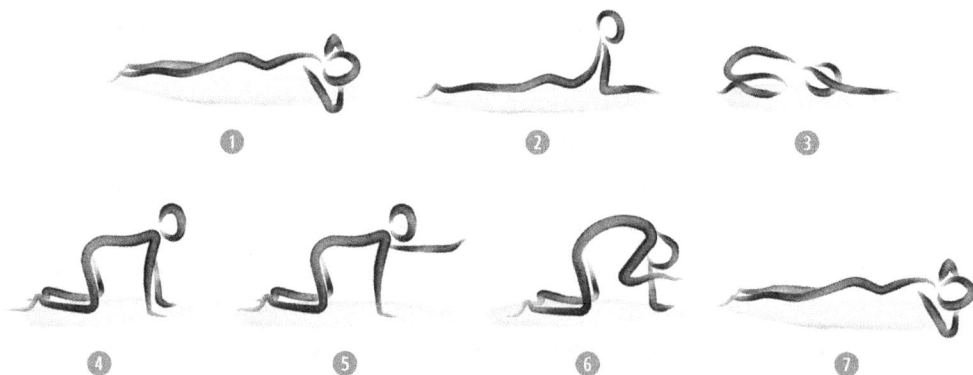

**Figure 5.43** Round 5: Yield-Push-Reach-Grasp/Pull-Release

*Depicts Round 5: Yield-Push-Reach-Grasp/Pull-Release—Repeat Round 5, and finally release back to Lying on Belly. How do you feel differently now?*

## Chapter Summary

- In YTCT, yoga tools are applied using the panchamaya kosha, gunas, and a somatic psychology intervention known as the *six fundamental movements*.

- The fundamental movements are yield, push, reach, grasp/pull, and release. They are closely associated with one's attachment style.

- *Yield* is the first movement that allows one to feel safe and protected. A healthy, sattvic expression of *yield* is a state of relaxed alertness.

- Yielding is *not* the same thing as collapse, a state of dissociation that occurs when a person does not feel safe and protected. Because collapse can mimic yield, it is important that the YP use Look-Feel-Sound to determine what state the client is actually in.

- *Push* is the second movement in the fundamental movements, when a child learns to push against gravity. A healthy, sattvic expression of *push* allows a client to cultivate independence and create boundaries.

- *Reach* is the third movement of the fundamental movements. When a baby is curious about the people and objects in their world, they reach. A healthy, sattvic *reach* is associated with curiosity and satisfying needs.

- *Grasp/Pull* are the fourth and fifth movements of the fundamental movements. These two actions are so intertwined that they are usually presented together. When a child can successfully grasp and pull an object or person toward them, they experience connection—the sattvic expression of these actions.

- Ruella Frank (2013) introduced the idea of a sixth developmental movement—*release*—that completes the fundamental movements. Whereas the first five movements allow a child to explore their desires, this sixth action of release helps the child move on to the next thing. This is a critical step in healing from trauma, especially complex trauma.

- When a child is raised in a chaotic, unpredictable, and/or unsafe environment, the fundamental movements are disrupted. These disruptions show up in an individual's patterns of relating in their life as hyper-arousal (a *rajasic* state of too much mobilization) and/or hypo-arousal (a *tamasic* state of collapse or numbing).

# Defining Yoga Therapy— The Gunas and Panchamaya Kosha

In Chapter 6, our last chapter of Part I, we review the two most essential parts of our model: the gunas and panchamaya kosha. Our goals in this chapter are to:

- Highlight an alternative vocabulary of healing that YTCT and other schools of yoga therapy offer to both YPs and clients

- Differentiate between yoga and yoga therapy

- Explore two more vital components of our model: the gunas and panchamaya kosha

## Expanding the Vocabulary of Healing

In the introduction, we mentioned that yoga and yoga therapy are different, and that these differences are covered in this chapter. We also mentioned that yoga therapy in general, and YTCT in particular, offers an alternative language for describing the symptoms of complex trauma. This new vocabulary is meant to enhance (and not replace) commonly used psychological and medical terms. In essence, it destigmatizes complex trauma by offering different terms that give clients options about how they define their struggles and their healing. The newness of these terms means that clients do not have previous (and potentially negative) associations with them. For instance, Sullivan (2020) observes that when she substitutes the names of the gunas for terms like anxiety, depression, or pain, "[c]lients may be able to reflect more openly on their current experience, separate from their analysis of the 'stories' that arise" (p. 65). Mental health terms like "anxiety" and "depression" are loaded with the implication that an individual's behavior, and therefore the individual, are "abnormal" (Petrow, 2021, para. 1).

**When the YP uses terms from the gunas or fundamental movements (FM) to describe a client's symptoms, the client can choose how to describe their symptoms and make new meaning of their experience.** A client who complains of debilitating panic attacks may feel more empowered when they label their anxious energy as rajasic. A client who re-labels depressive symptoms like lethargy and lack of motivation with a "tamasic energy" may have an easier time depersonalizing these symptoms. When we as YPs invite clients to view their symptoms and states of mind as one or a few of the FM, they may more easily see the transitory nature of these states.

Sullivan (2020) says that using new terms can help clients "step back" (p. 65) and take a wider view of themselves. Clients who rewrite their narrative with new terms may more easily recognize that symptoms and dysfunctional behaviors were adaptations that made sense and served them well at one point, though they may not any longer. As you continue reading, notice how using the language of panchamaya kosha, the gunas, and FM changes *your* perspective of complex trauma. But right now, let's differentiate between yoga and yoga therapy.

## Yoga Versus Yoga Therapy

Yoga and yoga therapy seem so similar. Yoga itself is very therapeutic, and the authors have described how we each used yoga to heal from trauma even before we knew we had it. As Bhavanani et al. (2019) point out, "Yoga therapy nests inside the larger yoga and is therefore neither separate from nor greater than yoga" (p. 44).

So, what's the difference?

## Yoga

A modern-day yoga class (as opposed to yoga therapy) covers general themes, practices, and tools appropriate for a wide range of students. Well-trained yoga teachers have broad understanding of anatomy and physiology as it applies to yoga asana and pranayama, knowledge of how to weave yoga philosophy into themes throughout practice, and a basic knowledge of how to modify all practices to the needs of students. But yoga is not prescriptive—in other words, a yoga teacher offers yoga techniques suitable for a variety of different students, not for highly individualized needs. Of course, the philosophy and practice of classical yoga spans millennia. And some of its profound concepts and practices carry over to yoga therapy, so we will now review a brief history of this multifaceted tradition.

In his ground-breaking book *Light on Yoga* (1979), the great yoga master Sri B. K. S. Iyengar used his entire introduction to answer the question "What is yoga?" The Sanskrit root of "yoga" is *yuj*, which means to join, attach, yoke, or unite (Iyengar, 1979). These varied meanings show that the word *yoga* defies simple definition. In fact, historically it has had a multitude of meanings and been used in many different contexts (Feuerstein et al., 1995). In the modern sense, yoga is a system of practice, a philosophy, and a way of life.

The system of yoga was first codified by Patanjali in the *Yoga Sutras*, composed between 200 BC and 200 AD (Feuerstein et al., 1995). **Yoga's aim is to unite the individual with the highest truth about oneself and the world** (Iyengar, 1979). The truth, from the yogic standpoint, is that each human's essential nature is joyful, and full of a sense of awe—an understanding that we will see is echoed in the panchamaya kosha. Yet this is not common knowledge or lived experience for most humans, let alone those who have endured complex trauma. Interestingly, Iyengar (1979) points to a quote from the *Bhagavad Gita* which says: "**This is the real meaning of Yoga—a deliverance from contact with pain and sorrow**" (p. 19). It appears that the purpose of yoga has always been tied to alleviating the deepest of human suffering.

Yoga itself has therapeutic aspects that are not necessarily considered *yoga therapy*. Of these many aspects, we focus on two that are commonly used in many modern schools and traditions of yoga therapy: 1) the eight limbs of yoga that the YP chooses from to provide practices in a client's treatment plan, and 2) the gunas, which help the YP determine where a client is struggling with a surfeit or a deficit in their body, behavior, and life.

One aspect of yoga we don't cover in this volume is the *chakras* (wheels of energy in the body). As we have said at the beginning, this volume assumes basic knowledge of yogic concepts. Thus, if you currently use the chakras in your work with clients, we encourage you to continue to do so. For instance, given that the gunas permeate the chakras (M. Orpaz-Tsipris, personal communication, September 24, 2024), a YP could integrate the information about the gunas supplied in this book with their working understanding of the chakras. This applies to any other yogic or Ayurvedic concepts or practices you may already use; our CPTSD-informed model is flexible. We invite you to integrate whatever aspects you find helpful from our model into your current yoga therapy practice.

## Eight Limbs of Yoga

The eight limbs comprise the practical application of yoga, and so they are used in both yoga and yoga therapy. In YTCT, the YP draws from the eight limbs to prescribe individualized yoga tools to clients. While Chapter 5 highlighted them in relation to the fundamental movements, the limbs of yoga were not fully defined. As a refresher, here is a description of each:

- *Yama*—one's personal moral code (what NOT to do)

- *Niyama*—social observances with others (what TO do)

- *Pranayama*—breathing practices

- *Asana*—physical postures

- *Pratyahara*—sense withdrawal (such as Yoga Nidra)

- *Dharana*—focusing techniques (such as a body scan)

- *Dhyana*—meditation

- *Samadhi*—the result of practicing the other seven limbs; a state of connection to oneself and all living things

## The Gunas

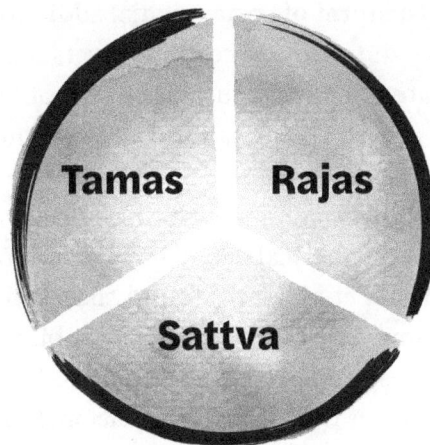

**Figure 6.1** The Gunas
*Depicts the interdependent and holistic nature of the three gunas—sattva, tamas, and rajas.*

The gunas (see also Chapter 3) are the key to understanding the psychology of yoga (Mohan & Mohan, 2004). Like the eight limbs of yoga, the gunas are employed in both yoga and many modern traditions of yoga therapy, including this one. To review, the gunas make up the phenomenological world, from the outer environment to our inner thoughts, emotions, and perceptions (Sullivan, 2020). The three are intertwined, interdependent parts of the whole, as shown in Figure 6.1.

When we integrate the concepts of the gunas and the six fundamental movements, we can view the symptoms of CPTSD in a new light. As we have seen, trauma at any level causes disruption in the rhythms of human life (Holzer, 2022), and this can be observed as imbalances in the gunas.

CPTSD survivors who suffer from depressive symptoms like fatigue, brain fog, and even chronic illness are expressing a tamasic, or collapsed, relationship to the fundamental movement of *yield* (Chapter 5). Devin (Chapter 4) exhibited a lot of tamasic imbalance because of CPTSD: they "zoned out," felt lack of motivation, and at first dissociated in downregulating yoga practices like deep breathing and savasana. This tamasic state of dissociation and collapse is also known as hypo-arousal.

CPTSD survivors who suffer from hypervigilance, anxiety, panic attacks, and/or anger and rage show an excess of rajas. Teresa (Chapter 2) showed a rajasic relationship to *yield*, because she felt panicked when she tried to relax. "High functioning" individuals like Teresa who suffer from excess rajas may not even know they have an imbalance, because our modern world operates on excessive rajas in the form of social media, addiction, and the constant need to be productive and/or to succeed. And yet, as we saw in Chapter 3, excessive rajas is a state of hyper-arousal that cannot be sustained without health consequences (physical, mental, and/or emotional), because it is not a balanced state of homeostasis.

Perhaps not surprisingly, clients with rajasic psychological symptoms often struggle with rajasic physical disorders such as stomach irritation and hypermobility. Silvernale et al. (2024) found that patients suffering from Ehlers–Danlos syndrome (EDS) and joint hypermobility who had comorbid stomach irritation as well reported more childhood trauma than patients who did not have stomach irritation. The relationship between hypermobility and psychological distress is so prevalent that Smith and colleagues (2014) conducted a systematic review and meta-analysis on the topic. They found that individuals with joint hypermobility commonly presented with symptoms of hyper-arousal and other rajasic emotional responses such as anxiety, fear, and panic.

Survivors of CPTSD often suffer from an imbalance of both rajas and tamas in a roller coaster ride of continual emotional dysregulation. For instance, when Devin wasn't lost in a dissociative state, they complained of high anxiety that often resulted in panic attacks.

Lastly, yoga and Ayurvedic experts agree that when there is an excess of sattva, one may avoid difficulty and the messiness of needed change (Frawley, 1999; Sullivan, 2020; Wheeler, 2021). Many individuals begin yoga practice or seek out a yoga therapist to find relief from their suffering. But when yoga practice becomes a way to avoid, rather than face, psychological pain and suffering, they are not progressing so much as avoiding.

Clearly, this kind of avoidance is harmful in CPTSD-informed yoga therapy. If a client seems overly reliant on their yoga tools or avoids other important activities and people in their life in favor of yoga practice, the YP can gently suggest new and slightly more activating (rajasic) yoga tools.

So far we have covered concepts (the gunas) and practice (eight limbs of yoga) shared by both yoga and yoga therapy. Now let's explore in more definitive detail what makes yoga therapy different from classical yoga.

## Yoga Therapy

While classical yoga is not prescriptive, yoga therapy is. Yoga therapy is an emerging healthcare profession grounded in yogic techniques and philosophy, offering a client-centered and evidence-informed approach to health and well-being. It recognizes the intrinsic interconnectedness of all aspects of being, understanding that restoring balance in one area fosters harmony in the whole. Drawing on medical knowledge, psychotherapeutic skills, psychophysiology, behavioral change science, and yoga's subtle energetic principles, yoga therapy unites the wisdom of tradition with the rigor of evidence-based practice while empowering individuals to take an active role in their healing (H. Mason, personal communication, 2024). Owner and founder of the Minded Institute, Heather Mason, emphasizes that any yogic practices used in yoga therapy treatment should also be grounded in scientific understanding (personal communication, 2021).

Bhavanani et al. (2019) also note that "yoga therapy is a practice that focuses on salutogenesis and eudaimonic well-being" (p. 44). *Salutogenesis* is a term associated with positive psychology and is defined as an "orientation focusing attention on the study of the origins of health, contra the origins of disease" (Mittelmark & Bauer, 2016, para. 1). In other words, yoga therapy interventions promote health and optimize well-being, rather than focus on a client's problems and pathologies (Bhavanani et al., 2019).

*Eudaimonia* is a Greek word that can be translated as happiness, welfare, or sometimes well-being (Moore, 2019). Aristotle first proposed this kind of happiness that arises not from momentary pleasure, but from living a balanced life in line with one's virtues, such as following the yamas and niyamas (Bhavanani et al., 2019). "The yoga therapist is uniquely situated to facilitate a process in which—regardless of condition, illness, or pain—the primary focus is the cultivation of eudaimonic well-being" (Sullivan, 2020, p. 25).

Other elements that distinguish yoga therapy include:

1. Using assessments (such as an intake assessment and range of motion assessment)

2. Setting measurable goals and objectives with the client

3. Tracking progress

4. Regularly reassessing goals and objectives to determine progress

Doctor of Occupational Therapy, yoga therapist, researcher, and lecturer Michal Orpaz-Tsipris adds that measuring goals and objectives "can be qualitative and/or quantitative. But [they] should be measurable" (personal communication, September 24, 2024). See our sample Intake Form in Appendix 1.

Presently, yoga therapy is used in a variety of physical and mental health issues such as anxiety and depression, eating disorders, neurodiversity, and of course, trauma. Yoga therapy can also be beneficial for physical health issues like chronic pain, autoimmune diseases like fibromyalgia, and perimenopause (Cleveland Clinic, 2024).

In this book and model, we use yoga therapy to treat an individual's complex trauma. And while there are increasing numbers of trauma-informed yoga approaches, none targets the symptom cluster unique to complex trauma. In addition, few address the specific needs of children and adolescents. As we have seen in Part I of this book, this is crucial to the safe, effective delivery of yoga therapy for youth, and even adults who suffered CPTSD in childhood.

## Panchamaya Kosha

The last and most important component of our CPTSD-informed yoga therapy model is panchamaya kosha, first outlined in the second chapter of the

*Taittiriya Upanishad* (6th century BC). Panchamaya kosha is the conceptual framework most often used by yoga therapists, according to Diane Finlayson, former Yoga Therapy Chair at Maryland University of Integrative Health (2018).

In Sanksrit, *pancha* means five, *maya* means illusion, and *kosha* can be translated as sheath, layer, or body. Thus, panchamaya kosha is the five layers or sheaths of human experience. Because the word "maya" is included in each of these sheaths, the implication is that the koshas are layers of illusion covering our true nature. When one pierces through all five of these layers, the yogis say one finds freedom from all suffering (even if there is still a thin veil of illusion at the innermost layer of anandamaya kosha).

When there is so much suffering in the world, this may seem naive or avoidant. Famine, war, oppression, abuse, mistreatment, and neglect are all very real. The authors know firsthand just how real these issues are from their lived experience. Children and vulnerable persons do not get to decide whether they are subjected to these atrocities. However, we as adults, parents, caregivers, and those with power have a choice and a responsibility to pierce through the layers of our own illusions to help not only ourselves but also others, especially vulnerable others. Thus, doing one's own work—that is, working with and healing one's own mental and emotional wounds—is imperative when working with others.

The different sheaths, or layers, of our being can be seen as "parts" of ourselves. Internationally renowned meditation teacher Sally Kempton wrote beautifully about having an identity crisis in her early 20s in which she became aware of different parts of herself. When she began studying yoga years later, she learned that "my confusion about the multiple parts of myself wasn't so strange," and that panchamaya kosha describes a human being "as having five sheaths, or *koshas*, that interpenetrate each other" much like the layers of an onion (Kempton, 2020, para. 4).

Another apt metaphor for panchamaya kosha is that of nesting dolls, where the outermost sheath represents the physical layer, with the progressively deeper layers nested within, as pictured in Figure 6.2.

Whereas allopathic medicine tends to split the human experience into parts, panchamaya kosha helps us understand these different layers of ourselves in a more integrated, holistic way. By using panchamaya kosha as the framework for healing, the YP can "assist as a sort of 'generalist' who can aid in discovery of disconnection and effective (re)integration of these sheaths" (Finlayson, 2018, para. 5). This is invaluable for survivors of CPTSD, whose experience is often splintered into parts.

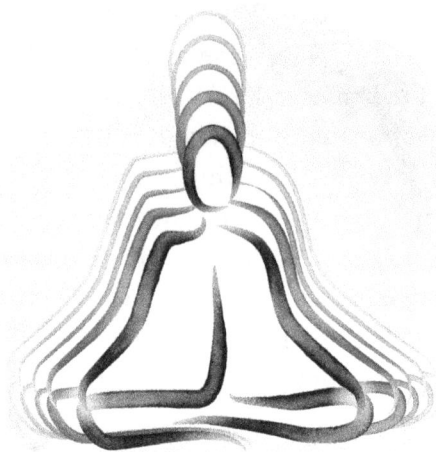

**Figure 6.2** Panchamaya Kosha

*Depicts panchamaya kosha, which is commonly depicted as five nesting dolls, where the outermost layer is representative of the physical body (annamaya kosha) and the innermost layer as anandamaya kosha.*

Some models of modern psychotherapy also recognize the existence of "parts" within human beings, including internal family systems and gestalt (Goldstein, 2023). This understanding is often used in trauma therapy for clients who experience deep internal conflicts, lapses in memory, and/or behavior inconsistent with their sense of self. As discussed in Chapter 1, these are examples of *dissociation*—a way of splitting off painful experiences from one's conscious awareness. The aim of "parts work," as it is sometimes called, is to integrate these disenfranchised parts of oneself. The beauty of panchamaya kosha is that it can help normalize and cultivate the experience of and further integration of one's sense of self. The next five sections cover the five sheaths of *panchamaya kosha*, according to yoga therapy experts (Finlayson, 2018; Gibbs, 2021; Kempton, 2020).

## Annamaya Kosha

Annamaya kosha is the outermost sheath, which includes all physical elements of our body such as muscle, bone, and tissue. It is "our size, shape, gender identification, race and ethnicity, anatomy, and physiology, and even extending to our homes and the planet we all share" (Gibbs, 2021, "Annamaya kosha" section). Sometimes it is referred to as the food sheath or "bread basket" (Finlayson, 2018, para. 2) because it is literally made up of what we eat.

Each sheath is said to have a main attribute, which is helpful in assessing where a client is stuck. For instance, annamaya kosha's main attribute is stability. When a client says they feel the opposite—unstable, insecure, or unsafe in their life—the YP knows to start yoga therapy treatments at the physical level. This aligns with Phase 1 of CPTSD treatment that recommends creating safety, stability, and engagement in a client's life.

## Pranamaya Kosha

Pranamaya kosha refers to the energy or breath sheath. *Prana* is the vitality of all life. Within a human, the breath carries our life force, or prana. The breath is like the car, and the prana is the person in the car. So, while prana and breath are closely linked, they are not synonymous. Finlayson (2018) says these first two sheaths are the most tangible of the five. They are also very much intertwined. For instance, both yoga and meditation are aimed at "toning" the physical body, as well as moving "stagnant energy, or *prana*, through the body" (Kempton, 2020, "Pranamaya kosha/vital energy body" section).

The main attribute of the pranamaya kosha is vitality. A client who complains of exhaustion, depression, chronic illness or pain (which often deplete one's energy), or other symptoms of hypo-arousal may suffer from problems at the pranamaya kosha level. We can see that a lack of vitality also relates to dissociation or "collapse" triggered by trauma.

## Manomaya Kosha

Manomaya kosha is the next, progressively subtle sheath that houses mental/emotional awareness. Finlayson (2018) says this is the lower mind, where our instinctual drives reside. It is the storehouse of beliefs, opinions, and assumptions accumulated over life that "cause your perceptions of yourself and your life to run in certain fixed patterns" (Kempton, 2020, "Manomaya kosha/mental sheath" section). Our sense of individuality arises from this sheath (Sullivan, 2020).

This kosha is associated with the *samskaras* (Kempton, 2020, "Manomaya kosha/mental sheath" section). Samskaras are "conscious or unconscious patterns of thought, communication, and behaviors" (Wheeler, 2021, p. 72) that are created by activity of the mind, or *vrittis*. Once a conscious thought (an activity of the mind, and therefore a vritti) is forgotten, it may remain dormant or latent as a samskara, deeply embedded in our consciousness.

Here's a simple example: Let's say you eat a juicy mango for the first time on a beautiful summer day. Your reaction, barely registered as a thought, is "Mango is delicious!" This is a vritti. The next year you notice a craving for mangoes, whether you remember the thought or not. In this case, this is a positive samskara—the impulse to eat a mango is pleasant and healthy. But if you later develop an allergy to mangoes, or instead of mangoes you develop a penchant for an addictive substance, the samskara reverberates in harmful ways. Even if mangoes are healthy for you but you can't get one, the yogis say you'll suffer because you're attached.

A lot of human suffering emerges from this kosha. Yet the main attribute of the manomaya kosha is clarity, because when we clear our attachments and negative samskaras, we can use the faculties of mind, thought patterns, and perception in effective, positive ways. A client who suffers from confusion, overwhelm, lack of focus, or inattention may have blockages at this kosha.

## Vijnanamaya Kosha

Vijnanamaya kosha is translated as intuitive wisdom. Though all humans possess this layer, many are not aware of it. For this reason, it can be hard to define in words. Finlayson (2018) says it is the "higher mind." If manomaya kosha is awareness colored by individual perceptions, then vijnanamaya is discriminative awareness, sharing similar qualities to *buddhi* or intelligence (Sullivan, 2020).

"It can be thought of as the witness mind, or that aspect of our consciousness that is not *entangled in* what we are doing or thinking" (the Yoga Sanctuary, 2024, "Vijnanamaya kosha" section). Cultivating this level of awareness leads to insight. Kempton (2020) says that any time we focus creatively on activities like writing, math, painting, or problem solving we are tapping into this sheath.

Physiotherapist and yoga therapist Marlysa Sullivan (2020) says that vijnanamaya and anandamaya kosha lend themselves to the social domain of health. "From vijnanamaya kosha, insight into our habitual patterns may help us discover how thoughts, emotions, and behavior facilitate or hinder healthy social connection" (Sullivan, 2020, pp. 114–115). In this sense, vijnanamaya kosha can give the YP understanding of a client's attachment style. In our YTCT, we think of vijnanamaya kosha as the realm of personal relationships, and self-in-relationship-to-other.

When an individual with complex trauma has an "aha!" about a trauma trigger or negative self-belief, they are tapping into vijnanamaya kosha. For example, Teresa (Chapter 2) was frustrated that she continued to worry about making her ex-husband angry. She could not understand why she cared anymore when they had been divorced for a year. During a yoga therapy session in Phase 2 of her treatment Teresa was guided through a body scan. Afterward, she reported an epiphany that her ex-husband reminded her of her father, who intermittently exploded at Teresa when she was an adolescent. Though she continued to feel some degree of nausea in her belly when she interacted with her ex, she said she was not as triggered anymore because she understood the nauseous feeling in her belly was her body reacting to a past experience.

Vijnanamaya kosha's main attribute is wisdom. As we can see from the example above, Teresa gained wisdom (in other words, witness mind) when she was able to tie the nauseous feeling in her belly with the body "memory" of being afraid of her father. This was not simply a mental exercise, but an understanding that included her body, energy, mind, and insight (e.g., the first four koshas). Understanding the context of this sensation gave her insight, which in turn lessened the trigger when she felt it again while interacting with her ex. Reaching this level of wisdom and insight took months of rapport-building with her yoga therapist, and of practice in learning to feel her body sensations and identify her feelings. In general, clients suffering from lack of insight, unhealthy attachments, or confusion may have blockages at this level (May, 2022).

## Anandamaya Kosha

Anandamaya kosha is often translated as the bliss or joy sheath. However, Diane Finlayson says that this is a misnomer. She says that the experience of this kosha is a sense of awe. "[C]onnecting to Awe means we have the ability to connect to ALL of consciousness through this channel" (Finlayson, 2018, para. 2).

Psychologist Dacher Keltner says that awe takes us beyond our usual understanding of the world. In his book *Awe: The New Science of Everyday Wonder and How It Can Transform Your Life* (2023), Keltner writes about his research on the topic and suggests that awe has tremendous mental health benefits, including calming the nervous system as well as promoting trust and bonding.

Given Finlayson's interpretation and current research, we suggest that the main attribute of anandamaya kosha is a sense of awe. Almost all of us have had momentary experiences of it: graduating, winning a race, falling in love, having a baby, or achieving something important. We are tapping into this experience any time we feel a childlike and fresh sense of wonder.

While we tend to associate awe with momentous and life-changing events, it can also arise from simple, everyday experiences such as playing with a baby or watching a sunset. But sadly, 25% of the time awe is caused by gruesome events like war or genocide (Keltner, 2023).

Unfortunately, one who has suffered complex trauma may have little or no experience of awe of any kind—positive or negative. When this is the case, it is essential to meet clients where they are at and honor their current state. To do otherwise is to push a client aggressively toward a state they are not ready for.

In anandamaya kosha one also has awareness of one's true nature, and a sense of interconnectedness. Sullivan (2020) says this kosha allows one to practice prosocial values like compassion and empathy. In our model, we categorize connection to one's community and communal relationships (such as with a church, school, or other significant institutions in a client's life) within anandamaya kosha.

Though anandamaya kosha is the most refined of these five koshas, it is not in fact the core of our being, our true self. In *Light on the Yoga Sutras of Patanjali*, Iyengar notes two other koshas beyond it: *cittamaya kosha* (the body of consciousness) and *atmamaya kosha* (the body of the Self) (1993, p. 133). We will not delve further into these two subtlest of koshas, as they are beyond the scope of this book.

## Self-Care Practice: Balancing Your Koshas

We as caregivers often neglect ourselves. The very tools we know to offer our clients we rarely use ourselves. Here's a gentle reminder to do that now. Take a moment to consider Look-Feel-Sound for yourself. How do you look right now? How do you feel? What do the thoughts in your head sound like? Use this information to determine which of your koshas feels most out of balance:

- How is your annamaya kosha? What is your posture like at this moment? Are you slumped? Tense in places? Are you in physical pain?

- How is your pranamaya kosha? What is your energy level? Are you exhausted? Restless?

- How is your manomaya kosha? Are your thoughts clear, or do you feel foggy? Are you stuck on a thought? Is there any negative self-talk going on in your head?

- How about vijnanamaya kosha? Do you have an awareness of witness mind, your own inner wisdom? Do you feel indecisive or confused about something in your life? Do you feel like you can detach from your worries, or do you feel entangled in them?

- And how about anandamaya kosha? When was the last time you felt a sense of awe, in the positive sense, even if just briefly?

Choose one kosha to focus on—it could be the one that is most out of balance, or most frequently pestering you. What yoga tool(s) would help restore balance? Perhaps something comes to mind right away—trust your intuition, go with that. If not, refer to the recommended yoga tools for the imbalanced kosha in this chapter.

## Chapter Summary

- We offer an alternative language for describing the symptoms of complex trauma. This new vocabulary can help enhance commonly used psychological and medical terms.

- When the YP uses terms from the gunas or fundamental movements to describe a client's symptoms, the client can choose how to describe their symptoms and make new meaning of their experience.

- Yoga aims to unite the individual with their highest truth, and to heal from the pain and sorrow of life.

- Yoga *is not* prescriptive: a yoga class will cover general themes, practices, and tools appropriate for a broad range of students.

- Yoga therapy *is* prescriptive: it is the application of yoga practices in a holistic manner for the treatment of an individual's specific physical, mental, and emotional issues.

- Survivors of CPTSD often suffer from an imbalance of both rajas and tamas in a roller coaster ride of continual emotional dysregulation.

- Panchamaya kosha is the most important component of our CPTSD-informed model, and also the framework most used in other modern traditions of yoga therapy.

# Part II

# YOGA THERAPY FOR COMPLEX TRAUMA

## CHAPTER 7

# YTCT—A Model of CPTSD-Informed Yoga Therapy

In Part I (Chapters 1–6), we explored the theory and the rationale of our evidence-informed model of yoga therapy for complex trauma, or YTCT. We demonstrated that a body-based approach like yoga therapy can be enormously helpful in the treatment of CPTSD, because all trauma is experienced in the body (Ogden & Fisher, 2015; Rothschild, 2000; van der Kolk, 2014). We also presented the evidence for such an approach. We examined the five core components of this integrative model: the fundamental movements (FM) from somatic psychology, the phase-based approach of current trauma treatment, the gunas, and panchamaya kosha (PMK); the fifth component, community and self-care, will be covered in Chapter 12.

## Yoga Therapy for Complex Trauma

Part II (Chapters 7–10) covers the application of the model (including case conceptualization), and case studies for each age group covered in this book (Chapters 8–10). Here in Chapter 7 we introduce our model of CPTSD-informed yoga therapy called Yoga Therapy for Complex Trauma (YTCT). Figure 7.1 illustrates the five key components, where PMK lies at the center of the model.

We envision our model through the lens of assessment, treatment planning, and course of treatment. To start, when meeting with a client for the first time the YP gets a "snapshot" of who this client is as a unique individual, from what they tell us and through a process called Look-Feel-Sound. The YP then moves to a more complete assessment of the client in the PMK Overview, a core element of the initial intake interview. For every

PMK sheath, the YP explores the client's strengths, and investigates how the gunas impact the FM to determine the degree of balance or imbalance at that level of the koshas.

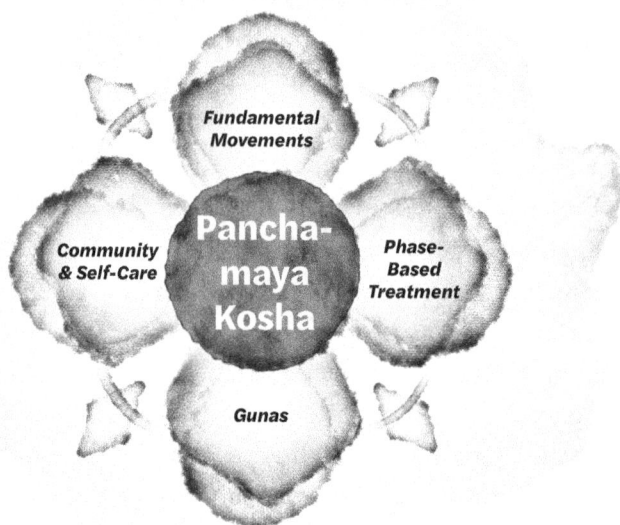

**Figure 7.1** YTCT Mandala

*Illustrates the YTCT Mandala, consisting of five key components, where PMK lies at the center of the model.*

Our rationale for integrating the FM into the more traditional yoga therapy of PMK is threefold. First, in modern mental health treatment, integrative approaches that marry two or more therapeutic modalities are common (Zarbo et al., 2016). Frank (2001) says that when integrative approaches are explored, "the resulting synthesis offers not only new knowledge, but new ways of looking at what is already known" (p. 7). Schwartz's *Complex PTSD Treatment Manual* (2021) is one such approach. In our model, we bring together the time-tested and ancient tradition of PMK with the modern somatic psychotherapy approach of the fundamental movements.

Second, PMK and the FM go very well together. The fundamental movements give the YP a tangible way to assess health and balance (via the gunas) at each layer of PMK. A client's body language and movements are readily observable to both you and them. In addition, trauma experts strongly advocate the use of body awareness as a therapeutic tool in trauma treatment (Ogden & Fisher, 2015; Rothschild, 2000), and of course both yoga therapy and the fundamental movements are body-based treatment lenses.

Finally, as we have emphasized throughout this book, one of the key features of CPTSD is interpersonal trauma. While a social and interpersonal element can be inferred in some of the koshas (Sullivan, 2020), there is no direct and explicit link. On the other hand, all the fundamental movements have interpersonal aspects related to attachment styles that echo throughout a client's life. In addition, the FM are not movement patterns that occur just in the body; they occur in the mind, emotions, and relational style of an individual as well. We find that integrating these two systems together allows the YP to assess clients more holistically. So now let's dive into an overview of the model, starting with Assessment.

## Assessment and Treatment Planning

The first step in creating a safe, effective treatment plan is assessment through the intake process. It is also during this stage that several other important elements of our model come into play, so they are bolded.

Assessment consists of:

1. *Snapshot*: Use a mindful technique called **Look-Feel-Sound** to capture a first impression of the client.

2. *Overview*: As part of the intake process, collect information from the Client Information Form and Intake Form (see Appendices) to create a **PMK Overview** that appraises the client's strengths and limitations for each of the five koshas; from the PMK Overview, determine the target kosha(s) to focus on in treatment.

3. *Goals*: To determine goals, consider how the **fundamental movements** and the **gunas** are impacting the target kosha(s).

4. *Objectives*: Create treatment objectives with **yoga tools**.

5. *Collaboration*: Confer with the client's care team.

Following these steps of assessment prepares the YP to create the treatment plan. Before considering each component, let's review Figure 7.2, which illustrates the entire process.

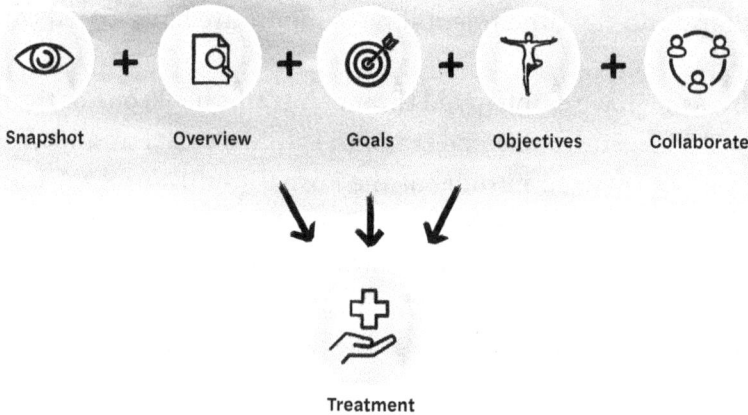

**Figure 7.2** Assessment Process

*Depicts the assessment process in YTCT—engaging in all the steps from getting
a snapshot of the client through Look-Feel-Sound through collaborating
with the client's care team ensures a complete treatment plan.*

## 1. Snapshot

### Presenting Problem

Sometimes referred to as the chief complaint, the *presenting problem(s)*
are the initial complaints and symptoms that bring a client to therapy
(Fritscher, 2023). When assessing a client, the YP considers the main issues
that the client has identified on their intake form. The client's assessment
of their presenting problem is key to ensuring that yoga therapy treatment
is client-centered.

### Look-Feel-Sound

Look-Feel-Sound describes a process that the YP uses whenever interacting with a client. Adapted from Rothschild's approach to trauma treatment
(2000), Michelle created this therapeutic tool to help herself and her clinical students attend to clients' nonverbal cues.

In Look-Feel-Sound, you attend to how the client:

- Looks (body language and facial expression)

- Feels (how they say they feel, and how you feel in the room or virtual
  space with them)

- Sounds (their tone of voice, cadence, words, volume of speech)

In Chapter 4, we learned that the body is a resource in trauma treatment (Rothschild, 2000), and that being well-regulated ourselves is crucial to establishing a positive rapport with clients (Perry & Winfrey, 2021). Thus, paying attention to both your client's and your own body language and signals is an excellent way to create safety and mindful rapport from the first moment of yoga therapy.

Practicing Look-Feel-Sound also cultivates a holistic view of the client. You note the client's physical body, tone of voice and cadence, behavior, presence in the room, interactions, beliefs, and perspectives. Be sure to learn the client's preferred name (which is not always the same as their legal or given name), pronouns, and cultural and gender identity.

Table 7.1 illustrates how to use Look-Feel-Sound to attune to clients' nonverbal cues and respond with the appropriate yoga tool(s). This not only helps the YP provide more accurate care to the client but also protects against vicarious trauma and compassion fatigue by helping the YP notice the nonverbal signs that a client needs to regulate (Rothschild, 2017). Table 7.1 is a useful reference guide throughout treatment to monitor a client's moment-to-moment state during sessions.

**Table 7.1** depicts attuning with the client—a summary of how to determine a client's state using Look-Feel-Sound, then how to respond with yoga tools.

| | Hypo-Arousal (Tamasic) | Calm/Alert (Sattvic) | Hyper-Arousal (Rajasic) |
|---|---|---|---|
| Client State | Lethargic, depressed | Well-regulated | Hypervigilant, anxious |
| LOOK | | | |
| Posture | Collapsed upper body | Upright yet relaxed | Tense, rigid |
| Movement/ Energy | Lack of movement, slack muscles | Smooth, rhythmic movements | Hyperactive, jumpy, fidgety hands and legs |
| Gaze/Eyes | Dull or far-off gaze | Responsive gaze | Darting eyes, possibly staring gaze |
| FEEL | | | |
| Client Report | Sad, numb, possibly irritation or anger | Normal range of emotions | Stress, overwhelm, possibly irritation or anger |
| Affect | Blunted, flat | Calm, steady | Nervous, hyperactive |
| Engagement | Low engagement to unresponsive | High engagement | Engagement varies |

*cont.*

| | Hypo-Arousal (Tamasic) | Calm/Alert (Sattvic) | Hyper-Arousal (Rajasic) |
|---|---|---|---|
| **SOUND** | | | |
| **Tone** | Monotone | Even tone | Irritated or tense |
| **Volume** | Quiet, silent | Average | Strained, yelling |
| **Cadence** | Slow | Average | Rapid |
| **YP RESPONSE** | | | |
| **Suggested Yoga Tools** | Rajasic, energizing practices | Continue current practice | Tamasic, calming practices |

## 2. Overview via PMK

The Initial Intake Assessment is part of best practice care (Chapter 4). In the YTCT model the intake process consists of requesting information from the client, gathering and documenting the essential elements during and after the intake session, and using this data to create the PMK Overview. In the Appendices we have provided several forms related to this process. First, we provide client information forms for both youth (5–18 years old) and adults (18 and older) found in Appendices 4 and 5. The client information form is completed by the new client and/or their guardian. Typically, the YP requests that this form be filled out (and hopefully returned) before the first meeting.

We also provide an all-ages intake form (Appendix 1), which is completed by the YP during and after the intake appointment. This intake appointment is the official start of yoga therapy, and therefore it is essential to obtain the client's (and/or their guardian's) written consent to treatment. The Consent to Treatment signature page is included on the last page of the intake form. These forms are examples of how to incorporate the YTCT principles into your intake process. It is entirely up to you whether and how you use them.

The next step is to assess the client's strengths and presenting problem(s) via the *PMK Overview*. While Look-Feel-Sound is a snapshot, the PMK Overview is a complete picture of all five sheaths, fundamental movements, and gunas. We created the PMK Overview worksheet (Table 7.2/Appendix 7) to help the YP consider how the fundamental movements and the gunas interact within each kosha. The worksheet was created in response to feedback from a focus group that met during the writing of this book that discussed and experimented with the model. It helps clarify the target kosha(s) and is a useful first step in conceptualizing a client's issues.

**Table 7.2** depicts the PMK Overview Worksheet that the YP can use to determine a client's target kosha(s) and subsequent treatment plan.

| Kosha | Client's Presentation |
|---|---|
| **Annamaya Kosha** (Stability) | What are the client's strengths and imbalances in annamaya kosha? |
| | When thinking about the client's Look-Feel-Sound, what fundamental movements seem most imbalanced? Do they push their arms into their seat, revealing a rajasic relationship to *push*? Does their upper body appear collapsed, revealing a tamasic relationship to *yield*? |
| **Pranamaya Kosha** (Vitality) | What are the client's strengths and imbalances in pranamaya kosha? |
| | Do they appear calm and alert (sattvic)? Tired and collapsed (tamasic)? Restless (rajasic)? |
| | How do the gunas express in their fundamental movements to reveal imbalances of energy, vitality, and health? |
| **Manomaya Kosha** (Clarity) | What are the client's strengths and imbalances in manomaya kosha? |
| | Do they appear anxious and restless (rajasic), or collapsed and disengaged (tamasic)? |
| | What is their quality of thought? Clear (sattvic)? Overwhelmed (rajasic)? Confused/unclear (tamasic)? |
| | What characteristics or roles does the client identify with? |
| **Vijnanamaya Kosha** (Wisdom/ Intuition) | What are the client's strengths and imbalances in vijnanamaya kosha? |
| | How insightful are they about their strengths and challenges? |
| | How is the quality of their personal relationships? |
| | In relationships, does the client seem to struggle with one or a few of the fundamental movements? |
| **Anandamaya Kosha** (Joy/Awe) | What are the client's strengths and imbalances in anandamaya kosha? |
| | What brings them joy or a sense of awe? |
| | Do they have community resources (school, work, affiliations, clubs, religion)? |

## 3. Goals

Once the target kosha has been established, the YP then collaborates with the client (and their guardian if they are a minor) to generate observable, measurable treatment goals and objectives. **Goals and objectives ensure that sessions stay focused and help both the client and YP track progress.**

Each goal aims to alleviate a *target problem*, which is the main issue identified in the target kosha. The gunas and the fundamental movements help define the target problem by indicating imbalance (areas that are over- or under-functioning). For instance, Devin's target problem (from Chapter 4) was a lack of body awareness that could lead to panic attacks and/or dissociation, making their target kosha annamaya kosha. These symptoms demonstrated an under-functioning of *yield*, the first fundamental movement. From the standpoint of the gunas, a lack of awareness is a tamasic state that needs to be increased. Thus, an appropriate goal for Devin was to "increase body awareness." (Whenever possible, state the goal with positive verbs like *increase, cultivate, generate, learn,* etc. Other possibilities include *alleviate, heal, maintain.*)

## 4. Objectives

Objectives in this model describe the yoga tools used to accomplish the treatment goal. Along with the PMK Overview and target kosha, two other factors are important when considering appropriate objectives: the client's *phase of treatment* and their *age.* The target problem/kosha, along with these two factors, help you determine the precise yoga tools for a client.

For instance, one of the objectives for Devin's goal was to "practice yoga sequences and coping strategies that cultivate body awareness and increase emotion regulation." Devin was in Phase 1 of CPTSD treatment, so the yoga tools Michelle suggested were ones that helped increase body awareness and alleviated stress. Because Devin was an adolescent, Michelle encouraged them to decide what practices and strategies they felt increased their body awareness the most, and they chose flowing yoga vinyasas. (While a child client should also be empowered to choose practices that work best for them, the YP may need to be more directive by offering two options from which the child chooses.) Practices like Sa Ta Na Ma and Five Senses Mindfulness also helped Devin alleviate stress.

## 5. Collaboration

During the process of assessment, you confer with your client's care team by obtaining written permission to speak with each member. As mentioned in Chapter 4, obtain written consent from a guardian to start treatment with a minor. Regardless of the client's age, the primary therapist is a key team member with whom to coordinate care. This ensures that the treatment plan you create with the client (especially the goals and objectives) complements their overall care plan. If your client is an adult, the primary therapist may be the only team member with whom you confer. If an adult client has a psychiatrist, you may want to obtain permission to consult with them as well.

Two other essential elements of a client's care to consider include what phase of treatment they are in, and how old the client is. As we've discussed, clients often don't know whether or that they have trauma (at any level). When a client hasn't reported trauma on their Client Information Form or in their intake session, it is fair to assume that they either don't have trauma or don't know they have trauma. In these cases, focus on Phase 1 tools and techniques to help build safety, stability, and engagement with the client.

## Phase

Let's review the three phases of CPTSD treatment (Courtois & Ford, 2016; Ford & Courtois, 2020; Schwartz, 2021):

- Phase 1: Build safety, stability, and engagement

- Phase 2: Process trauma

- Phase 3: Integrate new skills and knowledge

Here's an example of Phase 1 with a 14-year-old named Claudia. Claudia is an American (mother is Caucasian, father is of South Korean descent—adopted by an American family almost at birth), who struggles with anxiety and depression. She was referred to Michelle by her parents after she told her school counselor that she'd been cutting (a form of self-harm). In accordance with Phase 1, all yoga tools will support Claudia's emotional and physical safety, provide her a sense of stability, and cultivate engagement with her. In other words, Michelle did not use yoga tools to unearth or work through traumas yet. The primary work was safety and stability.

## Age

In Chapters 8–10 we will discuss in detail how age and developmental stage impact treatment. For now, simply bear in mind that the client's age determines how you present yoga tools. In the case of Claudia (age 14), Michelle presented yoga tools such as Five Senses Mindfulness, Yoga Nidra, and Sa Ta Na Ma. Whereas Devin (age 16) liked short yoga vinyasas, Claudia wasn't quite sure how she felt about yoga at first. This was because Claudia seemed to want to distance herself from her mother's interests, which included yoga. (Her mother mentioned she was considering an Ayurvedic teacher training during one of Claudia's sessions.) So, in the beginning of Claudia's treatment, Michelle offered her practices she could easily do on her own at school or at home. And other than Sa Ta Na Ma, Michelle avoided Sanskrit names for yoga tools. Claudia's need to differentiate from her mother's interests was natural and healthy for an adolescent. By noticing and honoring Claudia's desire to differentiate, Michelle was making therapy a safe space for her.

## Other Treatment Logistics

### Therapy Schedule

Within the first few sessions it is best practice to establish a therapy schedule. Frequency of sessions should be consistent, especially in the beginning. **Consistency of sessions is particularly important to establish safety and stability for those with CPTSD.** For example, you and your client may decide to meet weekly for the first 4–6 weeks to establish rapport and routine. Once a client begins to make progress on their goals and objectives, you can scale back the frequency of sessions based on the client's preferences.

### Client Education

**Educating clients about the kinds of interventions (e.g., yoga tools) you offer is an essential part of safe, effective treatment.** Regardless of age, clients benefit from understanding what techniques will be used, and why. When working with clients who are minors, invite parents/guardians to attend these education segments. In addition, provide clients with different intervention options. This allows them to exercise choice, which is part of empowering clients in their own treatment.

### Tracking Progress

**Working on goals and objectives is the core activity of yoga therapy treatment, because it is how you measure progress.** Review them on a regular basis with clients to ensure they are still applicable. We recommend reviewing goals every six sessions, especially in the first few months of treatment. Over time, objectives and goals will naturally change as the client progresses or other priorities become important.

Part of working on goals and objectives is yoga therapy homework. Usually, clients receive yoga therapy once a week at most. To truly see progress, clients need to practice the skills they learn with you in their daily life. From the first session, let clients and families know how essential therapy homework is to the therapeutic process.

Family involvement in homework depends on the client's age. Primary school children (5–12 years old) need a lot of support from caregivers. These clients and families benefit from individualized homework charts, or a hard copy calendar where they can place a sticker each time they complete practice.

For adolescents, almost the exact opposite is true: adolescents will feel offended if you give them a sticker chart or suggest that their caregiver remind them to practice. For instance, when Claudia became open to practicing Sa Ta Na Ma at home, Michelle asked if she'd like support from her mother. She adamantly refused. "This is my responsibility!" Still, adolescents may need a gentle nudge to create their own reminders. Both Devin and Claudia used phone alerts and emotion tracking apps to help them monitor progress. Adult clients benefit from these same apps and alerts.

## Communication

Expect to have regular communication with the caregivers of primary school children, since they provide transport, supervise therapy homework, and participate regularly in sessions. If several adults are involved in the child's life, determine who the main "point person" is for regular correspondence.

In adolescence, clients begin to rely less on caregivers and family and more on friends. As stated, this is natural and healthy. Whenever possible, allow the adolescent client to dictate the frequency of caregiver contact. When a client's health or safety is at risk, the YP is required to speak directly with or otherwise contact the guardian. Be sure to state this clearly in the intake session, so the adolescent is not surprised if the necessity arises. It is also important to define for the adolescent and their caregiver what constitutes a risk to health or safety. Every country/municipality defines this a bit differently. It is your professional responsibility to educate yourself about such laws for your area.

## Yoga Tools

Having charted a clear path through assessment and treatment planning, let's consider yoga tools. In Chapter 5 we considered yoga tools from the lens of the fundamental movements and went into detail for each of the eight limbs. This is because integrating the two systems is novel to this book and required a full exploration. Here we examine yoga tools from the lens of each kosha with a much broader brushstroke, since PMK and yoga tools are part of the same ancient system of yoga therapy. Throughout this section we use terminology from the FM, limbs, guna, and PMK to facilitate further integration of how they work together.

## Annamaya Yoga Tools

*Asana* is the main limb of yoga used to heal physical issues at the annamaya kosha level (Cook, 2024). A simple exercise to help clients feel stable is to bring awareness to the feet, or whatever part of their body is touching the floor, chair, or yoga mat. This is an example of *yield*, the first movement in the fundamental movements. Michal Orpaz-Tsipris points out that the same pose can be used for multiple reasons. Orpaz-Tsipris uses the Tree Pose as an example: "[I]f the person needs more... stability, then you'd focus on the roots of the tree... If the person is lacking inspiration and needs more of a sattvic quality... then the guidance would be to focus on the [leaves]" (personal communication, October 3, 2024).

## Pranamaya Yoga Tools

Not surprisingly, *pranayama* is often the yoga practice associated with issues at the pranamaya kosha level. Yet this is contraindicated in certain circumstances—namely, when a client associates deep breathing with hyperventilation, or when calming breathing techniques feel too much like a state of collapse for the client.

Recall that for Devin, relaxing yoga tools such as deep breathing felt too much like dissociation. Thus, even though the symptoms of dissociation and collapse indicated blockages at the pranamaya kosha level, breathing techniques were triggering at the beginning of treatment. Instead, Devin benefited from practicing short asana sequences to move the prana without Devin needing to be consciously in control of their breathing.

Of note, over time Devin was eventually able to practice deep breathing and calming yoga tools. As they transitioned from Phase 1 to Phase 2 of treatment, they began to identify body sensations in yoga asana. They reported feeling more aware of and safer in their body (increased healing at the annamaya kosha level). As a result, Devin reported no longer dissociating in relaxing poses. Once they developed the ability to stay present to sensations and feelings (i.e., not dissociate), Devin could differentiate between relaxing and dissociating. Rather than the "flowy" sensation of dissociation, Devin reported feelings of "peace" and being present. We will cover what worked (and didn't) for Claudia in detail in Chapter 9.

## Manomaya Yoga Tools

Many of the limbs of yoga are helpful for healing blockages at this level. Mantra and mudra can help with creating new patterns of thinking. For instance, many of Michelle's clients have benefited from using the Sa Ta Na Ma mantra with its hand mudras (Appendix 8). Asana (with or without spoken affirmations) is also healing for the manomaya kosha, as it helps regulate the nervous system during physical yoga practice (Cook, 2024). Think about how often yoga clients say they feel more clear-headed after yoga asana. Lastly, meditation for clients who are not triggered by calming yoga tools is another powerful way to help clients focus the mind and create new patterns of thinking.

Many of the current evidence-based psychological treatments target issues in the manomaya kosha, since it is the level of mental/emotional awareness. As such, yoga therapy integrates beautifully with treatment modalities such as cognitive behavioral therapy (CBT), mindfulness-based stress reduction (MBSR), dialectical behavioral therapy (DBT), and acceptance and commitment therapy (ACT). All incorporate mindfulness and sometimes even yoga-based tools into their interventions to relieve mental and emotional suffering (Khalsa et al., 2015; Lundgren et al., 2008; Pascoe et al., 2017; Riegler et al., 2023).

## Vijnanamaya Yoga Tools

To cultivate vijnanamaya kosha, Patrinos (2021) recommends *pratyahara* (withdrawal of the senses through techniques like body scans and Yoga Nidra), *dharana* (focusing practices like visualization or a mudra/mantra practice like Sa Ta Na Ma), and *dhyana* (mindfulness and meditation practices). Treatment is highly individualized at this layer of awareness.

In our YTCT model, vijnanamaya kosha also encompasses personal relationships—that is, one-on-one relationships. As such, santosa and svadhyaya are excellent tools to help clients with relational challenges. For children, and even adolescents and adults, the mindfulness poem *All Is Well* in the *Yoga Pretzels*© card deck (Guber et al., 2005) is very effective for cultivating santosa (acceptance) and ahimsa (nonviolence) for self and others.

## Anandamaya Yoga Tools

So how do we help CPTSD survivors cultivate a sense of awe in their lives? Two clues seem to be simplicity and repeated practice. While doing a study at San Quentin Prison in 2016, psychologist Dacher Keltner said he overheard prisoners talking about finding awe in small things like the air or light (2023); Keltner says seeking out these small moments of awe allows the negative voices in one's head to quiet down. In the same way, we can encourage clients who lack a sense of awe to start small. Find a small moment of awe in taking a deep breath, or simply drinking tea. As we have seen, all layers of the PMK are interwoven.

Anandamaya kosha encompasses communal relationships in our YTCT model. Yoga tools that cultivate compassion and empathy for all help with blockages at this level. Clients suffering from climate anxiety may benefit from practices like *Green Breath Meditation* from Michelle's first book *Using Yoga Therapy to Promote Mental Health in Children and Adolescents* (2015, p. 110).

## Case Conceptualization

Another incredibly helpful tool to use during a client's treatment is the case conceptualization. A *case conceptualization* is a summary of the key findings from a clinical evaluation that helps mental health professionals generate treatment plans and recommendations (Gaines, 2022). In the YTCT model, the PMK Overview worksheet (Table 7.2 and Appendix 7) is a building block toward the creation of a case conceptualization. So, the YP begins to construct this during and/or after the formation of goals and objectives. Sperry and Sperry (2020) say that creating a case conceptualization is second only to building a safe and trusting therapeutic rapport. This is because creating one deepens the YP's understanding of the client's overall strengths and needs, which helps set the course of treatment.

Michelle first learned about case conceptualizations during her internship at the Rape Assistance and Awareness Program (RAAP, now called the Blue Bench), where she would present them to her supervisor to better understand her clients. She later learned how to turn her conceptualizations of clients into case presentations while working at Children's Hospital Colorado. In YTCT, we use the case conceptualization in both ways: to help the YP understand their clients and needs better, and as an effective communication tool to use with other professionals on a client's care team.

Table 7.3 (also in Appendix 6) shows an example of a case conceptualization format that consists of four main categories: client's background and referral information, client strengths, client limitations, and overall impression. This form allows you the YP to easily distill information from a client's intake evaluation (and PMK Overview worksheet) into a case presentation. As with all forms offered in this book, you may use the form as is or retrofit for your clinical needs.

**Table 7.3** depicts the Case Conceptualization Form, which can also be found in Appendix 6.

| Client Background | Background: Client's age, stated gender, level of education, and/or vocation |
| --- | --- |
| | Look |
| | Feel |
| | Sound |
| **Strengths** | Review PMK Overview to identify strengths |
| | Client's stated strengths |
| **Limitations** | Review PMK Overview to identify limitations |
| | Target kosha(s) |
| | Fundamental movements impacted (rajasic, tamasic, sattvic) |

*cont.*

| Overall Impression | Diagnostic impression (including DSM/ICD reported by client and/or referral source) |
|---|---|
| | |
| | Current goals and objectives (including yoga tools) and progress |
| | |
| | Future directions/questions for team |
| | |

## Self-Care Practice: Letting Go After a Session

Witnessing clients' pain, struggles, and ongoing problems through the intake process and ongoing sessions takes a toll on a YP. It's important to develop a quick, easy routine that helps you release the burden you take on by doing this work. There are many ways to release this burden after a difficult session or day:

- Splash either cold or hot water on your face

- Starting at the top of your head, literally "brush off" that last session or intake. Continue by brushing the shoulders, arms, chest, belly, front of legs, backs of legs, and feet

- Take deep breaths, and with each exhale, imagine releasing the pain, tension, and storyline of what you just heard and observed

- Take a walk and practice Five Senses Mindfulness

- Talk to a colleague

We recommend doing this practice after each intake and difficult session. The more you practice this on a regular basis, the more it becomes a habit. And making these short, simple self-care practices a habit helps reduce and eliminate burnout.

## Chapter Summary

- Look-Feel-Sound is a therapeutic tool that helps YPs attend to clients' nonverbal cues.

- The first step in creating a safe, effective treatment plan is assessment through the intake process.

- The YTCT Assessment process consists of:

  - *Snapshot*: Client's presenting problem(s) and Look-Feel-Sound

  - *PMK Overview*: Appraises the client's strengths and limitations for each of the five koshas, including how the fundamental movements and gunas interact

  - *Goals*: Considering the PMK Overview, what kosha(s) seem to be most impacted?

  - *Objectives*: Create treatment objectives with yoga tools

  - *Collaboration*: Confer with the client's care team

- The PMK Overview provides a roadmap for treatment planning, including clarification of the target kosha/problem.

- Goals and objectives ensure that sessions stay focused and help both the client and YP track progress.

- Consistency of sessions is particularly important to establish safety and stability for those with CPTSD.

- Educating clients about the kinds of interventions (e.g., yoga tools) you offer is an essential part of safe, effective treatment.

- Working on goals and objectives is the core activity of yoga therapy treatment, because it is how you measure progress.

- In YTCT, we use the case conceptualization: 1) to help the YP understand their clients and needs better, and 2) as an effective communication tool to use with a client's care team.

## CHAPTER 8

# CPTSD-Informed Yoga Therapy for Children

## Evidence and Rationale of YTCT for Children

There is increasing evidence that yoga on its own (without a therapeutic component) is helpful for primary school children (5–12 years old). Two US-based studies found that yoga provides stress relief and decreases emotional dysregulation for children in urban school settings (Beltran et al., 2016; Centeio et al., 2017). Centeio and colleagues (2017) also reported that children find yoga fun and easy to do at home. Beltran and associates (2016) found that children with ADHD showed increased ability to self-soothe and de-stress compared to their peers.

While both studies focused on yoga (versus yoga therapy) for children's general mental health, Beltran et al. (2016) noted that yoga may be a promising intervention for children who have experienced trauma, because yoga helps increase self-regulation and internal awareness.

## Case Study: Iryna

This is a case study of 7-year-old Iryna. She was introduced to yoga as part of a ten-week after-school yoga club Ayala offered, and then later received individual yoga therapy sessions from Ayala. The group yoga session is a common place for children to first encounter yoga. Typically, schools call these sessions yoga clubs, programs, or classes, and not yoga therapy. Yet YPs have shared with the authors that the school staff expect a mental health benefit from these yoga sessions (E. Cochrane, personal communication, May 3, 2024; A. Homossany, personal communication, June 8, 2023).

When the YP is able to provide a safe, welcoming environment in a group, it increases the likelihood that each child will enjoy and benefit from yoga.

Thus, we offer this case example in the school setting for two reasons: 1) to show how useful CPTSD-informed yoga skills can be in a group; and 2) to demonstrate the transition from group yoga (which may or may not be labeled by the institution as "yoga therapy") to individualized yoga therapy.

First, let's focus on Ayala's main goal for the group, which was to establish safety and trust with all of the children. Her objective for this goal was to foster children's psychological resources (Chapter 4) by using yoga tools in creative and imaginative ways. Creativity is recognized by the WHO (1994) as one of the ten essential life skills. Kumar et al. (2024) say that creativity plays a vital role in human development by fostering resilience, sparking joy, and contributing to a sense of personal growth, ultimately contributing to overall well-being.

Creating a therapeutic environment that prioritizes creativity and curiosity is essential for effective healing, because it promotes safety and control (Sullivan, 2020; van der Kolk, 2014). By allowing children to express themselves creatively, the YP provides a means of regaining agency over their experiences. Levine and Kline (2006) found that creative expression leads to better emotional regulation and coping strategies, particularly for those affected by trauma.

One of the practices that Ayala used to foster creativity and curiosity through yoga tools was Paintbrush Circles. This practice encourages children to use their palms, elbows, and knees as imaginary paintbrushes, drawing circles while choosing colors and strokes; they may choose to draw circles while sitting up or lying down.

Body awareness practices such as this help children integrate their brain's responses, fostering emotional regulation by engaging with the body's signals (Siegel & Bryson, 2012). Treleaven (2018) emphasizes that cultivating sensitivity to bodily sensations can enhance interoceptive awareness, a critical component in trauma recovery and overall emotional well-being. In addition, the Paintbrush Circles practice integrates repetitive and rhythmic movements, which Bruce Perry (2020b) says are calming for children.

Another group practice that helped create group cohesion and collective creativity was the 'Yoga Dance' game from the *Enchanted Wonders A–Z Cards* (Homossany & Calo-Henkin, 2015). Ayala divided children into groups of three. Each group received 5–6 cards with different poses and was asked to combine them into a yoga sequence, a "yoga dance." This exercise encouraged teamwork, imagination, and communication. During this activity, Ayala noticed that Iryna seemed to interact positively with her peers without the pressure of direct verbal communication. Ayala introduced the group to many more CPTSD-informed yoga tools, all of which are featured in the next section on individual yoga therapy.

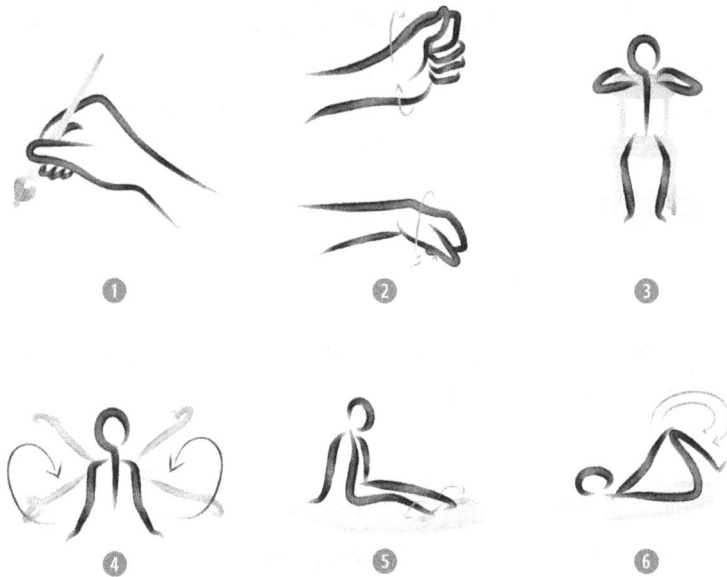

**Figure 8.1** Paintbrush Circles Range of Motion (ROM)

*Illustrates the Paintbrush Circle Sequence, where one imagines holding a paintbrush with different body parts to create circular motions. This exercise can be performed as a ROM practice or as a preparation for relaxation on the floor, functioning as a pre-yield activity.*

As the ten-week course progressed, a few students showed interest in learning more about how these practices could help them individually. Iryna was one of them: her mother reached out to Ayala to share that Iryna seemed much more regulated and relaxed on the days she'd attended yoga club. After getting in trouble during her lunch period one day, Iryna's mother asked Ayala if she could see Iryna individually.

What follows is individual work Ayala did with Iryna. Many of the practices Ayala chose to do with Iryna individually were ones that she learned in the group yoga setting. With some of these practices we provide two variations of sequences, depending on a child's physical mobility.

While Ayala was unable to do a full assessment, she used her observations from group sessions, including Paintbrush Circles, which can double as a ROM assessment for the YP. Ayala observed that Iryna struggled in this practice to generate movement in her shoulders, with most of the motion coming from her arms rather than from the shoulder girdle itself. Additionally, Iryna's foot movements were limited, with minimal ability to achieve full flexion and extension. These limitations in Iryna's movements were another indication of her tamasic relationship to *push*.

## Snapshot
### Presenting Problem

Iryna, a 7-year-old girl, joined at the beginning of the school year an after-school yoga club led by Ayala. The yoga club ran throughout the school year where children can sign up per term (ten weeks). While Iryna expressed enthusiasm and arrived each session, her behavior revealed underlying distress which mainly manifested as disruptive behavior toward her peers. She frequently arrived early and stayed late, yet struggled with concentration during challenging activities, often disrupting her peers by teasing or pushing them. After such incidents, Iryna would withdraw from the group, sometimes tucking her head between her knees.

Iryna was born in Ukraine and abandoned at the hospital by her biological mother. She lived in a foster home until age 2, after which she was adopted and relocated to the UK. She shared openly that she was adopted, which at times appeared to create discomfort for her peers.

During yoga sessions, Iryna displayed rajasic behavior, characterized by an inability to follow instructions, maintain attention, or manage her energy, especially during asanas and games. However, she favored end-of-session relaxation and reflection, where her rajasic behavior transformed into focused attention. After one session, she confided in Ayala that she had few friends and felt misunderstood by her teachers. She said that yoga was her favorite time of the week because it made her feel welcomed. And she liked relaxation, which helped quiet the noise in her head.

Behavioral challenges in children often mask deeper emotional and psychological issues, such as trauma, anxiety, and unmet emotional needs (Greene, 2014). In *The Boy Who Was Raised as a Dog* (2007), Bruce Perry and Maia Szalavitz explain that children exposed to trauma may display aggressive, impulsive, or withdrawn behaviors, which often stem from internal emotional chaos rather than deliberate defiance or misbehavior. These outward behaviors can obscure underlying emotional distress, emphasizing the importance of addressing the root causes rather than just the symptoms (Greene, 2014; Perry & Szalavitz, 2007).

### Look-Feel-Sound

- **Look:** Iryna is a 7-year-old girl. She is well-groomed, appears her age, and has a slim body type. She presents with balance and coordination issues. She has rounded shoulders and a forward-tilted head, indicating disengagement and collapse. She exhibits hypervigilance, as demonstrated by constantly scanning the room when other children are present.

- **Feel:** Iryna says she feels happy and welcome in yoga and is generally engaged in the practice. However, when she struggles with a pose or does not want to participate in a group activity, she gives up easily and can become disruptive. She may invade her peers' space or become aggressive. If a child reacts with surprise or fear to her erratic boundaries, she either becomes aggressive or isolates herself.

- **Sound:** Iryna speaks clearly, but her speech volume fluctuates based on her emotional state. At times, she speaks quickly and loudly, interrupting others, while at other times she speaks softly, especially when anxious or feeling misunderstood.

In the following sections, we'll explore how creating a safe and supportive environment allowed trust to grow, making it easier for Iryna to engage positively with the group. Ayala observed her unique needs and used grounding and centering techniques to help her feel secure and connected. This approach encouraged Iryna's comfort in expressing herself while gently integrating her into group dynamics.

### Assessment with PMK Overview

For Iryna, much of the information came from observing her in sessions and conversations with her parents, along with a permission/registration form completed by her parents prior to the after-school club.

### Annamaya Kosha

Iryna presented with a posterior pelvic tilt and rounded shoulders that seemed to impact her balance and coordination in yoga poses. These postural imbalances indicated a tamasic expression of *push* (Chapter 5), and what appeared to be a lack of proprioceptive awareness. *Proprioception* is the body's ability to sense position, movement, and location in space, allowing one to coordinate actions without constantly looking at the limbs (WebMD, 2024). These body alignment issues and lack of proprioception affected Iryna's balance and coordination, and possibly her breathing patterns too.

Iryna also exhibited *rajasic-push* behaviors, such as restlessness, agitation, and a reluctance to fully engage with her peer group; and she demonstrated an acute lack of interoceptive awareness (Chapter 4), as evidenced by her inability to recognize internal bodily cues like hunger or the need to use the bathroom. Her challenges in attuning to these signals suggested that her body was communicating in ways she could not fully interpret, as described by Rothschild (2000) in Chapter 4 of this book.

Physical and yoga therapist Rachel Krentzman poignantly states in her book *Yoga for a Happy Back* (2016), "Our bodies tell the story that we are trying to hide" (p. 46). Iryna's collapsed physical posture and the discomfort she expressed specifically during standing postures appeared to be outward expressions of her unprocessed early life experiences, including pre-verbal trauma from abandonment at birth and the subsequent instability of foster care.

Despite these challenges, Iryna seemed to benefit from the contrasting experience of relaxation followed by a group conversation at the end of sessions. Her mother told Ayala that after yoga sessions, Iryna continued to demonstrate calm and focused behavior at home.

## Pranamaya Kosha

Iryna exhibited erratic energy levels, often alternating between bursts of hyperactivity and sudden fatigue. Pranayama kosha refers to the life force (prana) body and is associated with the organs of respiration, as well as speech. Although Iryna was articulate, especially after the relaxation part of the session, she sometimes spoke rapidly and slurred her words, particularly when she was anxious or excited. This made her difficult to understand and often led to frustration when she felt misunderstood. In addition, her teachers described her as "wild and unpredictable in her behavior," indicating a rajasic energetic pattern.

Her posture may have contributed to her shallow breathing pattern, manifested as tightness in her accessory muscles, and no movement in her lower ribcage. Her shallow breathing potentially led to an increased stress response (Sullivan, 2020). Iryna also exhibited mouth breathing and reverse breathing (Chapter 1).

## Manomaya Kosha

Despite being a bright and creative child, Iryna had difficulty concentrating in school and during yoga, a manifestation of excessive rajas. In yoga sessions, Iryna became frustrated when she was unable to perform a yoga pose. She would quickly lose her temper, saying things like, "I hate this pose!" or "This is boring!" Subsequently, she would isolate herself, sit apart, and utter harsh criticisms like calling herself "stupid." These behaviors again illustrated *tamasic-push* tendencies, characterized by self-criticism, withdrawal, and feeling inadequate. Interestingly, her mother observed that Iryna's negative self-view was less prominent in music, where she displayed confidence and persistence. This suggested that her strengths in activities like music helped mitigate some of the negative self-perception observed in other contexts.

## Vijnanamaya Kosha

Iryna participated in a variety of diverse activities such as football, art classes, and music lessons. In particular, she said her favorite school subjects were art and violin. She once shared a piece of art she'd made with her peers in a yoga club. This act of sharing highlighted her enthusiasm for creative expression, her identification with it, and her desire to connect with others through her artistic achievements.

Yoga also appeared to offer Iryna a valuable creative outlet. Activities like creating her own "nest" or experimenting with poses gave Iryna chances to express her creativity and individuality, encouraging innovation and adaptation in line with her artistic nature. However, her negative self-perception hindered her ability to fully embrace new experiences outside of her comfort zone.

Iryna's unpredictable behavior often left her peers uncertain about how to interact with her. Teachers said that some children avoided her, and some children bullied her. This social isolation manifested in frustration and conflict with her peers. For example, she had a physical altercation with another child, which resulted in the headteacher calling her parents in for a meeting.

Despite difficulties with peers, Iryna demonstrated a strong desire to form meaningful relationships with caring adults. She established bonds with her adoptive parents, her art teacher, and with Ayala, her yoga instructor. These attachments created a foundation of security and acceptance, essential for her entire well-being. To reinforce this foundation, Ayala made a point of saying how happy she was to see Iryna at the beginning of each yoga session. This simple interaction seemed to make a positive impact on Iryna, who once responded, "You are my first teacher at school who is so kind to me." While she found it challenging to establish friendships with her classmates, the supportive relationships she was forming with adults served as a stabilizing force in her life.

## Anandamaya Kosha

Due to her negative self-perceptions and her erratic behavior that isolated her from her peers, young Iryna seemed to struggle to find a sense of joy in life. Yet there were many glimmers of hope: Iryna's creative expression, her love of playing the violin, her enjoyment of relaxation during yoga, and her strong, meaningful attachments with caring adults all indicated her ability to access joy.

Anandamaya kosha is also the kosha of community support, as defined by YTCT. Iryna's main community support was school and the group she played violin with outside school.

## PMK Overview

Iryna's challenges spanned physical, energetic, emotional, and social domains, reflecting unprocessed trauma and inconsistent emotional regulation. Her struggles with posture, energy, self-criticism, and social isolation were balanced by her creativity, support from adults, and moments of calm after yoga, indicating her capacity for healing and personal growth.

**Table 8.1** depicts the PMK Overview for Iryna, a 7-year-old child.

| Kosha | Client's Presentation |
|---|---|
| **Annamaya Kosha** (Stability) | Physical challenges, including poor posture, balance issues, and difficulty with proprioception and interoception. A *tamasic-rajasic push* imbalance is present throughout the yoga session. |
| **Pranamaya Kosha** (Vitality) | Iryna presents with reversed and shallow breathing. Changes in speech expression during stress highlight imbalances in rajasic-tamasic energy. All contribute to her physical and emotional stress responses. After relaxation she presents with a *sattva-yield* state, where she is articulate and enjoys sharing her thoughts. |
| **Manomaya Kosha** (Clarity) | Emotionally, in the *manomaya kosha*, Iryna battles self-criticism and frustration, especially when tasks don't come easily, a clear sign of *tamasic-push* energy. However, her confidence in music suggests areas of emotional strength. |

*cont.*

| Kosha | Client's Presentation |
|---|---|
| **Vijnanamaya Kosha** (Wisdom/ Intuition) | The *vijnanamaya kosha* reveals Iryna's creativity and insight, especially in art and music, but her negative self-view limits her ability to fully engage with new experiences. Iryna presents with *tamasic-reach* expressed as her struggle to connect with her peer group. While Iryna struggles with social relationships, particularly among her peers, supportive adult connections provide her with much-needed emotional security and stability. |
| **Anandamaya Kosha** (Joy/Awe) | Playing her violin, creating art, and connecting with adults seem to give Iryna much joy. |

## Treatment Planning
### Target Koshas

It was clear, from the Paintbrush Circles ROM and Ayala's observations of Iryna through Look-Feel-Sound, that both annamaya and pranamaya koshas were the most impacted. By targeting annamaya kosha, Ayala could address Iryna's physical instability and the imbalances in the *push* state. For instance, improving her physical posture would most likely help Iryna with balance and coordination. This in turn would help her to relate with the physical action of *push* in a sattvic way. And by addressing Iryna's postural imbalances, Ayala sought to help Iryna improve her breathing (pranamaya kosha).

Had Ayala seen Iryna long term, the next kosha to focus on would have been vijnanamaya kosha, given Iryna's strained relationships with herself and with her peers. Beyond that, Iryna would later benefit from a focus on anandamaya kosha, to foster feelings of joy, connection, and sense of belonging.

### *Goal 1: Iryna will develop safety and stability through body awareness.*

Ayala used a system of short term (6–10 weeks), mid-term (10–16 weeks), and long term (6–12 months) stages to guide her planning for Iryna's goals and objectives. She learned this method through her training at the Minded Institute. This system of different stages of treatment is supported by evidence from the American Psychological Association (APA, 2017), which recommends two of these three stages (mid-term and long term).

The initial, short-term goal focused on Iryna's evident lack of interoceptive and proprioceptive awareness to help her develop safety and stability in her body. Re-patterning Iryna's imbalance between *yield* and *push*—in particular toggling back and forth between *rajasic-push* and *tamasic-push*—was crucial. Director of the BodyMind Centering® Program in Montreal, Mariko

Tanabe, explains: "*yield* and *push* is the pattern that enables the baby to find themselves, to feel where their body begins and ends, and to start to embody that" (Kemble, 2018, 36:28–36:45). Without this re-patterning of the first two FMs, Iryna's ability to *reach* would have been unsupported.

**Objective 1a: Iryna will practice yoga tools that stabilize and strengthen her core muscles.**

Iryna needed to strengthen and stabilize her core to improve her posture and breathing patterns. A stable and strong core is essential for the FM of *push* (Chapter 5). Yoga therapist Doug Keller (2016) emphasizes that "core stability has to be established for any neck and shoulders action to work" (p. 32). Yoga master Donna Farhi and yoga therapist Leila Stuart (2022) assert that core stability is important across all five koshas because "the core is a multifaceted experience of self that is centered in the present" (p. 4). This involves maintaining balance and alignment with the ground, gravity, and space, while using awareness to effectively activate core muscles. To this end, Ayala introduced Iryna to the Cuddly Cat Sequence.

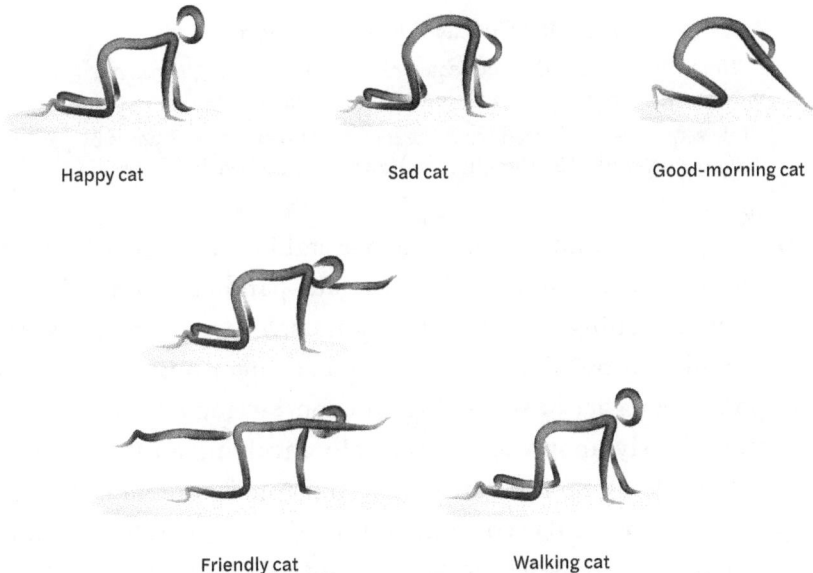

Happy cat          Sad cat          Good-morning cat

Friendly cat          Walking cat

**Figure 8.2** Cuddly Cat Sequence

*Illustrates the Cuddly Cat Sequence, a vinyasa that integrates all FM movements to stabilize the core.*

This sequence is adapted from the *Enchanted Wonders A–Z Cards* by Homossany and Calo-Henkin (2015), and reprinted with permission.

This sequence was featured in group yoga sessions. Some children with limited mobility found the seated version more accessible. We provide that option as well.

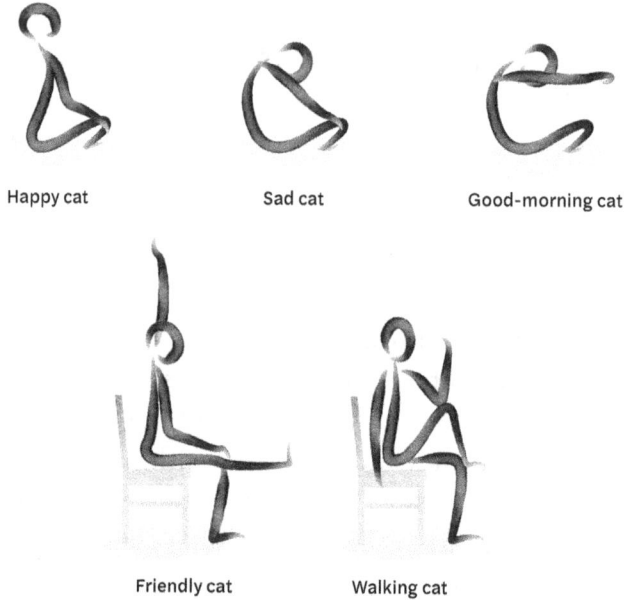

Happy cat           Sad cat           Good-morning cat

Friendly cat        Walking cat

**Figure 8.3** Cuddly Cat Seated Variation

*Illustrates the Cuddly Cat Sequence (seated variation), a vinyasa that integrates all FM movements to stabilize the core.*

This sequence is adapted from the *Enchanted Wonders A–Z Cards* by Homossany and Calo-Henkin (2015), and reprinted with permission.

Both variations of the Cuddly Cat Sequence stabilize core muscles through vinyasa. The sequences also provide conscious pandiculation—the mindful process of stretching and contracting muscles with awareness (Warren, 2022)—which allowed Iryna to create a stronger push into the floor; it is the spontaneous act of stretching and contracting muscles that often occurs unconsciously upon waking, typically involving a full body stretch and yawn. The role of pandiculation is to release chronic muscle tension and improve neuromuscular control, and in addition, it relieves pain and chronic tension, where muscles remain involuntarily contracted due to stress or trauma (Warren, 2022).

In the Cuddly Cat sequence, pandiculation also helped Iryna create a stronger *push* into the floor. As Iryna flowed through the sequence, Ayala asked, "Is there an area that feels tense?" and "Which movement made the tight feeling worse or better?" These questions cued greater body awareness and insights into how movements affect tension levels. By engaging consciously in a supportive environment, Iryna became more aware of her core muscles.

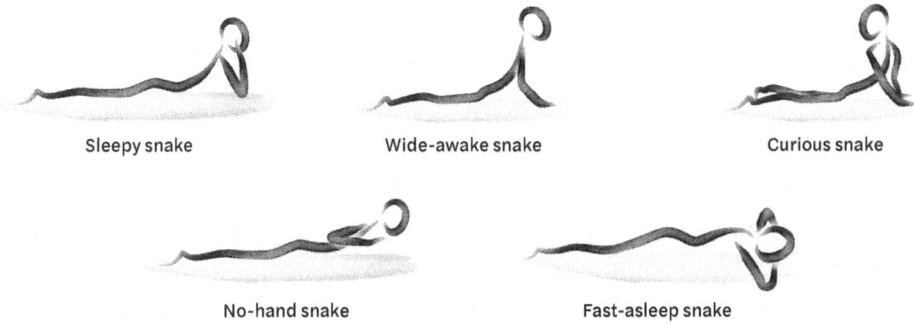

Sleepy snake    Wide-awake snake    Curious snake

No-hand snake    Fast-asleep snake

**Figure 8.4** Sleepy Snake Sequence

*Illustrates the Sleepy Snake Sequence that may balance tamasic and rajasic qualities of push.*

This sequence is adapted from the *Enchanted Wonders A–Z Cards* by Homossany and Calo-Henkin (2015), and reprinted with permission.

Next, Ayala reviewed with Iryna the Sleepy Snake Sequence, which stabilized and strengthened Iryna's core muscles. Transitioning from the active *yield* of Sleepy Snake to the *rajasic push* of Wide-Awake Snake provided a gentle way to re-pattern her tendencies. Sleepy Snake was also taught in the group class. Thus, a seated variation is offered here.

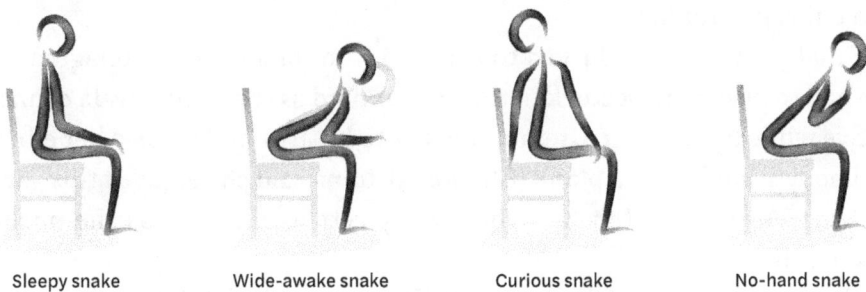

Sleepy snake    Wide-awake snake    Curious snake    No-hand snake

**Figure 8.5** Sleepy Snake Sequence—Seated Variation

*Illustrates the seated variation of the Sleepy Snake Sequence. Invite children to focus on their contact points with the ground and the chair before beginning the sequence to establish a stable push movement.*

This sequence is adapted from the *Enchanted Wonders A–Z Cards* by Homossany and Calo-Henkin (2015), and reprinted with permission.

Since Iryna exhibited reverse and mouth breathing, a sequence like Sleepy Snake Pose helped her use the ground as feedback for the movement of her diaphragm. In addition, playfully moving her tongue and making sounds could potentially help her establish a supportive breathing pattern. In Sleepy Snake Pose (makarasana), Iryna can dynamically explore how it feels to collapse and lift through her shoulders while resting on her elbows and playing between tamasic and rajasic yielding. Annie Brook (n.d.) calls this exploration an active *yield*, where one's muscles are engaged without being tense or totally relaxed.

Tongue exercises also offer significant benefits for children, especially in addressing mouth breathing issues. Rothenberg (2020) notes that over 50% of primary school children exhibit mouth breathing, leading to various physical and cognitive issues. "A floppy tongue can potentially set up a situation for mouth breathing as the child develops" (Rothenberg, 2020, p. 128). Incorporating tongue exercises may help promote proper oral posture, supporting healthy facial development and mitigating the negative effects of mouth breathing.

In Curious Snake Pose, Ayala invited Iryna to hiss and move her tongue in all directions, pretending to explore their surroundings. Iryna was then invited to create her own Fast Asleep Snake Pose. Ayala asked her which of the five movements she enjoyed the most. Iryna hesitated, struggling with No Hand Snake Pose, but chose to continue with Curious Snake Pose. By making the sequence repetitive and exploratory, Ayala created a welcoming environment for Iryna to participate in whatever way was accessible and enjoyable for her.

Finally, Ayala invited Iryna to stand in front of a wall and imagine that she had to push a truck stuck in the mud as hard as she could. Ayala counted to five while Iryna pushed, reminding her to breathe and to keep her elbows and body straight like a plank (Chapter 5). Iryna said she enjoyed this game, and shared that she felt her whole body getting stronger as she pushed against the wall.

For the Nourishing-Nest Sequence, Iryna was asked to imagine her body transforming into a nourishing nest filled with positive actions, ideas, and foods. Once full, she was invited to bring her knees closer to her chest, balancing on her hips and imagining herself as a cosmic egg floating in space. Ayala then invited Iryna to roll back and forth and explore if there was something she was happy to send out into the world. Although she struggled to return to sitting after rolling backward, Iryna kept trying. This practice helped her connect to deep core muscles while also engaging her vestibular system, providing a soothing refuge.

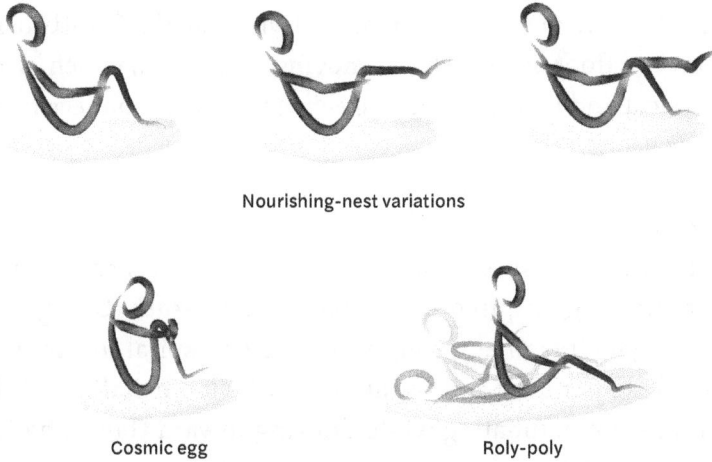

Nourishing-nest variations

Cosmic egg                                    Roly-poly

**Figure 8.6** Nourishing-Nest Sequence

*Illustrates the Nourishing-Nest Sequence, transitioning through balancing variations that symbolize inviting goodness into one's space, holding it in cosmic egg pose, and sharing it with the world through a gentle rocking "roly-poly" movement.*

This sequence is adapted from the *Enchanted Wonders A–Z Cards* by Homossany and Calo-Henkin (2015), and reprinted with permission.

**Objective 1b: Iryna will practice yoga tools that increase her body and breath awareness.**

## Yield and Pre-Yield

To help Iryna build interoceptive awareness, Ayala first introduced her to two kinds of guided mindfulness practices. Practices like a guided body scan help clients attune to the body in various postures and activities, identify tension or misalignment, and improve physical imbalances. Louise Goldberg (2016) says that learning to recognize subtle body signals helps "students develop a sense of control over their response to the world around them" (p. 150).

The first guided mindfulness practice came from Ayala's observation of how much Iryna liked the relaxation and reflection at the end of group sessions. Ayala emphasized this in Iryna's individual sessions: she invited Iryna to choose a comfortable position, where she could feel as if receiving a cozy hug from an imaginary friend or resting on a soft pillow. This kind of imagery empowered Iryna to choose what worked for her and encouraged a mental form of *yielding*. Ayala also gave Iryna a scarf to use as she wished—either as a pillow, a blanket, or simply to hold. Iryna opted to lie on her side with the scarf under her head. Offering Iryna a physical object like a scarf was a form of anchor for her (Chapter 4).

Another effective yielding practice for Iryna was the Paintbrush Circles practiced on the floor. It served as a moving body scan, which also helped create a physical and mental state of *yielding* as well as connecting with her physical sensations.

## Spiral Breath

The Spiral Breath exercise enhances Iryna's bodily awareness by integrating breath with drawing, inspired by the book *Draw Breath* (Granger, 2019). In this practice, Iryna imagines or physically draws a spiral in two ways: first, inhaling while expanding the spiral outward then exhaling while drawing it inward; second, inhaling while drawing inward then exhaling while expanding outward. Iryna particularly enjoyed this exercise, as her passion for drawing allowed her to express herself creatively, deepening her engagement with the practice. In her experience, Ayala found that for children who love art, like Iryna, this type of breath practice led them in and opened a door to try other breathing practices.

To help Iryna foster a deeper sense of safety and presence within her body, she was also introduced to yoga tools that incorporated breath awareness along with her physical sensations. For example, the Hot Drink Mindfulness practice was aimed at enhancing Iryna's bodily awareness through the comforting experience of imaging or holding a favorite warm beverage.

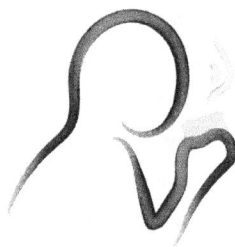

**Figure 8.7** Hot Drink Mindfulness Practice
*Illustrates the Hot Drink Mindfulness practice—a commonly used practice in mindfulness groups across all ages.*

Iryna was asked to imagine holding a cup of hot cocoa, tea, or soup. Inhaling, she could imagine smelling the aroma of the hot drink she chose. Exhaling, she visualized cooling the drink by breathing softly over it. This imaginal practice helped Iryna tune into how the warmth and aroma affected her emotional state, while also practicing deep breathing.

At the end of her session, she received a handout to draw her favorite hot drink. Ayala did this exercise with Iryna's group as well. Handouts are a great way to provide children an opportunity to share their creations with their caregivers and repeat the practice at home.

### Goal 2: Iryna will cultivate self-compassion and social skills.

Upon completion of goal #1, Iryna started her mid-term goal of cultivating self-compassion to decrease her negative self-talk, as well as her feelings of guilt and shame. Chris Germer (2021) says these feelings arise from "the belief that something is wrong with me that renders me unlovable, that somehow we are too flawed to be accepted or approved by others" (4:03–4:17).

### Objective 2a: Iryna will learn and practice self-compassion.

Mindfulness exercises in the form of self-compassion were introduced to help Iryna recognize her strengths, encouraging a kinder inner dialogue while gradually reducing negative self-talk. Self-compassion is the act of offering oneself the same kindness that one would extend to a friend during tough times (Germer, 2009; Neff, 2011). Lovingkindness meditation focuses on directing positive thoughts and well wishes toward oneself and others.

This practice entails mentally repeating phrases for oneself, someone you love, a neutral person, and all living beings, such as "May you be well," "May you be happy," and "May you live with ease" (Brach, 2019; Kabat-Zinn, 2005; Kornfield, 2008; Nhat Hanh, 2017). Engaging in this meditation can shift our perspective, fostering a sense of connection and reducing feelings of isolation. Meditation master Sharon Salzberg (2018) says that through this practice we begin to understand that all beings, regardless of their differences, share a fundamental longing for happiness.

By incorporating hand movements, Mantra Wishes is a form of self-compassion for children which makes the practice more tangible and accessible to them. Notice these are the same hand movements as Sa Ta Na Ma. In Iryna's case, the purpose of the practice was to develop kinder self-talk where the affirmations were replaced with a wish style affirmation to create a vision of a change. By encouraging her to create her own wishes, this practice also empowered Iryna to come up with solutions for herself in the future.

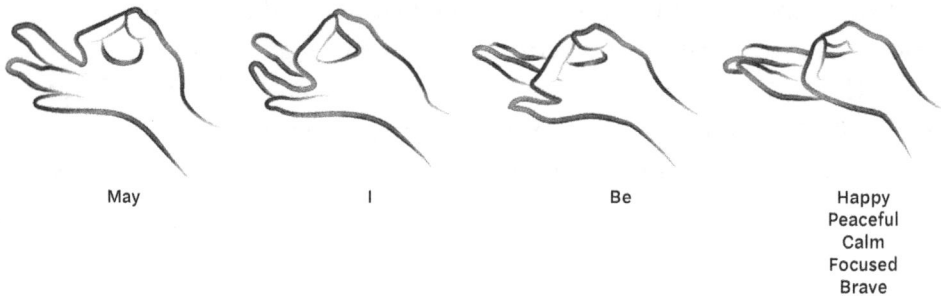

| May | I | Be | Happy |
| | | | Peaceful |
| | | | Calm |
| | | | Focused |
| | | | Brave |

**Figure 8.8** Mantra Wishes

*Illustrates the Mantra Wishes practice. Children create their own affirmations with words like "Happy," "Peaceful," "Calm," "Focused," and "Brave," or other words that resonate with the child.*

## Course of Treatment

*Note to the Reader: The semester came to an end before Ayala could introduce Iryna to this objective and the following goal #3. However, for a child like Iryna these goals and objectives would have been the next natural step. Thus, the authors felt it important to include them.*

**Objective 2b: Iryna will learn and practice positive social interactions through group activities.**

Iryna's second objective aimed at increasing her social interactions with peers through the FM of *reach*, which represents the wish to explore and connect with others. After increasing her interoceptive awareness in goal #1 through *yield-push* yoga tools, she was ready to join a group game, such as the Let's Plaoga Dance described earlier in the chapter. The objectives of this group interaction for Iryna would have been to help her build trust, improve communication, and develop cooperation skills.

**Goal 3: Iryna will develop emotional regulation.**

Building on the progress from goals #1 and #2, an appropriate long-term goal for Iryna would be to develop emotion regulation, a manomaya kosha goal. Goal #1 had helped Iryna learn to become aware of her internal sensations—this is the first step to identifying and labeling emotions.

**Objective 3a: Iryna will learn to identify and label emotions.**

Primary school age children like Iryna benefit from colorful visual tools to learn new concepts. Amy Wheeler's Mental/Emotional State Assessment Feelings Chart for children featured in Chapter 4 is an excellent tool, because it features faces showing each emotion. Using such a tool could expand Iryna's emotional vocabulary and develop better emotional control.

In her young life, Iryna had endured a lot. The unspoken trauma of being abandoned and living in foster care from birth to 2 years old had an enormous impact on her nervous system. These traumas echoed through her inability to notice her own body signals, self-regulate, and relate with peers. Yoga therapy opened a door for Iryna to relate with herself, others, and her world in a new way. By learning to pay attention to her body's signals, Iryna found her first taste of empowerment. Ayala was able to capitalize on her strengths—her creativity and her ability to bond with adults—through their yoga therapy sessions. Early intervention like this is invaluable.

## Specific Considerations for Children
### Musculoskeletal

Children's flexibility often exceeds their strength, making it essential to introduce yoga practices that align with their capabilities while modifying poses to prevent strain (Chapter 2). Poses should be held for shorter durations to avoid over-extension. In addition, the YP should encourage curious exploration of poses rather than strict adherence to form. Core stability is often weaker in children who do not participate in sports or spend extended time sitting, which can weaken core muscles necessary for good posture and movement (Tiwari et al., 2024). Incorporating core-strengthening practices is vital for overall development, not just for trauma recovery.

Yoga therapist and Somatic Experiencing™ Practitioner Shawnee Thornton-Hardy (2023) says that "having a child explore movement closer to the ground when they are less coordinated or their sensory system is underdeveloped, will give them more of a felt sense of safety and stability" (p. 49).

Similarly, children's vascular systems continue to develop through the age of 8 (MacGregor, 2008). Thus, when introducing breathing practices, it's important to consider a child's stage of development. Before the age of 8 years, children should not be introduced to formal pranayama practices but should instead learn breath awareness practices in an exploratory manner that sparks their curiosity and sense of play, such as Hot Drink or Sleepy Snake sequence.

## Social/Emotional

See Chapter 2 for a more general overview of social/emotional needs for children 5–12 years of age. Here, we focus on the impact that adoption has on children.

### Effects of Adoption

Iryna's adoption trauma is a crucial consideration in her treatment. Children who experience adoption trauma often struggle to form secure attachments due to past disruptions and traumatic events (Shafir, 2024). Shafir adds that adopted children "may struggle with forming stable, safe, and secure bonds with caregivers due to traumatic events or being moved to a different home. These challenges can also lead to attachment disorders in adulthood" (2024, para. 9). As an adopted child, Iryna needed a supportive, consistent approach in her yoga practice to help her develop emotional stability.

Another key aspect when working with adopted children is the role of a regulated adult. Jyoti Manuel, founder of Special Yoga Ltd, states: "Children adopted at an early age, especially pre-verbal, will struggle with healthy attachment in their lives. If the primary caregiver isn't solid, there is nothing for the child to hold onto to give them any sense of attachment" (personal communication, September 23, 2024). Given these factors, Iryna's therapeutic environment needed to be grounded in consistency and emotional attunement, with regulated adults offering stability to help her heal.

## Cognitive and Neurobiological

Children's ongoing brain development, particularly in areas related to attention, self-regulation, and emotional control, is influenced by the maturation of the prefrontal cortex and anterior cingulate cortex (Perlman & Pelphrey, 2010). Both play crucial roles in executive functions such as attention, self-regulation, and emotional control. During childhood, these brain regions continue to mature, making it an opportune time for children to increase their cognitive abilities. Studies both by Chaya et al. (2012) and Gothe et al. (2013) emphasize that yoga, by engaging mindfulness and body awareness, enhances activity in these brain regions. Specific practices like mindful breathing and dynamic movement encourage children to maintain attention and self-regulate their emotions, supporting cognitive development (Sample et al., 2010).

Activities that promote body awareness, such as yoga sequences involving transitions between poses, enhance cognitive flexibility and memory, fostering a better understanding of spatial awareness and body control (Diamond & Lee, 2011). Engaging in sports during late childhood has been shown to have a positive impact on both cognitive and emotional development (Bidzan-Bluma & Lipowska, 2018). This is particularly important in an age characterized by high screen time and sedentary behavior, which can negatively affect attention and learning (Hillman et al., 2008).

Teicher et al. (2016) found that trauma can lead to a reduction in both the size and integrity of the corpus callosum, which connects the left and right hemispheres of the brain. This reduction disrupts effective communication between the hemispheres and contributes to difficulties in emotional regulation and coordination (Teicher et al., 2016). Research indicates that children and adolescents who have experienced maltreatment often exhibit reduced corpus callosum volume compared to their non-maltreated peers (Ayre & Krishnamoorthy, 2023).

Engaging in activities that require *crossing the midline*—such as reaching across the body in the Seated Walking Cat (Figure 8.3) or performing *contralateral*, coordinated movements such as in Walking Cat or Friendly Cat (Figure 8.2)—stimulates both hemispheres and may help strengthen this communication pathway (Blackmore, 2020; Stapella, 2023). Hardy explains that "*Contralateral* movement is a dialogue movement of one upper limb with the opposite lower limb. This is a necessary skill in being able to walk with smooth, rhythmic, and coordinated movement" (2023, p. 55).

## Caregiver Engagement and Provider Collaboration

Children with trauma, lack of interoceptive awareness, and physical challenges often exhibit behavioral challenges as with Iryna. This requires integrated collaboration among parents, schoolteachers and staff, and the YP. Unfortunately, it is often up to the YP to ensure that good communication occurs among staff and family. For instance, Iryna's teacher and parents were not present during the after-school group yoga sessions, which could make coordination with both more challenging. Additionally, the pick-up time at the club doesn't provide enough privacy to discuss any situations that may have occurred during the session with the parents, making it even more difficult to address any concerns.

Despite these challenges, effective ways to engage both her parents and teacher exist. One approach that Ayala uses during her after-school sessions is providing handouts at the end of each session, detailing the activities and practices covered that day.

These handouts serve multiple purposes: explaining the benefits of the practices, offering suggestions for continuing activities at home, and encouraging parental involvement.

Ayala provided Iryna and her group with a few handouts over the course of their ten-week yoga club. As a result, Iryna was able to share what she learned with her parents. She even reported teaching some of the yoga tools she'd learned at home! This role reversal was powerful, as it reinforced Iryna's learning, empowered her to become the leader/teacher, and gave her a unique opportunity to engage with adults meaningfully.

Handouts also promote continuity of practice outside the after-school program, extending the benefits beyond the classroom. This engagement can also foster a deeper connection between children and parents, as they participate together in activities that support emotional and physical well-being. Stewart-Henry and Friesen (2018) suggest that when children are encouraged to teach or share what they have learned, it enhances their understanding and confidence while strengthening the parent–child bond.

Finally, handouts open a channel for ongoing communication with both teachers and parents. They give parents the opportunity to be actively involved in a child's progress in yoga. And handouts can help the teacher better support children during school hours by using some of the yoga tools in class, even if they aren't directly involved in the yoga program. In *Best Practices for Yoga in School* (Yoga Service Council, 2015) the authors speak of the importance of collaborating with school staff, saying that YPs "should work to understand and respect the responsibilities and needs of classroom teachers and other school staff" (p. 67).

When 1:1 yoga therapy sessions are part of the school day, collaborations can expand to include the child's teacher, the student support coordinator, occupational therapist, speech therapist, educational psychologist, counselor, and social worker, all of whom can adapt to different educational systems and cultures. Fostering this collaboration creates a more supportive and integrated approach that benefits the child involved.

## Self-Care Practice: Yoga and Creativity

As previously mentioned, Bessel van der Kolk emphasizes the pivotal role of creativity in trauma recovery, providing a vital, nonverbal means of processing complex emotions and experiences (2014). For practitioners supporting individuals in this process, self-care is essential for maintaining emotional resilience and sustaining their ability to help others.

Before diving into this chapter's self-care practice, let's first acknowledge the potential internal barrier of the inner critic. Penman (2012) says, "When your inner critic is in full flow, it can sap your energy and enthusiasm for life. It becomes impossible to think clearly or creatively" (p. 33).

To help students guard against this in her yoga and mindfulness for children teacher training, Empowering Children Through Yoga and Creativity, Ayala uses the following strategy. Prior to tapping into your creative nature, visualize your inner critic and place it on a small, decorated stool, perhaps adorned with comforting colors or ribbons. This symbolic act of inviting the inner critic to sit aside creates mental space, allowing creativity to flow more freely.

Next, invite yourself to explore a new or familiar environment. Choose a place, perhaps one you visit regularly or somewhere new. When you arrive, put on your "beginner's mind" glasses and observe the surroundings as if you're seeing them for the first time. How does being in this space affect your mood? What new details or shapes can you recognize? How does the texture of surfaces feel when you touch them? What sounds can you hear, and how do they influence your experience of the environment? Are there any smells that stand out? How do they make you feel? Stay in the space for as long as you feel comfortable, taking mental notes about your experience.

Afterward, take a few moments to reflect on your exploration. What insights or feelings did it evoke? Nurturing your creativity is essential—not only for your well-being but also for those you are helping. Engaging in such practice strengthens the connection between your self-care and your capacity to hold space for others' healing. Your creativity, like that of the children you support, can be a powerful source of renewal and resilience.

## Chapter Summary

- Yoga helps primary school children, including those with ADHD and trauma, by reducing stress, enhancing emotional regulation, and promoting self-soothing. It also provides benefits to staff by alleviating vicarious trauma.

- Group yoga sessions for children additionally also provide mental health benefits when facilitated in a safe and supportive environment.

- Children's disruptive behaviors often mask underlying trauma and emotional distress, which can manifest in lack of concentration, agitation, and negative social interactions. Yoga and yoga therapy offer a supportive environment where children are empowered to build internal body awareness, self-regulate, and possibly find a sense of belonging.

- Children frequently encounter yoga (and possibly yoga therapy) for the first time in group settings, like school or a recreation center.

- When children learn yoga tools that help calm and regulate them, they often share this with a parent or caregiver.

- Usually, a parent or caregiver reaches out to the YP to inquire about individual yoga therapy for a child, as Iryna's mother did for her.

- When working in group settings, such as a school, YPs should gather information from whatever sources are available to tailor sessions to the children's individual needs.

- Yoga and yoga therapy that foster curiosity and creativity in children can promote emotional regulation, resilience, and build agency.

- Yoga practices stabilizing core muscles and improving bodily awareness boost children's posture, proprioception, and emotional regulation.

- To effectively support adopted children experiencing trauma, it is crucial to create a nurturing and consistent environment led by regulated adults that fosters secure attachments and emotional healing.

- Collaboration among parents, teachers, and therapists is crucial in supporting children in yoga classes who experience trauma, as it enhances emotional regulation, strengthens the parent–child bond, and fosters a more integrated approach to their healing and growth.

## CHAPTER 9

# CPTSD-Informed Yoga Therapy for Adolescents

## Evidence and Rationale of YTCT for Adolescents

Yoga therapy is tailor-made for adolescents in the prevention and/or minimization of complex trauma. This assertion stems from the authors' understanding of the importance that emotion regulation plays in the healthy development of adolescents. While emotion regulation is an important skill for all humans regardless of age, adolescents are at a particular disadvantage. As previously discussed, due to significant changes in the brain during adolescence many struggle with emotion regulation (Siegel, 2014). And research now suggests that yoga helps adolescents increase emotion regulation (Daly et al., 2015; Frank et al., 2017). Though there does not appear to be any research regarding the efficacy of yoga *therapy* for adolescent complex trauma, we provide what we believe is compelling evidence for its use.

Let's explore the role that emotion regulation (or dysregulation, in this case) plays in the development of CPTSD for adolescents. First, consider substantial changes that occur both externally and internally during adolescence. Externally, adolescents depend less on family and caregivers, rely more on friends for emotional support (who may also struggle with their own emotion regulation), and take on new challenges like increased academic pressure, a job, and perhaps romantic relationships (Young et al., 2019). Internally, adolescents experience substantial changes in neurobiology, physiology, and even immunity (Frank et al., 2017; Schwartz, 2021; Siegel, 2014). The brain changes can impair an adolescent's judgment and emotion regulation (Frank et al., 2017; Siegel, 2014).

Defined as the capacity to manage one's own emotional responses, *emotion regulation* is a critical element in all relationships (Young et al., 2019). Adolescents' impaired judgment and decreased emotion regulation put them at risk for a host of mental health issues, according to Young et al. (2019). But as we have discussed in previous chapters, they are particularly vulnerable to interpersonal trauma (Schwartz, 2021), a defining factor of complex trauma.

Now research suggests yoga helps adolescents increase emotion regulation (Daly et al., 2015; Frank et al., 2017). Specifically, Frank and colleagues found that yoga helps adolescents think more positively and engage in "cognitive restructuring" (2017, p. 544). As discussed in Chapter 2, Feldman Barrett (Corrigan, 2022) says that simply moving the body helps with emotion regulation, because it changes perception. These positive outcomes make yoga and yoga therapy a potential protective factor in adolescents' development.

## Case Study: Claudia

In the last chapter we explored how to apply CPTSD-informed yoga therapy when working with a child in a school setting. For our adolescent case study, let's explore a private practice setting, in which 14-year-old Claudia is referred for yoga therapy by her parents to alleviate anxiety, depression, and increase emotion regulation. We will pay particular attention to how yoga tools help Claudia to regulate her emotions and think differently about her problems. And we will consider how to work with an adolescent's developmental need to exercise choice, which sometimes presents as resistance.

Of note, neither Claudia nor her parents realized that her symptoms might be signs of complex trauma. Her case provides a good example of how useful CPTSD-informed yoga therapy skills are in working with a client who potentially has trauma or complex trauma but doesn't know it. If diagnosis is outside a YP's scope of practice, certainly the YP would not make a diagnosis or even suggest one. Still, these tools allow the YP to work with the client in a safe, relational way. Using CPTSD-informed skills won't hurt a client who does not have complex trauma but will greatly benefit a client who potentially does. In addition, knowing CPTSD may be part of a client's symptoms, and being able to respond to that need with appropriate care, can greatly reduce the YP's own compassion fatigue, burnout, and vicarious trauma.

If a client's presenting issues are outside your scope of practice, you may also want to consider supervision from a YP or other therapist with a specialization in trauma. Through supervision, you can determine whether to refer the client for additional psychotherapy services (if you yourself are not a licensed psychotherapist). Lastly, supervision is a great way for YPs to practice self-care by receiving support and guidance on difficult cases. As stated throughout this book, self-compassion and self-care are paramount skills for a YP working with all levels of trauma.

## Snapshot
### Presenting Problem

Margaret referred her daughter Claudia for therapy due to self-harm (cutting on her arms and legs), suicidal ideation, panic attacks, negative self-talk, and social issues at school. Margaret found Michelle on the website Psychology Today, and said she liked the fact that Michelle also offered yoga therapy.

Mother and daughter attended the virtual intake appointment together. During this initial session, Margaret said the trigger for Claudia's mental health issues seemed to be tension with school friends at the end of last school year, and Claudia agreed. Margaret also mentioned that she and Claudia's father divorced a few years ago when Claudia was still in primary school. While Claudia said she was very sad her parents divorced, she said she was also happy her parents weren't together anymore, because the fighting was "bad at the end." She said the hardest thing now was traveling back and forth between their houses.

The presenting problems reported by Claudia and her mother do not necessarily add up to complex trauma—though it is true that divorce in and of itself is very stressful on children. It was not until several sessions into treatment that the pervasive stress Claudia endured became more apparent to Michelle. Clients' core and/or biggest issues often don't present themselves until after several sessions. This is for a few reasons. First, building rapport takes time, which means that clients don't open up right away about their biggest stressors and fears. As such, we may not learn right away about a client's most acute struggles. This is natural. It is our job as YPs to earn our clients' trust.

Second, like many clients, Claudia didn't know she was suffering from complex trauma. Clients tend to have a stereotyped view of what trauma looks like. They may assume complex trauma only arises as the result of childhood abuse or other severe circumstances. Younger children may assume that their circumstances are just like everyone else's, and that their symptoms are somehow their fault.

Finally, CPTSD is not recognized as a formal diagnosis in all countries. For instance, in the US complex trauma is not included in the DSM-5. The way that Michelle worked with this was to consider the component parts of Claudia's CPTSD symptoms, such as anxiety, depression, and relational issues, and treat these.

## Look-Feel-Sound

- **Look:** Claudia is a tall, thin 14-year-old Korean American girl (she/her) with dark hair who wears heavy eye make-up, baggy black clothes, and lots of jewelry that cloak her like a layer of armor. She exhibits a lot of rajasic movements: hands flutter around her face, her eyes dart around the room, and she frequently shifts in her seat.

- **Feel:** Claudia says she feels happy, but her rajasic body movements give the impression of anxiety and hypervigilance. She readily engages with her YP Michelle but looks to her mother for reassurance.

- **Sound:** Claudia speaks quickly and interrupts her own thoughts. She says "I don't know" a lot, and then looks pleadingly at Michelle or her mother. Sometimes she speaks so quickly that Michelle must ask her to slow down and repeat herself.

### Assessment with PMK Overview

Though Margaret was enthusiastic about her daughter trying yoga therapy, Claudia herself seemed resistant to yoga asana at first. Yet she didn't mind trying a variety of other yoga tools (breathing, visualization, affirmations, and Yoga Nidra touch). Michelle realized Claudia's resistance could be a way to differentiate from her mother, who loved yoga. Or perhaps Claudia's resistance had something to do with her lack of interoceptive awareness. Lastly, Claudia might feel self-conscious about her changing adolescent body. Many adolescents feel reluctant to move, because it reminds them of these changes.

Regardless of the reason, Michelle prioritized building safety and trust in the therapeutic rapport first. Research shows that the therapeutic rapport (or, alliance, as it is sometimes called) is an essential ingredient to the success of any relational therapy (Stubbe, 2018). So, Michelle focused on strategies and mindful yoga techniques other than asanas. In addition, Claudia learned about the window of tolerance, and how they'd use it in sessions to ensure that she felt safe and well-regulated.

## Annamaya Kosha

Annamaya kosha represents all aspects of one's physical existence, such as the body, physical functioning, and even one's home. Its core quality is stability. As previously mentioned, Claudia was a tall, thin, 14-year-old girl of Korean American descent, who presented with rajasic body movements and goth style of dress.

One of Claudia's annamaya kosha imbalances was a history of cutting—a problem stemming from the manomaya kosha that impacted the annamaya kosha. She said her suicidal ideation and self-harm behaviors were triggered by peer relationships in the previous school year. She said she was in therapy to find other means of coping with her social stress. Her motivation to not self-harm was a protective factor that meant Michelle did not need to prioritize this as a safety goal.

A second was that Claudia split her time between her parents' two homes, and said this was her choice because "I love them both and I don't want either to miss me too much." Alternating houses from week to week since her parents' divorce created instability in Claudia's annamaya kosha. Michelle suspected that this weekly change of home might also contribute to a rajasic relationship to yield. Far from looking relaxed and alert, **Claudia presented as anxious and distracted in sessions**.

Finally, **Claudia reported sleep issues that began when she heard her parents fighting before the divorce**. This led Michelle to believe that personal stress was a contributing factor to Claudia's sleep difficulties. Another possible factor was that Claudia spent over three hours a day during the week on some sort of digital devices between school and social activities. Michelle told her that the blue light from electronic devices can cause sleep problems (Harvard Health Publishing, 2024).

## Pranamaya Kosha

Annamaya and pranamaya koshas are inextricably linked (Kempton, 2020)—whereas annamaya kosha is the stability of one's physical existence, pranamaya kosha is the breath and energy that give the body vitality. As such, Claudia's rajasic body movements (annamaya kosha) appeared to be a bodily expression of too much energy (rajas) in her pranamaya kosha. She also struggled with two other **pranamaya kosha imbalances: ADHD (diagnosed by her nurse practitioner) and migraines**.

## Manomaya Kosha

Recall that manomaya kosha is the sheath of mental/emotional awareness, and its core quality is clarity (Chapter 6). It is also awareness colored by individual perceptions. In this sense, it is the realm of the ego. When the mind lacks clarity, feelings of overwhelm and confusion are not far behind. Claudia exhibited manomaya kosha imbalances such as negative self-talk, hypervigilance, panic attacks, past suicidal ideation, and past self-harm. Notice how four of these symptoms (hypervigilance, panic attacks, self-harm, and suicidal ideation) demonstrate Claudia's inability to *yield*. That is, her hypervigilance and panic showed that she didn't feel safe.

Additionally, all four symptoms have physical, annamaya kosha qualities and implications: hypervigilance and panic attacks cause increased heart and breathing rates; self-harm causes physical damage to the body; and suicidal ideation has severe implications for the health and survival of the body. The koshas are indeed intertwined. Lastly, note that hypervigilance and panic attacks are rajasic symptoms—there is a surfeit of energy in the body. Conversely, self-harm can be thought of as a tamasic symptom because it represents clouded judgment about how to solve one's psychic pain.

During her panic attacks Claudia said she cried a lot, couldn't breathe, and felt a sense of dread. She also felt confused about what brought the panic on. Margaret gently suggested that tensions with school friends were one trigger, but Claudia said she wasn't sure. Michelle recognized that Claudia didn't yet have enough body (interoceptive) awareness to notice the body sensations of panic like increased heart rate and breathing. Yoga asana can be a great way to help clients develop interoception. But, of course, Claudia didn't want to do asana at first. To help Claudia increase her interoceptive awareness, Michelle decided she would offer body-centered and mindfulness yoga tools without using Sanskrit names and that didn't require a yoga mat.

Claudia said she didn't like school and struggled to keep her grades at a passing level. She had a very hard time focusing in school. Her mediocre grades and focus seemed to be a function of her ADHD.

As mentioned above, Claudia reported significant "screen time"—not just for school but on social media as well. The US Surgeon General Vivek Murthy recommends no more than three hours a day, because youth who spend more than this amount of time seem to struggle with sleep and suffer more mental health consequences, according to his 2023 US Department of Health and Human Services report. Murthy says that adolescence and childhood represent critical stages "in brain development that can make young people more vulnerable to harms from social media" (US Department of Health and Human Services, 2023, para. 2). Think about how much social media can alter children and adolescents' perceptions of themselves and the world. To help Claudia not only with her sleep issues but her negative self-talk and peer struggles too, Michelle recommended to Claudia and her mother that she limit her time on social media.

## Vijnanamaya Kosha

If manomaya kosha is the domain of one's individual knowledge, vijnanamaya kosha is one's wisdom and insight that sees beyond personal perceptions. For a 14-year-old, Claudia was perceptive: she chose to see her school counselor regularly and was an engaged participant in yoga therapy with Michelle. When she noticed friends were being mean and divisive on social media, she blocked them. She also showed a lot of empathy toward others—a quality that requires insight and introspection.

In this sense, vijnanamaya kosha can also be seen as the domain of social awareness and personal relationships: "From vijnanamaya kosha, insight into our habitual patterns may help us discover how thoughts, emotions, and behavior facilitate or hinder healthy social connection" (Sullivan, 2020, p. 115).

The divorce of Claudia's parents when she was 11 years old was a painful rupture in her most important personal relationships—her family. D'Onofrio and Emery (2019) note that "parental divorce/separation is associated with an increased risk for child and adolescent adjustment problems, including academic difficulties (e.g., lower grades and school dropout), disruptive behaviors (e.g., conduct and substance use problems), and depressed mood" (para. 5). Luckily, Claudia thought of her dog Mookie like a sibling. He traveled back and forth with her between houses, making him an important personal relationship and protective factor for Claudia.

Claudia appeared close to both parents. Her mother appeared to be a solid emotional support for her. But as for her father, she said, "sometimes he seems a little lost to me." Claudia explained that her father was of Korean descent and adopted as a baby by a White American family. She said he seemed to feel like an outcast. When Michelle heard this, she began to suspect intergenerational trauma, a form of CPTSD (Chapter 3).

Claudia had two best friends she'd known since early childhood. But at school she struggled with friends. Margaret said Claudia was a very empathic person, who put others' needs before hers. (Michelle wondered if Claudia did the same with parents—going back and forth between their houses to make sure they both felt loved, even though this constant moving was hard on her.) She seemed to choose school friends who were "wounded puppies," as her mother put it. Sometimes these friends were mean or hurtful. Her mother worried that others would take advantage of her kind nature.

Claudia was also a talented artist. She dreamed of being a fashion or interior designer. She loved to draw yet admitted her tendency to be a perfectionist about it. "I don't really worry too much about my grades, but I get frustrated when my art doesn't turn out the way I want." In this way, Claudia's artmaking could be a protective or risk factor, depending on how she felt about it.

## Anandamaya Kosha

Anandamaya kosha is one's awareness of joy, or sense of awe, in life. Claudia found joy in hanging out with friends, art, expressing her fashion sense, and interior design. This is also the kosha in which YTCT considers a client's *community relationships* (such as school, work, religious/spiritual organizations, and any other community resource important to that individual). Claudia's main community support was school. She said her family didn't practice any religion, but she said she did often contemplate the meaning of life. Adolescence can be a time of spiritual awakening for those who are so inclined.

## PMK Overview

Several patterns emerged from Claudia's PMK Overview: first, imbalances in Claudia's annamaya kosha (panic attacks, self-harm, and sleep issues) were related to and influenced by imbalances in her manomaya kosha (negative self-talk, hypervigilance, lack of emotion regulation). In addition, Claudia struggled with migraines and ADHD (pranayama imbalances).

Finally, Claudia reported feeling unsafe due to parents' fighting before their divorce, and then unstable due to alternating homes after the divorce. Her symptoms of panic, inability to relax (including sleep issues), self-harm, and suicidal ideation all pointed to a rajasic relationship to the first fundamental movement of yield.

Michelle used the PMK worksheet to get a clearer idea of what the target kosha was at the beginning of treatment (Table 9.1).

**Table 9.1** depicts the PMK Overview for Claudia, a 14-year-old girl.

| Kosha | Client's Presentation |
|---|---|
| **Annamaya Kosha** (Stability) | Claudia's main annamaya kosha imbalances include panic attacks, self-harm, and sleep issues. She seems to have a rajasic relationship to the fundamental movement of yield, as evidenced by her anxious presentation. |
| **Pranamaya Kosha** (Vitality) | Claudia's main pranamaya kosha imbalances include migraines and ADHD. Her breathing seemed shallow, and at times she almost seemed to hold her breath, then let it out with a sudden exhale. Her energy was hyperactive.<br><br>Her inability to sleep shows how entrenched her rajasic relationship with yield is in that it straddles the anna/pranamaya koshas. |
| **Manomaya Kosha** (Clarity) | Claudia's main manomaya kosha imbalances include negative self-talk, hypervigilance, and lack of emotion regulation. She often appears overwhelmed, and interrupts herself.<br><br>Claudia is a middle-school student. She is friendly, artistic, and enjoys expressing her own sense of style. |
| **Vijnanamaya Kosha** (Wisdom/ Intuition) | Claudia has a lot of strengths in vijnanamaya kosha: she's insightful, seeks out support/advice from trusted adults, and forms meaningful friendships and bonds.<br><br>She appears to have intergenerational trauma, along with her father, who is of Korean descent but was adopted by a White American family.<br><br>Especially with her father, she seems to struggle with creating healthy boundaries (tamasic push) that possibly translates into choosing friends with whom she has blurry boundaries. |
| **Anandamaya Kosha** (Joy/Awe) | Claudia found joy in hanging out with friends, art, expressing her fashion sense, and interior design. |

In summary, Claudia was having difficulty feeling safe and stable in her world. This overview revealed some forms of acute distress that cued Michelle to work with Claudia in a safe, supportive way—that is to say, in a CPTSD-informed manner. Later in treatment this approach helped uncover the hard truth that Claudia did indeed suffer from complex trauma.

## Treatment Planning

Michelle decided that the best way to help Claudia achieve safety and stability was to help her get in touch with her body, making annamaya kosha the first target kosha. Developing interoceptive awareness was the first step to emotion regulation (Chapter 4)—a manomaya kosha issue that seemed to be at the root of many of these symptoms.

**Goal 1: Claudia will increase her body awareness.**

Michelle discussed the PMK Overview with Claudia in terms that made sense to a 14-year-old, which meant not using Sanskrit or other jargony terms. For instance, Michelle used the term "body awareness" instead of "interoception." She explained to Claudia that recognizing the body sensations of stress could help her ward off a panic attack or the impulse to cut. Talking to the client in language they can understand is key to creating trust in the relationship and empowering clients of all ages in their own treatment.

**Objective 1a: Claudia will practice mindfulness skills and use a mood tracker.**

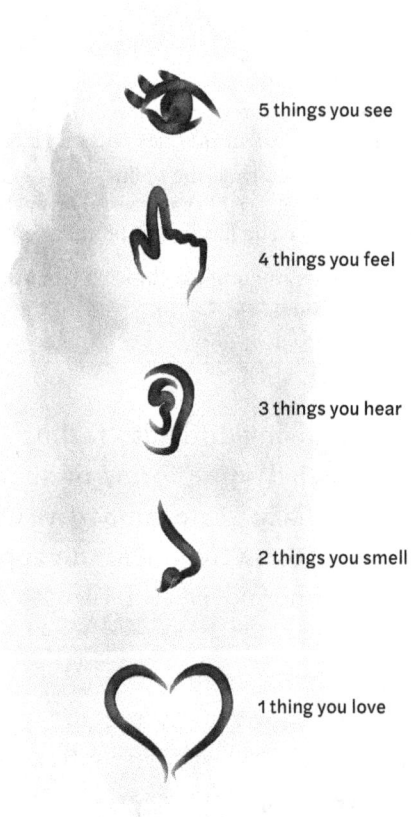

5 things you see

4 things you feel

3 things you hear

2 things you smell

1 thing you love

**Figure 9.1** Five Senses Mindfulness Exercise

*Illustrates the Five Senses Mindfulness Exercise—a commonly used practice in yoga therapy, psychotherapy, and mindfulness groups. It is great for all ages, especially children.*

In YTCT, we believe in meeting clients where they are at. Like Teresa (Chapter 2), Claudia had a rajasic relationship to the first fundamental movement of *yield*. This meant offering Claudia yoga tools that matched her hyperactive, anxious energy. Later in treatment, she would learn yoga tools to gradually calm and relax. So first Claudia learned the Five Senses Mindfulness Exercise, which allowed her to focus attention very briefly on each of the five senses. Focusing in this way can be a powerful way to help clients with ADHD to find brief moments of focus.

Once Claudia experienced slowing her mind down by paying attention to her five senses, Michelle introduced her to box breathing, where she used her finger to draw a box in the air where each "side" of the box was an inhale or exhale. This was a bit of a risk, since it has a Sanskrit chant. Like Sa Ta Na Ma, this breathing technique is an excellent "bridge" for clients with ADHD and anxiety, because they can draw the imaginary box and breathe very fast to match their rajasic energy, and slow down gradually as they feel comfortable. Afterward, Claudia said this breathing technique really helped—and even reported in a later session that she taught it to her mother. Success!

Lastly, as part of this objective, Michelle encouraged Claudia to upload a mood tracker on her phone to track her moods and progress. When working with adolescents, incorporating technology in this way helps them relate to the practice and feel empowered to take charge of their own healing.

**Objective 1b: Claudia will learn and practice good sleep hygiene.**

*Sleep hygiene* describes a set of tools and practices that aid in proper sleep. Adolescents need eight to ten hours of sleep per night, yet often report getting seven hours or fewer on a regular basis (Children's Hospital of Orange County [CHOC], 2016). CHOC offers an informative handout outlining sleep hygiene guidelines for adolescents at https://choc.org/wp-content/uploads/2016/04/Sleep-Hygiene-Teen-Handout.pdf.

Claudia's sleep hygiene protocol included putting away all electronic devices an hour before bed and going to bed around the same time every night (10pm). She also received a Yoga Nidra recording with Michelle's voice that contained minimal Sanskrit words. Recording meditation, visualization, and relaxation tools with the YP's voice is an excellent way to cultivate and strengthen therapeutic rapport. (One caveat to visualizations is that not all clients can visualize—ask a client whether they like to visualize before automatically assigning them.)

Sleep plays an essential role in emotion regulation for clients of all ages, but especially for youth. Feldman Barrett (Corrigan, 2022) says that **getting enough sleep is one of the best ways to teach both children and adolescents emotion regulation**. This is because proper sleep is key to dealing with emotional stress in everyday life (Vandekerckhove & Wang, 2017).

## Course of Treatment
### Phase 1: Cultivating Safety and Stability
**The most important ingredient to successful yoga therapy treatment is establishing a safe, trusting rapport with the client.** It is also the number one predictor of successful therapy (Chapter 4). While this is true in any therapeutic rapport, it is especially true when a client suffers from CPTSD, which involves relational trauma. Michelle suspected some level of relational/intergenerational trauma when Claudia shared that her father was adopted, of a different ethnic background (Korean) than his adoptive parents (Caucasian), and that he felt like an outcast. But establishing a safe, nurturing therapeutic rapport with Claudia was the priority.

To this end, Michelle paid close attention to Claudia's nonverbal cues. When did she seem extra antsy? What seemed to help her relax? Sometimes Michelle noticed Claudia doodling on her arm with a pen. Michelle gave her some colored pencils and paper and invited her to draw as much as she liked when they were chatting between yoga practices. Drawing was one of the first *oases* Michelle and Claudia created in her treatment. Discussed in Chapter 4, oases help reduce hyper-arousal and quiet the mind (Rothschild, 2000).

Yoga tools are also natural oases for clients. Within the first few months of treatment, Claudia reported regularly using her yoga tools (which she referred to as "coping skills") in her life outside sessions to help her regulate her mood. For instance, in her math class she was given an accommodation to draw because it helped her focus more. When she felt anxious or insecure, she could silently repeat the Sa Ta Na Ma mantra in her head while doing the hand motions under her desk. And if she felt panicky or depressed, she could redirect her attention by practicing Five Senses Mindfulness.

Claudia also reported listening to the Yoga Nidra recording several nights a week. As a result, she reported an increase in her awareness of her body sensations after doing Yoga Nidra regularly. And importantly, the frequency of her panic attacks decreased to once every few weeks rather than at least once a week.

## Phase 2: Processing Trauma

About six months into treatment, Claudia began sharing more about home life, both before and after her parents' divorce. She said her parents fought "like cats and dogs" toward the end of their marriage. They didn't fight in front of her, but she said she could hear their screaming from her room at night when she was trying to get to sleep.

In addition, Claudia said she felt responsible for her father's well-being. "Sometimes I feel like he treats me like his therapist." She said she listened to his struggles with mental health and worried about his drinking, much like a parent would. She had taken on the role of a parentified child. Also known as *parentification*, this is when a child takes on the role of parenting their parent by offering developmentally inappropriate emotional support or other adult responsibilities (Dariotis et al., 2023). Claudia's relationship with her father helped explain her tendency to caretake friends.

It is not uncommon for a client to divulge their pain first in yoga therapy before sharing it in other therapeutic settings. Though in Claudia's case Michelle was the primary therapist, Michelle has also had the experience of clients opening up about trauma to her first when she was not the primary therapist. Other YPs have shared similar experiences with Michelle in her trainings on yoga therapy for youth mental health.

Working with the body as we do in yoga therapy has a way of helping clients open up. This is why, of course, we are writing this book—yoga therapy can be an invaluable tool to helping clients recognize and heal their traumatic pain. It is also why YPs should establish communication with other key providers early on. Doing so allows individual providers to work as an integrated team to support the client when and if they share traumatic material. In addition, working with a team helps the YP and other providers decrease the likelihood of burnout and vicarious trauma by supporting one another.

Because she was the primary therapist in this case, Michelle educated Claudia on intergenerational trauma and how it seemed to be impacting her family. They then scheduled a family meeting with her father, during which Michelle gently explained the impact his drinking and oversharing was having on his daughter. Claudia's father said he understood and would change his drinking around her. He also agreed to see a therapist. He said he wanted nothing more than for his daughter to be happy. As with Teresa (Chapters 2 and 3), Claudia's case of CPTSD and intergenerational trauma did not easily fit the stereotype of trauma and family conflict often portrayed in the media.

***Goal 2*: Claudia will increase emotion regulation.**

Around this time, Claudia said she was open to incorporating yoga asana into her sessions. Her panic attacks had increased a bit after sharing such tough family information, and she said she wanted more tools to actively regulate her emotions. As noted above, her therapy goal changed to reflect this. And with her goal change, the target kosha also shifted to both anna-maya and manomaya koshas.

***Objective 2a*: Claudia will learn and practice yoga tools to regulate emotions.**

While the first yoga tools she'd learned did in fact help Claudia regulate her emotions, the primary objective had been to help her notice present moment body sensation. Now Michelle was excited to offer Claudia yoga tools that helped her actively change her experience. Feldman Barrett says that one of the best ways to "master feelings in the moment" (Corrigan, 2022, 50:20–50:23) is to move the body, and that's what Claudia was going to learn to do.

As mentioned in Chapter 5, the fundamental movements are used in the beginning stages of assessment and then again throughout the client's treatment process. In the PMK Overview, Michelle focused on Claudia's rajasic relationship to *yield*. Claudia's symptoms of anxiety, panic, and inability to relax reflected her feelings of lack of safety. Now, Michelle wanted to get a better sense of how Claudia related to all six of the fundamental movements.

Michelle showed Claudia the yoga vinyasa (Figure 9.2), in which each yoga pose represents a movement in the fundamental movements sequence. Creating such a yoga vinyasa allows the YP to see not only how the client relates with each of the fundamental movements, but also how they transition from one to the next. Bear in mind that this is not a set or fixed sequence. Different clients have different needs. A YP is free to select whichever yoga poses work best for a client's abilities, limitations, and needs. For instance, if a client uses a wheelchair, a YP should select a sequence of yoga poses that help the client explore the fundamental movements and that they can perform easily in their chair.

As an able-bodied, 14-year-old girl, the above sequence was easily accessible to Claudia. She said she loved lying on her belly. "It feels open and protected." Relaxing easily into the floor demonstrated a comfortable relationship to yielding. Yielding—like rest and relaxation—is a tamasic action, in that it is stable and unmoving. Michelle was somewhat surprised that Claudia liked it, since she exhibited such rajasic symptoms. But then Michelle reflected on how she'd observed Claudia easily relax into her mother's shoulder during the intake and other family meetings. It was possible that Claudia had difficulty relaxing on her *own* but had the ability to relax with the support of the floor and the support of *others*, especially trusted adults.

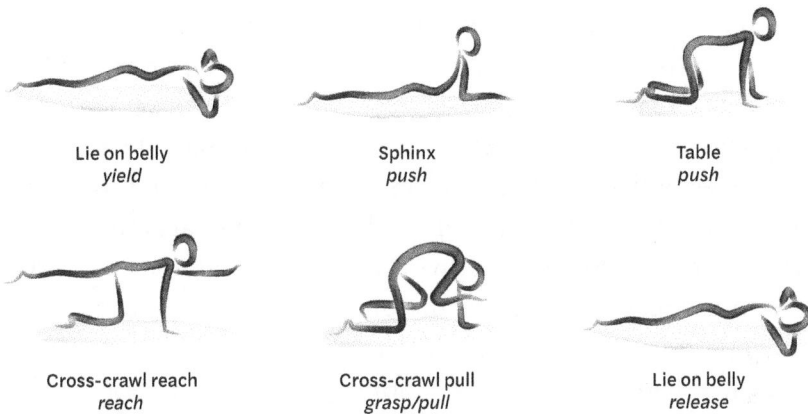

| Lie on belly | Sphinx | Table |
|:---:|:---:|:---:|
| *yield* | *push* | *push* |

| Cross-crawl reach | Cross-crawl pull | Lie on belly |
|:---:|:---:|:---:|
| *reach* | *grasp/pull* | *release* |

**Figure 9.2** Claudia's Fundamental Movements Vinyasa

*Illustration depicts a series of yoga poses Michelle showed Claudia to assess her relationship with each of the six fundamental movements.*

Being able to trust others is an expression of secure attachment, which Claudia seemed to share with her mother. In the same way that a newborn baby can actively rest on their parent's chest, Claudia was able to receive the support of the floor when resting on her belly. As we have seen, the period of 0–3 years old is critical to the healthy growth and development of a child (Chapter 2) for this very reason: when a client has had the experience of regularly being held and nurtured, they can more easily relax into yoga poses that embody *yielding*. Claudia's ability to relax and trust seemed to extend beyond her enjoyment of the pose and into relationships. This ability was mirrored in her ability to trust and receive support from Michelle.

Claudia also said she liked Sphinx. Sphinx is an interesting pose that combines two seemingly opposing actions: the tamasic, restful stance of *yielding* to the floor with the rajasic, active movement of *pushing* the arms against the floor. In this way, Sphinx Pose is a supported push—it has qualities of tamas (the lower body is relaxed and supported by the floor) and rajas (actively pushing with the upper body, especially the arms).

In contrast, Claudia said she didn't like Table Pose because it felt "too exposed." Sphinx and Table Pose share the action of push but differ in the placement of the belly—in Sphinx the belly is on the ground, whereas in Table Pose the belly is suspended in the air. Claudia used the word "protected" to describe how she felt in Sphinx. In Table Pose Claudia said she felt "exposed." This indicated to Michelle that Claudia would benefit from yoga poses that replicated the supported push action of Sphinx. Sphinx also allows spinal extension that seemed enjoyable for Claudia.

Claudia said she also didn't like the cross crawl at all. The cross-crawl movements relate to the fundamental movements of *grasping* and *pulling*. Both grasping and pulling are rajasic (active, energetic) movements, and this pose requires a lot of core strength. Michelle noticed that when Claudia was doing it, she wobbled a lot due to a lack of core strength and stability—not surprising for a 14-year-old who reports limited physical activity.

Physical therapist Kelly Dean says that weak abdominal muscles can be caused by emotional and physical disconnection, which in turn are caused by trauma (2023). While there is not hard scientific evidence to back this claim, Michelle had observed this pattern in past clients. To test out this theory, Michelle offered Claudia practices that tied her preferred movements of yielding on the floor (Lying on Belly) and supported push (Sphinx) with yoga tools that could increase awareness and strength in her core (belly breathing and Locust Pose A and B), which can be seen in Figures 9.3–9.6. Of note, Sphinx Pose is considered a modification of Locust Pose B in the Ashtanga system of yoga (Swenson, 1999, p. 137).

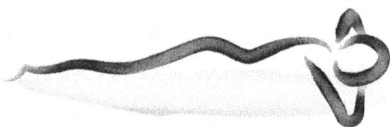

**Figure 9.3** Lying on Belly with Hands Under Head
*Depicts lying on the floor face-down with hands below forehead to support the neck as a form of yield.*

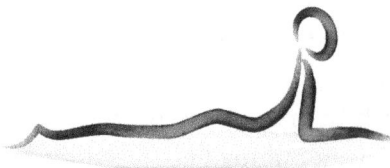

**Figure 9.4** Sphinx—Salabhasana Prep
*Depicts Sphinx Pose, which encourages a supported form of pushing into the floor.*

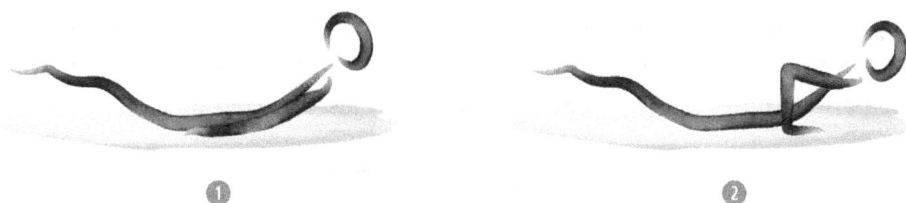

**Figure 9.5** Locust A and B—Salabhasana A and B

*Depicts Locust Poses A and B. Locust A helped Claudia explore a backward reach while Locust B helped her explore push, while respecting her preference to have her belly supported by the ground.*

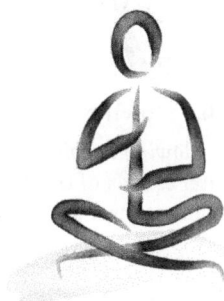

**Figure 9.6** Belly Breathing

*Depicts hands resting on the belly and chest to feel the movement of the breath. For those like Claudia who lack interoceptive awareness, belly breathing can be very helpful to increase this internal awareness.*

Michelle also wanted to continue offering Claudia yoga tools that didn't seem like yoga tools. So, during one session, Michelle invited Claudia to grab one of the colorful bubble wands she kept in a basket and go outside with her. Blowing bubbles engages the core muscles (Figure 9.7). Claudia enthusiastically grabbed the purple wand and followed Michelle outside. Once standing in the late summer sunlight, Michelle invited Claudia to join her in a patch of grass and take off her shoes. The two walked around a small patch of grass blowing bubbles and chatting. Walking is a form of the fundamental movement *push* through the legs that simultaneously stimulates the bowels (Figure 9.8).

In the year since Claudia started therapy, she has made significant progress. She is not only more aware of her body sensations; she can also use them to help regulate her emotions in several contexts. Her panic attacks have decreased to an all-time low of about twice a month. And she is also making healthy boundaries with her father when he wants to share too much. There is still a lot of work to do—she is not yet ready to fully examine the impact that intergenerational trauma has had on her family and her. She may not be for years. But she has come a long way. She even says she likes yoga and teaches it to her friends when they are stressed out!

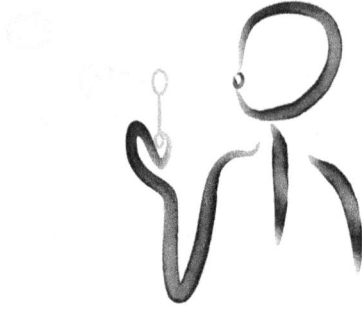

**Figure 9.7** Blowing Bubbles

*Depicts someone blowing bubbles. Blowing bubbles is a great practice for all ages. For children it teaches them greater control of their breath. For adolescents and adults, it does the same and reminds them of the playfulness of childhood.*

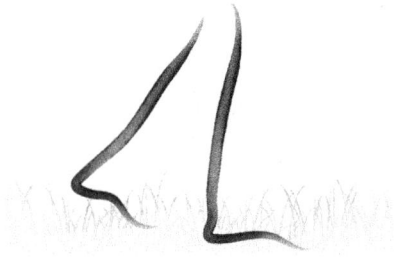

**Figure 9.8** Walking in Grass

*Depicts walking in the grass. This is a great practice for clients of all ages—it brings awareness to the present moment through the sensation of grass on the soles of one's feet. It also helps clients slow down, and is a wonderful first step toward walking meditation.*

## Specific Considerations for Adolescents
### Musculoskeletal: Importance of Regular Reassessment

Adolescence is a time of incredible change and growth—a client at age 13 will have significantly different needs than at age 18. Thus, it is important to do a range of motion assessment regularly. For instance, Michelle showed Claudia a yoga vinyasa that mimicked the fundamental movements sequence about six months into treatment. In that time, Claudia had grown a bit taller. The yoga sequence doubled as both an assessment of her movement patterns, as well as assessment of her current strength, flexibility, and endurance.

In addition, adolescent bodies are still growing even if they appear fully grown. They should not hold individual poses for as long as adults. When in doubt, a good rule of thumb is to hold poses no longer than 10 counts, and/or about half of what you would instruct an adult. Be sure to offer pose modifications for poses, especially those that require flexibility. This is because bones grow faster than muscle, and so both adolescents and children will experience more inflexibility when going through growth spurts.

Finally, adolescents are self-conscious about their developing bodies. In a group yoga therapy setting, be sure to arrange mats and carefully plan poses in such a way that clients won't feel uncomfortable. For instance, when doing Standing Wide-Legged Forward Bend Pose (prasarita padottanasana) ensure that mats are staggered, so no client feels like a peer is staring at their backside!

## Social/Emotional

Relating with adolescents in a developmentally appropriate way is vital to forming a trusting, effective rapport with them. Michelle did this with Claudia in a few ways: 1) Michelle respected Claudia's request not to do formal yoga asana, and instead offered her other yoga tools that met her therapeutic needs; 2) Michelle used plain-spoken language, absent of jargon and with a minimum of Sanskrit terms; and 3) Michelle used technology in a way that Claudia could relate with when she suggested a mood tracker phone app.

It is also important to educate both adolescents and their families about the detriment that too much screen time and social media can have on their sleep and mental health. Tell them about the US Surgeon General's recommendation of spending less than three hours a day on social media (US Department of Health and Human Services, 2023). Emphasize the importance of good sleep hygiene and help them navigate their social media use.

## Cognitive and Neurobiological

The YP can support adolescent clients' cognitive and neurobiological development in yoga therapy sessions in several ways. As mentioned above, using language that is developmentally appropriate is important. In addition, having a variety of fidget toys and art supplies available helps clients with attention issues. Michelle tries to find fidget toys and supplies that are colorful and pleasing to the eye. Using visual aids in general (such as a dry erase board and handouts) can also help adolescent clients absorb concepts discussed during sessions.

## Caregiver Engagement and Provider Collaboration

Adolescents are in a challenging transitional period of development where they are becoming more and more independent from family and caregivers but are not yet adults. While every adolescent's needs are unique, a good general rule is to include the guardian(s)/parent(s) in the initial intake. During that initial session, the YP can ask the adolescent and family members present how often caregivers should be involved in treatment. And while caregivers may be involved in developing initial goals, most adolescents will want the independence to choose their treatment objectives with the support of the YP (and without the guardian/parent).

The younger the adolescent, the more likely the YP is to want/need a release of information to speak to other providers, such as a school counselor, a favorite teacher, a psychiatrist, and possibly an occupational or physical therapist. See Chapter 11 for more information.

## Self-Care Practice: Your Inner Adolescent

Working with adolescents who have CPTSD, or have acute symptoms like Claudia's, is as taxing as it is rewarding. In this moment just after you've finished reading about her case, notice your body sensations, your state of mind, your mood. Have you "picked up" any of the tension, panic, or sadness that Claudia expressed?

First, we invite you to wash it off—literally. You may want to go to the bathroom sink and splash some cold water on your face. Or maybe drinking a cold glass of water would help.

Next, take a moment to get in touch with what *you* were like as an adolescent. Were you feisty and rebellious? Or did you follow all the rules? Did you enjoy laughing fits with friends? Perhaps you were a parentified child, like Claudia. Whatever your experience, pick a moment in your adolescent experience when you felt hope, excitement, possibility, and/or accomplishment. Recall a moment when you felt awe. It could be an intimate, quiet moment when you felt seen and understood by a friend, date partner, or teacher. Or maybe it was a pinnacle moment when you nailed that solo performance in a choir concert, got asked to the prom, or won an award. Whatever it is, close your eyes and really picture it. And then *feel* it. Feel that moment in the cells of your body.

Now notice what the body wants to do. Do your arms want to reach up?

Do you want to collapse with joy into a feather bed? Do you want to do a happy dance?

Go ahead, do it! Act out that movement with everything you've got. And then ask yourself, which fundamental movement or movements are you enacting? This is your adolescent self coming to life through the cells of your body and your actions. Enjoy the feeling of reconnecting with that part of yourself. And the next time you see an adolescent—whether it's a client, a relative, or a friend's child—recall that you know something about the hope, trepidation, excitement, confusion, and experience they may be going through.

## Chapter Summary

- Adolescents often struggle with emotion regulation, and research suggests that yoga helps them increase emotion regulation.

- Several internal and external changes impact adolescents' difficulty with emotion regulation. Internally, adolescents' judgment and emotion regulation are impaired by significant brain changes. Externally, adolescents depend less on family, more on friends, and take on new challenges and responsibilities in life.

- Adolescents' impaired judgment and decreased emotion regulation put them at risk for a host of mental health issues, including complex trauma.

- Our case study Claudia typifies a lot of adolescents, who lack interoceptive awareness, which leads to confusion and overwhelm and results in dysfunctional behaviors like cutting, addiction, or other risky behaviors.

- Sleep plays an essential role in emotion regulation for clients of all ages, but especially for youth.

- *Parentification* is when a child takes on the role of parenting their parent by offering developmentally inappropriate emotional support or other adult responsibilities. Adolescent clients who are becoming more vocal about their desires for independence may be more likely to share details of family life that indicate parentification.

- From a musculoskeletal point of view, adolescence is a time of rapid change and growth. Thus, it is important to reassess adolescent clients' range of motion regularly.

- Relating with adolescents in a developmentally appropriate way is vital to forming a trusting, effective rapport with them.

- It is important to educate both adolescents and their families about the detriment that too much screen time and social media can have on their sleep and mental health.

# CPTSD-Informed Yoga Therapy for Adults

## Evidence and Rationale of YTCT for Adults

Studies on the effectiveness of yoga therapy for adult CPTSD survivors are still scant. Using the keywords "yoga therapy for complex trauma adults" (August 5, 2024) yielded five results. Several other results were offered with terms such as "therapeutic yoga," "trauma," and "adult survivors of childhood abuse."

Yet the extant research appears to promote body-based strategies for adults. Emmons et al. (2021) point out that "Complex trauma creates cognitive and physical disruptions in the body that significantly impact quality of life (QOL) that... may not respond well to mainstream PTSD treatments" (p. 266). Ong (2020) says the elements that make yoga therapy uniquely suited for complex trauma treatment include intentionally "developing self-awareness, self-regulation, and a benevolent relationship with their bodies" (p. 182).

## Case Study: Justin

Justin was a 33-year-old African American engineer originally from Texas. He moved to Colorado to be closer to the mountains and the outdoor lifestyle that Colorado is known for.

## Telehealth/Virtual Sessions

Clients of any age may request virtual sessions for a variety of reasons. Justin requested virtual appointments, due to his busy work schedule. Virtual sessions (or telehealth) make yoga therapy more accessible and convenient for many clients. For some, it may be the only way they can attend. Be sure to check your country/region's laws regarding telehealth. In addition, if you the YP have a license or other designated certification, you may also need to ensure that you abide by your governing body's rules and guidelines. For instance, in the US, licenses are regulated at the state level. This means that as a licensed professional counselor, Michelle can only see clients virtually when both they and she are within state borders.

Here are some other essential guidelines for virtual sessions/telehealth to communicate with your client:

- Ensure both your client and you have access to a private space where neither of you will be interrupted or overheard.

- Ensure that you both have ample space to roll out a yoga mat, or a towel, for practice.

- On the YP's end, ensure that you can adjust your computer camera so that the client can see your entire body as you move in yoga poses, and that the client can hear you well when you are on the yoga mat.

## Snapshot
### Presenting Problems

Justin reported a history of depression and anxiety (diagnosed in early adulthood by a psychiatrist). He reported problems with confidence, creating healthy boundaries with others, and speaking up for himself. One of Justin's goals was to "get out of my head and into my body." This statement demonstrated his desire to increase interoceptive awareness, which we've seen is a key component of CPTSD-informed yoga therapy.

Justin said he'd seen a talk therapist in the past. He also tried EMDR (eye movement desensitization and reprocessing therapy) and found it useful, so he wanted to continue with another somatic approach like yoga therapy. EMDR is often used to treat trauma symptoms (Cleveland Clinic, 2022). Justin understood this but wasn't convinced he had trauma. "I know other people who've had it a lot worse."

### Look-Feel-Sound

- **Look:** Justin is tall (he verifies later that he is 6'3"/190.5 cm) with an athletic build, and identifies as a gay man of color. For the intake, he is dressed casually in a light sage green shirt and cargo shorts. He presents slightly hunched over, as if trying to hide his height.

- **Feel:** Justin has a distant look in his eyes, which may be due to his depressive symptoms. Despite his blunted affect, he demonstrates a sharp intellect, and a desire to engage. He has a dry sense of humor that he delivers with a slight smirk on his face.

- **Sound:** Justin is soft-spoken and takes a lot of time to mull over questions. He has a slight stutter that shows up when it appears he's anxious or feels vulnerable.

## Assessment with PMK Overview
### Annamaya Kosha
As stated, Justin was a tall, African American man originally from Texas. Occasionally, he would speak with a slight twang—a remnant of his home. He identified as a gay man, and said he moved to Colorado to enjoy the outdoor life. He appeared athletic, and said he enjoyed running and CrossFit™, though he was feeling less motivated these days.

Justin reported a stable home life. He said he'd been living with two housemates in a beautiful old Victorian home that they rented in a historic Denver neighborhood since he moved to Colorado about a year and a half ago. He said they had monthly house meetings to ensure good communication. Despite this seeming stability, Justin reported a feeling of apprehension, wondering if tensions would build with his housemates.

### Pranamaya Kosha
Even on video, Justin appeared slightly hunched over resulting in a collapsed upper chest. His affect was flat and his energy low. He reported breathing problems, migraines, sleep issues, and lack of motivation. Justin's descriptions of how hard it was to motivate himself demonstrated his tamasic relationship to the fundamental movement of *push*. Since the six fundamental movements are so intertwined, Michelle now got a clearer sense that he also had a tamasic relationship with the fundamental movement of *yield*.

### Manomaya Kosha
As we have discussed, manomaya kosha is the sheath of mental/emotional awareness. In Justin's PMK Overview, his manomaya kosha issues showed up clearly in his body and energy level: because of his depressive symptoms (manomaya kosha issues) he found it hard to go to his CrossFit workouts. His hunched shoulders (annamaya kosha) most likely impacted his breathing

(pranamaya kosha) to further exacerbate his low mood (manomaya kosha). He said he'd yo-yo'ed between antidepressants and anti-anxiety medications for most of his life and found it hard to strike a balance of even mood.

Manomaya kosha also houses the ego, or the *ahamkara* (Sullivan, 2020, p. 114). It contains our individual identity including race, age, sexual/gender identity, identification with our job or career, and our unique attributes like intelligence, creativity, confidence, and the like. From this lens, Justin exhibited a sharp intellect and quick wit. Because his company was based overseas, he worked from home for a start-up that made massive batteries for solar and energy companies. His dream was eventually to work more directly on climate change issues. In his current job, he traveled domestically and internationally regularly to conferences and work meetings. Despite his tamasic tendencies in the annamaya and pranamaya koshas, he exhibited more rajasic tendencies in this aspect of manomaya kosha.

And yet Justin struggled with confidence, and speaking up for himself. He recounted an instance recently when he took his partner's dog for a run, and received a reprimand from a woman who suggested this was bad for the dog. He said he was so taken aback he said nothing but then later had a lot of negative thoughts about what he wished he'd said to the woman. He said he felt very guilty about his "mean thoughts."

Justin realized he was gay as an adolescent when he didn't want to "get physical" with his girlfriend at the time. While this realization gave him the freedom to explore his sexuality and express an important part of his identity, it also posed a challenge: he felt the need to distance himself from his family, who held heteronormative values on sexual identity. As Kempton (2020) points out, manomaya kosha "holds the voices of our personal and cultural programming, the powerful, mental structures formed by the beliefs, opinions and assumptions that we've brought in from our family and our culture" ("Manomaya kosha" section, para. 2). Let's consider the impact of Justin's coming out to his family in vijnanamaya kosha, where we examine personal relationships.

## Vijnanamaya Kosha
Vijnanamaya kosha is one's wisdom and insight that sees beyond the individual perceptions of manomaya kosha (Chapter 6). In general, Justin showed a lot of strengths with regards to his intuition: he'd trusted his gut to embrace his sexuality, moved to Colorado, and chosen his housemates.

But Justin still had to contend with what it meant to be a gay man in his family. He said he first came out to them when he was about 21 years old, and at the time he thought they'd been accepting. He said his brother was, and continued to be, the most supportive, asking him questions and showing interest in his dating life. Yet his parents ignored the topic after their initial conversation as if it had never occurred.

As a Black man, Justin said his family was extremely important to him. "Since society doesn't have our backs, we need to have each other's." But when it came to his sexual identity, he felt like he was on his own. This was so painful for him, so he decided to move to Colorado. "I still talk to my family every week; I just can't live too close to them."

Right before moving to Denver, Justin decided to come out to his paternal grandparents, who were fairly accepting. In some ways, this didn't surprise him. He said his grandparents had been more like parents, because his mother suffered from schizophrenia. Though she could keep an outer appearance of normalcy in her work life, his brother and he had witnessed her mental breakdowns and hospitalizations throughout their childhoods.

"Sometimes she was a loving mother, and sometimes she was completely out to lunch. And sometimes she ranted that Jesus Christ our Lord was speaking to her through the toaster." He said his father had to work many odd jobs to support the family, so sometimes they didn't see him for days. As a result, Justin and his brother spent a lot of their childhoods staying with their grandparents, who lived close by.

All the adverse childhood experiences that Justin endured added up to complex trauma: being a Black man in the US experiencing systemic racism throughout his life, having a mother with acute mental health issues, and being gay in a family who ignored his sexual identity. Luckily, Justin exhibited several protective factors in his vijnanamaya kosha, including his intelligence, his resourcefulness in moving to a place (Colorado) that lifted his mood, and several supportive relationships (his housemates, dog, brother, and grandparents).

Despite these strengths, Justin said he felt like he didn't connect with others in the deep, authentic way he wanted to. He'd been dating his partner Bryce for about a year but felt a deep sense of insecurity about it. "I have this anxiety that I'm not good enough or not wanted." He said he couldn't tell if Bryce was as serious about the relationship as he was. This caused Justin anxiety, and he'd distance himself from Bryce, who would then feel hurt.

Despite these relational challenges, Justin seemed to find secure attachment with Bryce's dog, Clover, whom he'd take for runs when he had the energy.

### Anandamaya Kosha

In addition to not being able to connect to others the way he wanted to, Justin also said he rarely felt a sense of awe or joy. He described a layer of numbness surrounding him like bubble wrap, making it impossible to directly connect with other people or his own feelings of joy. His desperate desire to find satisfaction in relationships and life represented a rajasic association to the fundamental movement of *reach*. And the numbness that surrounded him when he did try to connect seemed to be an expression of his tamasic relationship to the fundamental movements of *grasp* and *pull*. He could reach, but he couldn't connect.

## Treatment Planning and Course of Treatment

Justin came to yoga therapy knowing he'd faced a lot of adversity in childhood and throughout his life, even though he did not describe his experience of it as traumatic. This awareness, and his fully developed nervous system as an adult, meant that treatment occurred more fluidly. He was able to process little bits of trauma (the second phase of CPTSD-informed treatment) within the first few months of starting therapy. While this happened in small moments at first, Justin was able to move into Phase 2 of treatment through his third goal of connecting with himself and with others more fully.

Bear in mind that this is not the case for all adult clients with CPTSD. Michelle has seen child and adolescent clients who were out of their traumatic situations and able to process some of their traumas. She has seen adult clients who needed years of therapy before they were able to move to Phase 2. And she has seen clients who stayed in Phase 1 for the duration of their treatment, which felt safe and nurturing for their situation. Every client is unique.

### Target Kosha

By doing the PMK Overview, Michelle could see that Justin's case was complex. As Table 10.1 shows, Michelle used the PMK Overview worksheet (Appendix 7) to get more clarity. Having a visual table with the koshas and fundamental movements helped her think about how the gunas interacted with the fundamental movements at each level of the koshas. This helped

Michelle build a summary to present to Justin so they could figure out his target kosha(s) and goals (his treatment plan) together.

**Table 10.1** depicts the PMK Overview for Justin, an adult.

| Annamaya Kosha (Stability) | In annamaya kosha, Justin shows a tamasic relationship with *yield* and *push* as evidenced by his hunched shoulders, flat affect, and sleep issues. |
|---|---|
| | He shows more of a sattvic relationship to *reach, grasp*, and *pull* given his stable, peaceful home life. |
| Pranamaya Kosha (Vitality) | In pranamaya kosha, Justin also shows a tamasic relationship with *yield* and *push* as evidenced above and through his lack of motivation and possible breathing problems. |
| Manomaya Kosha (Clarity) | On the one hand, Justin exhibits sattvic/rajasic tendencies with *push* as evidenced by his ability to embrace his identity as a gay man and engage in a meaningful career. |
| | However, he has symptoms (and diagnoses) of depression and anxiety, showing that his mood fluctuates from tamasic to rajasic. |
| Vijnanamaya Kosha (Wisdom/ Intuition) | Justin shows sattvic tendencies in vijnanamaya kosha with his ability to follow his intuition by moving to Colorado. |
| | With regards to relationships, Justin shows a rajasic tendency to *reach* out of a desire to connect. But he has tamasic tendencies with regards to *grasp/pull* because the connections don't satisfy him. |
| Anandamaya Kosha (Joy/Awe) | In the anandamaya kosha, Justin feels a lack of joy/awe, which is very frustrating for him. Again, his deep desire to connect to meaning represents a rajasic tendency to *reach* for joy/awe. But his inability to truly feel joy/awe represents a tamasic relationship to *grasp/pull*. |

Justin had clearly stated his presenting problem as wanting to "get out of my head and into my body." Michelle reminded him of this when she summarized her findings from the PMK Overview for him. Together they came up with three goals concentrating on four koshas. His first treatment goal was to increase body awareness (target kosha: annamaya). Within this goal, Michelle told Justin they'd work on his collapsed upper body which seems to be impacting his breathing, so there was some focus on pranamaya kosha as well. His second goal was to increase his confidence (manomaya kosha).

As we will see, Justin's third goal would come several months into treatment when Justin had successfully completed goals 1 and 2, and was ready to enter Phase 2 of CPTSD treatment, meaning he was ready to process some of his trauma. His third goal was to increase connection with others, and with his life (targeting both vijnanamaya and anandamaya koshas).

**Goal 1: Justin will increase his body awareness.**

Justin's tendency to be in his head (and lack body awareness) was no mistake—it was an adaptation developed at a very young age to a lack of safety and stability. To let go of this adaptation was to become aware of the very body sensations and internal cues Justin needed to avoid as a child.

As YPs, it is crucial to keep this in mind: Lack of interoceptive awareness is usually an adaptation from an earlier stage in the client's life. We must tread carefully when asking a client to let go of what was once a very useful skill. The prerequisite for a client to let go and allow themselves to feel their body sensations is safety and stability within the therapeutic relationship. As such, it can take some time for a client to develop that safety with the YP.

For Justin, this process took place over the course of several months. Sometimes he felt resourced enough to feel his internal body cues. At other times, he preferred to focus on the minutiae of a yoga technique or a problem with a co-worker (since Michelle was also his talk therapist) rather than his internal sensations. Having the freedom to move at his own pace was vital to the safety of the therapeutic rapport and his feelings of agency over his healing process.

**Objective 1a: Justin will learn and practice yoga tools that increase body awareness.**

Unlike Teresa (Chapters 2 and 3) and Claudia (Chapters 7 and 9), Justin seemed to have more of a tamasic relationship with the fundamental movement of *yield*, as evidenced by his collapsed upper body, breathing difficulties, general fatigue, and flat affect. But like Claudia, he lacked interoceptive awareness.

Due to his collapsed upper body, Michelle offered Justin some shoulder and neck release postures, such as shoulder rolls and yoga master Doug Keller's Forward Head Adjustment (Keller, 2021, p. 326), which is covered in detail in the next section. She also sent him an audio recording of Yoga Nidra to help with his sleep. After experimenting with these strategies, Justin became more aware of body sensations with two sets of vinyasas that were eventually tied together: first, through a grounding vinyasa that he said helped him feel his connection to gravity, and then through a gentle arm vinyasa with the breath that helped increase his awareness in his head, neck, shoulders, and spine.

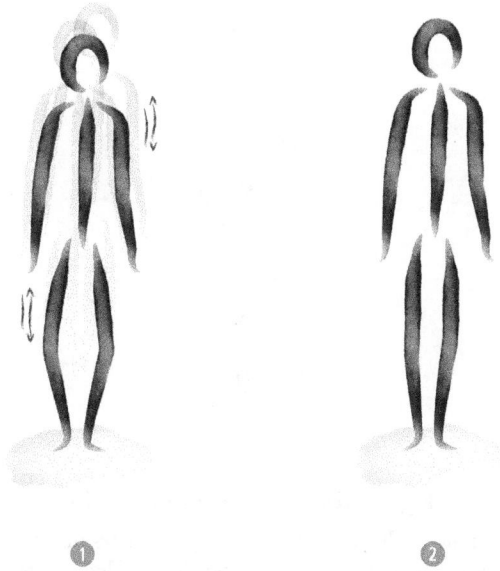

**Figure 10.1** Tadasana Shakes

*Depicts Tadasana Shakes: 1) stand in Mountain Pose and gently shake the body up and down, then 2) stand in Mountain Pose and notice the effect in your feet.*

1. Standing in Mountain Pose (tadasana), gently shake the body up and down, noticing the body's connection to the floor and gravity. Imagine patting the side of a sugar bowl to gently tap the sugar down to the bottom of the bowl.

2. Now stand still in Mountain Pose. Can you feel the connection with gravity more?

The purpose of this sequence was to help Justin feel his connection to gravity—he was pushing into the earth with his feet and legs, and this led to him feeling connection to it. He reported afterward that his feet felt heavy, and that he liked the sensation. In this way, Tadasana Shakes is a great sequence for clients who have a tamasic, collapsed relationship with the fundamental movements of both *yield* and *push*.

## Arm Vinyasa

This next Arm Vinyasa can be done sitting or standing. Because Justin was working on his connection to gravity, he decided to stay standing throughout the sequence, which helped him actively stay connected to the ground.

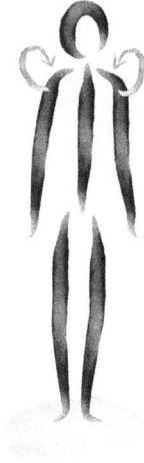

**Figure 10.2** Yogic Shoulder Rolls

*Depicts Yogic Shoulder Rolls: inhale and shrug shoulders up toward the ears, and then exhale the shoulders back down, sliding the shoulder blades down the back.*

1. Inhale, and shrug the shoulders up toward the ears.

2. Exhale, and roll them back and then down.

3. Repeat this breath vinyasa 3–5 times.

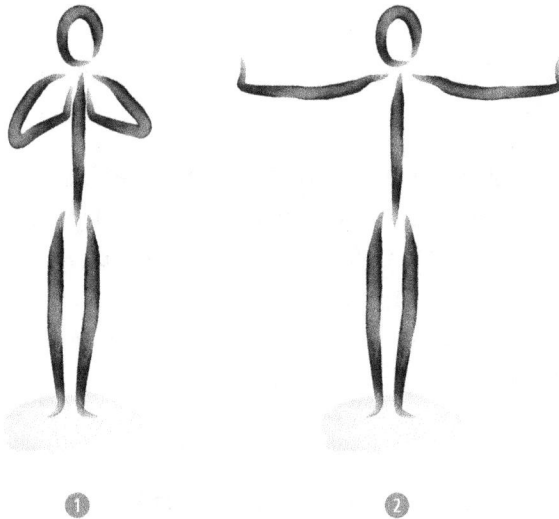

**Figure 10.3** Arm Extensions

*Depicts Arm Extensions: press hands together in Namaste. Inhale, and extend arms out to the side, pressing through the heels of the hands. Exhale, and bring hands back together.*

4. Press hands together in Namaste, and roll the shoulders back.

5. Inhale, and extend arms out to the sides pressing the heels of the hands away; feel the connection between the heel of the hand pressing out, and the shoulder rolling back.

6. Exhale, and bring the hands back to Namaste over the heart; as the hands come back together like magnets, feel the centerline of the body, the spine.

7. Repeat 3–5 times.

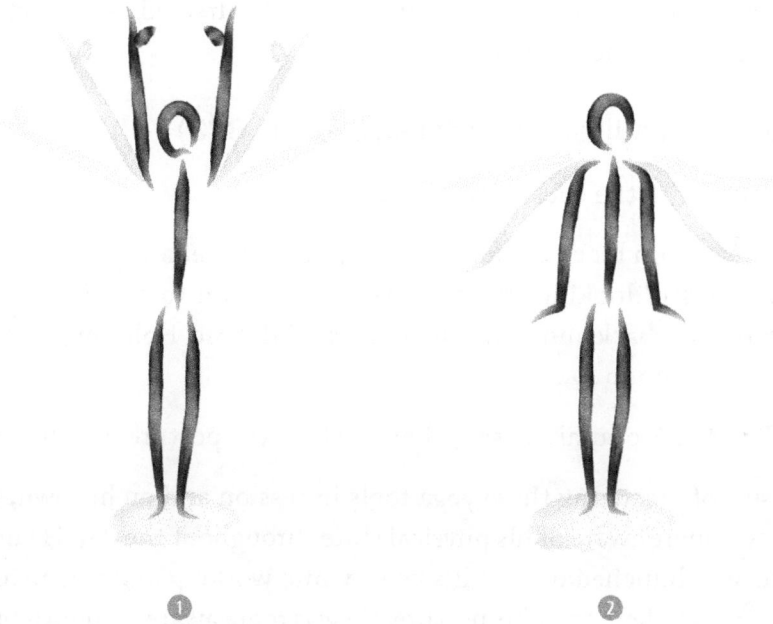

**Figure 10.4** Sweeping Arms

*Depicts Sweeping Arms: standing or seated, inhale and sweep arms up to the sky. Exhale, and sweep them back down to the sides of the body or lap.*

8. Inhale, and sweep arms overhead.

9. Exhale, and press hands down as if through thick water; feel the connection between the palms pressing down and the rhomboids (the muscles that pull the shoulder blades down the back).

The purpose of this vinyasa was to increase Justin's awareness of his head, neck, shoulders, and spine. When a client presents with a slumped posture as Justin did, they usually have little awareness of how they are holding their bodies. This exercise not only helps increase awareness but also improves posture.

***Objective 1b*: Justin will improve his posture to increase breathing capacity.**

To help Justin continue increasing his interoceptive awareness and improving his posture, Michelle taught Justin a technique from yoga master Doug Keller's book *The Therapeutic Wisdom of Yoga, Volume Two: Applications*. Keller (2021) explains that slumped posture is often caused by a "forward head" (p. 326), which causes neck flexion. The forward head posture can also cause symptoms like mouth breathing and sleep apnea, both of which Justin suffered from. Sitting at a desk, staring at a computer all day, were likely culprits for Justin's postural stress. Yet Keller also notes that, "More than any other foundation in the body, this one is acutely affected by the activities and tendencies of the mind" (2021, p. 323).

## Forward Head Adjustment (Keller, 2021, p. 323)

1. Stand with the back to the wall.

2. Place a yoga block behind the head, step the feet away from the wall. While still looking straight ahead, chin level to the floor, roll the shoulders back and down in Standing Fish Pose. Hold for 3–5 counts, working up to 10 counts.

3. Stand in Mountain Pose and notice how the posture has changed.

As a result of practicing these yoga tools in session and on his own, Justin said he was more aware of his physical state throughout the day. He noticed when he was hunched over in his chair while working and was using the shoulder rolls to help reset his posture. He was more aware of mouth breathing and adjusted that too. "I can't tell for sure, but I think I might have a little more energy." These were very encouraging signs. Justin's newfound body awareness also increased his sense of security in his physical body. From the perspective of the fundamental movements, he increased his sattvic relationship to *yield*—he felt safe enough to relax and pay attention to his body sensations. Much later, he also reported that the frequency of his migraines decreased from almost weekly to twice a month.

***Goal 2*: Justin will increase his confidence.**

Justin's second goal was to increase his confidence, a manomaya issue. He'd taken a few weeks to familiarize himself with the above yoga tools and practices before officially starting goal #2. And yet he reported that he was already feeling more confident. He said he noticed he trusted his judgment a little more and felt like he was making better boundaries with friends and housemates. Because yoga therapy is holistic, when Justin worked on his first goal that targeted annamaya and pranamaya koshas, his manomaya issues also improved.

**Objective 2a: Justin will learn and practice good boundaries.**

To increase his confidence more directly, Michelle suggested Justin learn to make better boundaries with others. In the intake, he'd reported that he didn't speak up for himself enough, which left him feeling resentful. Sometimes this resentment boiled over into anger when he'd allowed his boundaries to be crossed one too many times.

Michelle explained to Justin that from the fundamental movements perspective, blurry boundaries demonstrate a tamasic relationship with *push*. The remedy was to use rajasic yoga tools and strategies to increase his ability to push. To this end, Michelle taught Justin Lion's Breath (Chapter 5). Lion's Breath helps relax and strengthen the vocal muscles, and this was one of the most effective yoga tools for increasing his overall confidence.

Justin said Lion's Breath gave him the confidence to practice one of the psychotherapy tools Michelle also taught him: saying no to others, a common psychotherapy practice for clients who have a hard time speaking up for themselves. Justin said that learning and practicing Lion's Breath gave him the confidence to brave saying no to others, and he was amazed to find out he wasn't rejected the way he thought he would be. He also said he gained even more confidence.

**Goal 3: Justin will increase connection with others, and with his life.**

Justin struggled to feel connected to others (a vijnanamaya kosha issue), and rarely felt a sense of joy (an anandamaya kosha issue). For such a client, simply being in the therapy session can be intense and overwhelming. They may feel awkward not knowing how to connect, then feel easily rejected or criticized if they feel like they're doing the wrong thing.

Knowing this was probably the case for Justin, Michelle used something Pat Ogden calls "tracking statements" in the webinar series *Mastering the Treatment of Trauma* (Buczynski, 2023, p. 9)—simple observations that show the client that they are seen. For instance, when Justin was first learning the arm vinyasa, Michelle noted, "I noticed your shoulders relax after the arm sweeps!" Another time after a deep breathing practice, he seemed distant. Michelle gently said, "Hey, I noticed you got kind of quiet after that practice. It's okay if it brings things up. That's natural."

In both cases, Justin's response indicated that he felt seen. In the first case, he proudly rolled his shoulders back and smiled. In the second case, he looked Michelle in the eye and said quietly, "Yeah, I felt sad during that breathing practice. Feeling sad wasn't allowed when I was little."

Michelle suspected that Justin's inability to connect with others and his life had to do with the neglect he must have experienced because of his mother's acute mental illness. As we have seen in Chapter 5, neglect can cause a child not to *reach/grasp/pull*. Ruella Frank (2013) says that when a baby reaches for something, grasping soon appears. But if the baby (Justin, in this case) reaches, and the mother doesn't reach back enough, the baby stops trying. And that causes him not to fully learn the fundamental movements of *grasp/pull*.

About six months into yoga therapy sessions, Justin showed an increased readiness to move into Phase 2 of CPTSD treatment—processing trauma. Processing trauma means becoming aware of and talking about the body sensations linked to a trauma. While he'd done so in little moments throughout the previous six months, Justin demonstrated his readiness to more fully process a specific trauma by sharing the following memory. (As a reminder, processing trauma with a client requires a trauma therapist who is qualified to provide trauma-focused care—something that is beyond the scope of this book. However, as we will see, yoga therapy can be an invaluable addition to treatment at this stage.)

"I remember being a child, and hearing my mom outside my door, passing by my room," he recalled during a session one day. "It's not like it's one memory—it's like my whole childhood. She'd go right by my door. I wanted her so desperately to come in my room and check on me, say 'hi,' give me a hug. But she never did. She just kept going."

Justin's words demonstrate how devastating the silent trauma of neglect is. Psychiatrist and trauma researcher Dr. Ruth Lanius speaks to the physical signs of a client who has experienced the trauma of neglect: "They're shut down. They're slowed. Their movements are slowed. Often, their heart-rate is low, and they're completely disconnected from their inside world. They're disconnected from the (outside) world" (Buczynski, 2023, p. 1).

It is important for YPs to understand these physical signs of a client's neglect, since it is often overlooked and misunderstood. If you see this kind of physical presentation in a client who reports childhood experiences that sound like neglect, and primary trauma treatment is beyond your scope of practice, recommend that they see a therapist in conjunction with their yoga therapy treatment.

**Objective 3a: Justin will maintain interoceptive awareness while interacting with others.**

With his first two yoga therapy goals Justin learned to connect with what Lanius referred to as his "inside world" by increasing interoceptive awareness. But Michelle noticed that when he talked about wanting to connect with others, he'd say things like, "I need to put my feelings aside" or "I want to suppress my own stuff so I can be there for [so-and-so]." She realized that Justin was abandoning himself to try and relate with his partner, and in so doing, he could not connect. Now the objective would be to help him learn to stay rooted in his "inside world" while also learning to *reach/grasp/pull* his "outside world" toward him through a variety of new yoga tools. Like a lightbulb switching on in her head, Michelle realized that some of her basic yoga teacher training might help Justin do just that.

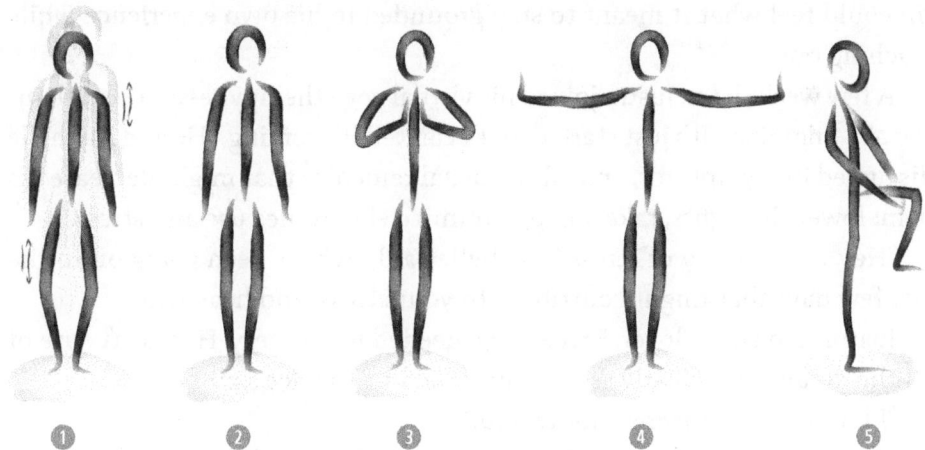

**Figure 10.5** Justin's Fundamental Movements Vinyasa
*Depicts a standing fundamental movements sequence tailored for Justin, a client who benefited from standing to feel his connection to gravity.*

Michelle suggested a vinyasa of three standing asanas to Justin that integrated the fundamental movements: Tadasana Shakes (a *yield* action), then Arm Extensions (a *push* action), and lastly a standing balance (Extended Hand-to-Big-Toe Pose), in which he *reached/grasped/pulled* his leg toward him. Along with the physical movements, Michelle cued Justin to imagine the following: as Justin shook in Tadasana Shakes, he thought of standing in his grandparent's house, feeling supported, nurtured, and cared for. Before starting Arm Extensions, he was asked to think of someone or something he wanted to distance himself from. He named a group of friends who made him feel not good enough. And then before he practiced Extended Hand-to-Big-Toe Pose, he was asked to think of someone or something he wanted to bring closer to him. He named his partner, Bryce.

The main purpose of this vinyasa was to help Justin stay connected to *yielding* while also *reaching/grasping/pulling*: that is, to learn the balancing act of staying connected with his own experience (by feeling gravity's pull on his feet) while also reaching for someone he wanted to connect with. Michelle added the *push* action of Arm Extensions in the middle of these two to allow Justin the full experience of the first five fundamental movements.

As usual, Justin said he enjoyed the feeling of the "heaviness in my feet" from Tadasana Shakes. He said he felt a "sigh of relief" as he pushed in Arm Extensions. "I felt like doing those poses first made the last balancing pose more holistic or balanced." At least on a physical level, it appeared that Justin could feel what it meant to stay grounded in his own experience while reaching out.

A few weeks later, Justin joined his virtual yoga therapy session complaining of a migraine. "It's just started, but I can tell it's coming." He and Michelle discussed his symptoms, and all the usual remedies that might decrease his pain: lower the lights, take a nap, minimize electronics use and stress.

"Hey, so speaking of stress," Michelle said, "what's been going on in the last few days that might contribute to your stress, and headache?"

Justin said that Clover, Bryce's dog, needed leg surgery. He wasn't sure of all the details, but clearly seemed upset about the dog's ailment.

"I know Clover means a lot to you."

"Yeah. I guess we're not going on any runs for a while."

There was a pause. Justin's gaze was far off. Michelle stayed silent, knowing this was a big step for Justin to allow himself to feel sad about his partner's dog.

"I went over there yesterday. The vet prescribed a pain med for Clover. It was an injection, and Bryce sounded kinda freaked out about giving it to him. So I went over."

"Oh wow. How did it go?"

"Actually, I was impressed with Bryce. He took a deep breath and did it."

"How did it feel to be there?"

For the first time since the pause, Justin perked up and looked at Michelle. "Good, actually. I know that sounds weird."

"No. No, not at all," Michelle said. And then she took a risk, "Hey, Justin, how connected did you feel to Clover—and to Bryce—while you were there?"

"Yeah, you know, I felt connected to both of them," he said, nodding with a perplexed look on his face. He laughed. "Man, it would be nice if that could happen when it wasn't because of an imminent surgery!"

They both laughed.

"Yes, for sure," Michelle chuckled. "But, you know, feeling connected is feeling connected. It doesn't really matter how it happens."

"I can see that," Justin said, still nodding and now smiling wryly.

Justin's newfound ability to connect with Bryce and Clover was a combination of many things—his willingness, bravery, and his dedication to his therapy practices (which combined both yoga therapy and talk therapy with Michelle). It's impossible to know how much of each created the final result, and obviously more work was left to be done. But that session showed that Justin was well on his way to feeling that connection he so desperately wanted.

## Oases and Anchors

Luckily, Justin had had the protective factor of loving grandparents who often took care of him and his brother. They were Justin's anchors (Chapter 4) that gave him a feeling "of relief and well-being" (Rothschild, 2000, p. 93). The important impact of his grandparents' care could be seen in Justin's ability to create a home with housemates, care for his partner (and helping to care for his partner's dog), and seek help and sustain a therapeutic relationship with Michelle.

Some clients are not so lucky to have the loving grandparents Justin did. It's important to remember each client is unique, as is their journey of healing. The most important thing is to meet each client where they are at.

## Specific Considerations for Adults
### Musculoskeletal

While adult clients may not need reassessment of their range of motion (ROM) with the frequency a child or adolescent client would, an initial ROM assessment is essential. As a reminder, *Structural Yoga Therapy* (2012) by Mukunda Stiles is an excellent resource for ROM exercises and assessment.

In addition, there is ample evidence that trauma at any level can have long-term health consequences (McFarlane, 2010). As such, adult clients presenting with symptoms of CPTSD will often have somatic complaints and health issues. This is another way yoga therapy can be instrumental to clients with CPTSD: if you have expertise in yoga for health concerns like fibromyalgia, migraine, or other disorders that commonly occur with complex trauma, you can seamlessly integrate your expertise into clients' treatment plans. Lastly, asking a client about their other health issues and offering resources when you have them create a more trusting and nurturing rapport with clients.

### Social/Emotional

Because complex trauma often occurs during the critical developmental years of childhood and adolescence, many (if not most) clients' social and emotional well-being is impacted (Chapter 3). As we have seen throughout this book, how CPTSD impacts a given client is unique. Thus, a comprehensive assessment is vital to understanding a particular client's struggles with social/emotional issues, regardless of age.

### Cognitive/Neurobiological

Complex trauma also impacts each client's cognitive/neurobiological functioning in unique ways. Your initial intake interview, PMK Overview, and ROM assessment are critical to understanding your adult client's unique needs.

## Self-Care Practice: Noting Practice

Sometimes working with adult clients is "easier" than working with children, and sometimes it is much, much harder. For instance, you may identify with an adult client's problems, because they are more like your own. While this can be good up to a certain extent, we as YPs can fall into the trap of over-identifying with a client and their issues.

How do you know if you're doing this? If you find yourself ruminating over the client's issues, scripting out conversations and planning multiple yoga sequences for them, wondering about how they're doing... you are over-identifying with them.

The first step is to create space. We invite you to use the commute from your office or studio to home to help disengage. If you work from home, try disengaging by taking a walk. Notice all the sights, sounds, smells, and landmarks you pass, creating distance between you and your workday, including your clients' problems.

Once home, you can continue the practice. Find a comfortable spot to sit for 10–20 minutes. Kristin Neff describes a mindful way to create space in her book *Self-Compassion: The Proven Power of Being Kind to Yourself* (2011) called *noting practice* (available in MP3 format at www.self-compassion.org). First, take a few deep, even breaths. Perhaps close your eyes if it feels comfortable. Neff recommends noting when a particular thought, feeling, or sensation arises—in this case, over-identifying with a client. When you notice the thoughts, become aware of the correspondent feelings and sensations. Is some part of your body tensing? Your jaw? Chest? Stomach? "This provides [you] with the opportunity to respond wisely to [your] current circumstances" (Neff, 2011, p. 89).

Continue to note the thoughts, emotions, and feelings within you, as well as the outer sounds, smells, and sensations around you. Do you hear the whir of a refrigerator? The sound of people talking in another room? Can you smell that candle you just lit? Or dinner being made in the kitchen?

"Every time you become aware of a new experience, acknowledge the experience with a quiet mental note. Then allow your attention to settle on the next experience it is drawn to" (Neff, 2011, p. 90). You might get lost in thought, Neff says. But this isn't a problem—it is the mind's job to think. And especially if you do this practice after a long day of work, it is natural. You can simply acknowledge the distraction and come back to your noting practice. Neff points out that this practice allows "us to be more fully engaged in the present" (2011, p. 90). And by being present, you re-engage with your own life and circumstances and let go of your client's.

## Chapter Summary

- Adults come to yoga therapy often knowing they've faced adversity, even if they don't label it complex trauma.

- On the one hand, adult clients' fully developed nervous systems may mean that treatment (especially the phases of trauma treatment) occur more fluidly. In other words, an adult may show more readiness to move into trauma processing (Phase 2) than a child or adolescent. Make sure to refer clients to a primary trauma therapist if this is not within your scope of practice.

- On the other hand, adults are as unique as children and adolescents. Some adult clients will remain in Phase 1 of treatment for the duration of their time in yoga therapy.

- While the YP should collaborate with clients of all ages, it is especially important to integrate adult clients' presenting problems/complaints into the treatment plan using their words and terminology as much as possible.

# Part III

# SUPPORT SYSTEMS— YOUR CLIENTS' AND YOURS

## CHAPTER 11

# Clients' Support System— Family, Providers, and Teachers

Almost all clients have a support system they rely on. Whether it be a 6-year-old's parent and favorite teacher, a 16-year-old's foster mother and case worker, or a 36-year-old's psychiatrist, clients often have trusted others who can offer valuable insights into how a YP works with the individual. Even clients who socially isolate or feel disenfranchised usually have at least one family member or agency representative who keeps tabs on them.

The younger the client, the more likely it is that obtaining permission and being in contact with a legal guardian is a necessity. But regardless of a client's age, developing alliances with key members of a client's support network can greatly support the client in their journey of healing from complex trauma.

In this chapter, we highlight two broad categories of a client's support system: family (parent/guardian) and providers/teachers. The first section of the chapter is dedicated to a client's family, most especially their parent/guardian. The second section explores interactions with both providers and teachers. Discussion of a client's support system brings up important related topics of confidentiality, consent to treat, and the YP's legal obligations with regards to protecting clients' safety and well-being. These topics are interwoven throughout the chapter as they apply. We cover the general protocol and best practices for interactions with a client's support system.

Lastly, the following information applies to yoga therapy treatment, but not yoga classes. There are many situations in which a YP is asked to offer yoga (and not yoga therapy) to an individual or group of children, adolescents, or even adults. For instance, Ayala saw 7-year-old Iryna in a school setting as part of a group yoga class (Chapter 8). As this case study showed, yoga is a promising intervention for children who have experienced trauma because yoga helps increase self-regulation and internal awareness (Beltran et al., 2016).

With her CPTSD-informed yoga therapy skills, Ayala was able to help Iryna learn how to self-regulate by building interoceptive awareness through the group yoga sequences and tools. Having these skills allowed Ayala to provide a safe, nurturing environment appropriate for a child who might be suffering from complex trauma, as it appeared Iryna was. Nonetheless, the group Ayala facilitated was labeled a yoga class and not yoga therapy. Thus, she was not required to offer individualized assessment for Iryna. However, most after-school programs such as the yoga program Ayala delivered typically require that parents sign a registration/permission form. Ayala's form gathered important details about the child's allergies and sensitivities and disclosed that the yoga sessions involved physical activity.

When a YP's services are labeled yoga therapy, more rules apply regarding interactions with clients' care teams, and whether legal consent is required. Numerous factors dictate what rules apply: the country/region, the setting (a school, recreation center, clinic, hospital, or private practice setting, for example), one's scope of practice, and whether clients are seen individually or in a group. Given the plethora of factors, **be sure to learn and abide by your country and/or region's specific laws and regulations, especially if the client is a minor.**

The advice given in this chapter mostly applies to the outpatient and/or private practice setting, where the YP bears a lot of responsibility with regards to how they interact with family and team members. It is in these settings that the YP must: 1) ensure written consent to treat from either the client or the guardian before the first session; 2) include the parent/guardian in the intake process; and 3) obtain written permission from the client/guardian before consulting with other team members.

We also offer guidance on yoga offered in group and institution settings in the "Level of Engagement" and the "Providers and Teachers" sections. As Ayala's case study showed, institutions like schools or recreation centers are common places for YPs to offer their services. Regardless of whether the YP offers yoga classes or yoga therapy in these settings, it is still vital to know how to interact with a client's family or other team members.

## Family: Parents/Guardians

When working with an adult client, the YP may likely only hear about family in passing from a client and may not meet any family members throughout the course of yoga therapy treatment. The exception to this is if the adult client has a legal guardian. For example, adult clients with developmental disabilities or traumatic brain injuries that impact their cognitive functioning may require help in major decision-making, and as such, may be appointed a legal guardian (who may or may not be a family member). In this case, follow your country/region's legal protocols for any individual who has a guardian—that is to say, obtain written consent from the guardian before starting treatment, and throughout treatment as necessary.

Now let's focus on clients who are children or adolescents. Interactions with guardians and other key family members are not only legally required in the case of minors; their input and insight are often invaluable to effective treatment of youth clients.

## Minor Clients: Initial Contact and Consent to Treatment

Written consent from a guardian is required before treating a minor (Chapter 4). In most cases, a minor's guardian is their parent, who initiates the child's yoga therapy treatment, signs and/or co-signs all forms, and readily engages in the intake process. In some cases, a child's guardian may not be their parent and may instead be a different family member or friend. In rare cases, a child may be a ward of the state with a *guardian ad litem*, a court-appointed person who makes legal decisions regarding a child's welfare.

Two additional factors are essential to understand when treating minors. First, yoga therapy is a self-regulated profession in many countries, including the US and the UK (which both have accreditation bodies). The Minded Institute in the UK (one of the most comprehensive yoga therapy training programs in the world) advises its trainees that "further legal advice would need to be drawn from guidance provided to yoga teachers and other therapists such as counsellors," according to Amanda-Jayne Crompton, Quality and Standards Manager at Minded (personal communication, August 19, 2024). In the next section, we offer some online resources on confidentiality for YPs practicing in the US and UK.

The second important factor to consider when treating minors is this: the *age of majority* and *a client's age of consent to treatment* are not the same thing in some countries. For instance, in the United States and England the age of majority is 18 years old. Yet as of 2019 in the State of Colorado, the age of consent for outpatient psychotherapy services is 12 years old as per Colorado HB 19-1120 (Colorado General Assembly, 2019). What this means is that a child of 12 years old can consent to mental health treatment with or without a guardian's consent, even though they are still legally a minor. In the UK, the age of consent for treatment is 16 years old; however, the *Gillick Competence* rule states that "Children under the age of 16 can consent to their own treatment if they're believed to have enough intelligence, competence and understanding to fully appreciate what's involved in their treatment" (NHS, 2022a).

Of course, yoga therapy spans a whole range of professionals with specialties in oncology, physical therapy, occupational therapy, and mental/behavioral health, and many more. However, increasingly yoga and yoga therapy are recommended to youth with mental health issues in school, clinics, and mental health settings. It is feasible that if yoga therapy were included as an integral part of a child's complex trauma treatment, and was formally recommended by the treatment team, it could be construed as a service that a youth would be allowed to consent to without guardian consent.

## Confidentiality

The confidentiality of a client's personal information is vital, regardless of the client's age and regardless of what country the YP practices in. When it comes to adult clients, this is a straightforward matter: keep all personal information about a client (also called *personal health information,* or *PHI*) confidential and secured. *Confidential* means that you keep the client's information private. *Secured* means that you keep the client's file (or any written information), whether it be in hard copy or electronic form, in a secure, password protected location.

When working with minors, confidentiality is a little more complicated. The rule of thumb is that **all information a child or adolescent client shares with you is confidential EXCEPT matters of health and safety**. It's vital to share this fact with children and adolescents, as well as their guardian, during the intake. Doing so avoids rifts in trust, because you have clearly communicated the limits of confidentiality.

Let's consider an example to clarify this complex topic: on the one hand if a client shares sensitive information that is NOT a matter of health or safety, it is your ethical duty to keep your client's confidence. For instance, if a 12-year-old client tells you he is bisexual, you may not share this with his parents/legal guardians, since no health or safety risks exist.

On the other hand, if that same 12-year-old client shares that he is bisexual and has been self-harming to manage his anxiety about telling his parents, you must let the parents know about the self-harm behavior. The best approach in this situation is to ask the youth if he wants to tell his parents, or if he wants you to tell his parents. Clarify for him that his parents needn't know he is bisexual unless he's ready to share that. But sharing the self-harm information with the parents in your presence is nonnegotiable. You've offered two choices, and in both you are present to witness that the guardians are told. Giving limited choices ("Do you want to do [this or that]?") offers the youth a sense of choice and control.

One other exception to confidentiality exists: **If a client who is a minor shares that they—or another minor—is being subjected to abuse or neglect, *or* the YP witnesses the child being subjected to circumstances that would reasonably result in abuse or neglect, the YP is legally required to report this to local authorities and/or to the local child-abuse reporting hotline**. The purpose of this legal exception is, of course, to protect youth from abuse and neglect. In the US, each state has its own individual law to address this federally mandated protection. In the State of Colorado in the US, the law is called *mandatory reporting* (Colorado Department of Human Services, 2024). While laws vary from state to state in the US, learn more about mandatory reporting laws throughout the US at www.childwelfare. gov/topics/safety-and-risk/mandated-reporting/?top=78. In the UK, this legal protection is referred to as *safeguarding children* (learn more at www.gov. uk/government/publications/working-together-to-safeguard-children--2).

## Level of Engagement

A caregiver's participation in their child's yoga therapy treatment depends on the setting, as well as the youth's age. In this section, we cover both the group and individual settings, as they each dictate different levels of contact between the YP and caregivers.

In the *group* setting—whether at a school, recreation center, clinic or outpatient setting—parents will most likely not witness the actual yoga therapy sessions, since other children are present. But the YP may have contact with parents via email, phone, or perhaps during pick-up. If the YP wants to assign home practice to children in these settings, having a master list of parents' emails is a great way to ensure that families are aware of it. As Mimi Felton of Mimi's YogaKids (Chapter 3) observed, children will often naturally share what they've learned in yoga therapy with their families, which helps to strengthen their grasp and mastery of it (M. Felton, personal communication, August 5, 2024).

A YP may also see a child or youth *individually* in any of the above settings. As discussed in Chapter 6, one of the big differences between yoga and yoga therapy is assessment. While assessment may be minimal in the group setting (perhaps just a Lickert scale gauging participants' mood before and after session), individual sessions require a more comprehensive assessment, such as an intake session with quantitative evaluation to determine the needs of the specific child (Chapter 7). Accordingly, the parent/guardian participates in the intake session at a minimum, and on an ongoing basis depending on the client's age, development, and preference. Let's consider this in depth.

## Family Participation in Individual Sessions

As children grow and mature, their relationships change. Nowhere is this more noticeable than in the parent–child relationship. It is understandable that parents get confused about how to relate with their growing children as they transition into their own individuality and independence. When considering how much involvement parents should have in a minor's individual yoga therapy session, it is helpful to use the following metaphor: parents of primary-school-aged children (5–12 year olds) are like their *managers*, who coordinate most aspects of the child's relationships, schedule, and activities of daily living; as the child enters adolescence, the parent's role slowly transforms into that of a *consultant*.

For clients aged 5–8 years old, a parent attends most if not all of the first session to see what the child is learning and to help facilitate home practice. In subsequent sessions, the parent will most likely attend some portion of each session to offer details about the child's progress, and ensure the child understands new home practice skills. Clients aged 9–12 years old will often want and need more autonomy. Parents are required to attend the intake session. Beyond that, the YP should work with the client and guardian to decide how frequently they will attend a part of the session on a regular basis (for instance, once every 4–8 weeks).

For adolescent clients (13–18 years old), a parent or guardian attends the intake session at a minimum. Thereafter, it is developmentally appropriate to allow the adolescent client to decide how frequently—if at all—they would like a parent or guardian to attend. In Claudia's case, she was clear she did not want parents involved regarding her *yoga therapy* practice. "I feel like this is something I have to do on my own," she said when Michelle asked if she wanted any help from her mother to remember to practice.

The process of the adolescent becoming more independent happens gradually over time, which can be challenging for both the parent(s) and the adolescent. The YP can assist in helping adolescent clients and parents work through this process by having discussions from time to time about how involved the youth client would like their parent to be.

These are some general guidelines for parental engagement in a youth's individual yoga therapy:

- 5–8 years old: parent present some of session, all sessions

- 9–12 years old: parent present for check-in on a regular basis (every 4–8 sessions)

- 13–18 years old: sporadic check-ins with parent, perhaps an occasional family session (which can be called by the adolescent, parent, or YP)

## Home Practice

Home practice is a great way for children and adolescents to integrate and master the yoga tools they've learned in sessions. The younger the child, the more support they will need from their caregiver to practice yoga tools at home. As mentioned earlier, the YP can communicate home practice instruction and tools with parents via phone, email, or verbally in session. Here are some general guidelines with regards to parental engagement in a youth client's home practice:

- 5–8 years old: parent directs home practice

- 9–12 years old: parent works with child to determine parental support

- 13–18 years old: parent knows about adolescent's practice, and may encourage it if adolescent asks or the YP recommends

Visual aids in the form of feelings charts, handouts, tracking forms, and pictorial yoga practice sequences are all essential tools for the YP working with youth. We offer Amy Wheeler's feelings charts in Appendices 2 and 3. But we encourage YPs to develop their own library of frequently used tools to offer clients and their families.

## Providers and Teachers

Care team members other than a client's parent/guardian can include school staff (like a teacher, school counselor, or coach) and medical and/or behavioral staff (like a primary doctor, psychiatrist, or occupational therapist). These individuals offer insights about a client beyond their home setting and can provide invaluable support in the care and treatment of the client. But before discussing a client with another team member, you must obtain consent.

## Confidentiality

Confidentiality with team members *other* than legal guardians is the same across the board: you only share information about a client when you have written consent from the client or their guardian to do so. In addition, this consent only extends to the specific team member(s) listed on the signed form. For instance, you may have signed permission to speak to the client's psychiatrist, but if you don't have it with their occupational therapist, you must obtain written permission from the client/guardian before speaking with them. This applies to all clients, regardless of age.

## Collaboration

Once written consent is obtained for a particular team member, the YP is free to contact them. In Claudia's case (Chapters 7 and 9), Michelle obtained written consent from her parents to speak to Claudia's school counselor, Ms. Bennett. Ms. Bennett shed more light on the friend group Claudia hung out with, noting that they were kids who had "rough home lives." Claudia had told her school counselor that she enjoyed being the kind of friend who listened to their troubles when others wouldn't. Ms. Bennett said unfortunately one or two of these girls had turned on Claudia, and been extremely hurtful to her by spreading rumors and lies about her on social media. This was about the time that Claudia began cutting.

Ms. Bennett clarified for Michelle that Claudia was dealing with the betrayal of close friends through online bullying—a very intense situation for an adolescent. Her school counselor's insights helped contextualize Claudia's self-harm behaviors.

Michelle was also able to shed light on Claudia's case for Ms. Bennett. Michelle explained that Claudia was learning to become aware of her body through various yoga tools, and as a result was better able to identify feelings and take action to stay regulated. Ms. Bennett asked how she could help support Claudia at school, and when Michelle shared the Five Senses Mindfulness practice, she said she was familiar with it. Ms. Bennett said she'd be happy to remind Claudia to practice her yoga tools, and even practice with her if it helped.

## You Are Part of a Team

As the collaboration between Ms. Bennett and Michelle shows, consulting with other team members can help the YP create a timeline and context for a client's behaviors. Such discussions also help the YP educate other team members about the application of yoga therapy in complex trauma treatment. These exchanges among team members are invaluable to the client, because care is more integrated. And they are equally helpful to team members, who feel more supported in their work together.

In this chapter we have discussed how to interact with a client's support team, and how to work collaboratively to support the client and one another. In our next and final chapter, we will explore the support that you the YP needs, to do this meaningful, but sometimes challenging, work.

## Self-Care Practice: Inner Allies

In anticipation of Chapter 12, we offer a self-care practice now that helps you contemplate what support you garner from your social network. In this moment, think about who lifts your spirits when you think of them. Who in your life inspires you, believes in you, sees the good in you (even when you struggle to)?

Perhaps your yoga teacher, a spiritual teacher, your best friend, a past professor, or a colleague comes to mind. Write their names down. If thinking of a person is difficult, recall your dog, cat, bearded dragon, or any pet who is special to you. Write those names down. These are your inner allies.

As you read over the list, stop at each name and notice how you feel when you're with each person or pet. Notice how your body responds. Are you smiling a little? Do you chuckle thinking about a funny look or an inside joke? Does your heart feel warm? Do your shoulders relax a bit?

Now, think of a secret, a problem, or a question you're currently struggling with. Who on this list would you want to talk to, confide in, about your worry? Close your eyes and bring this person (or pet) fully to mind. Imagine them sitting right next to you, noticing something is bothering you. Visualize their face, body posture, and movements that cue safety and support for you. A friend might move in a little closer, tilting their head, before asking what's wrong. Your dog might place its head in your lap to indicate support.

Imagine sharing your worry with them, and how they'd respond. What would they say? What would they do that feels supportive, nurturing, and validating to you? You're not going to try and solve your problem. Just notice what it feels like in your body to receive support. Notice how your body sensations change. Do you feel looser in the shoulders? Does your belly relax? Does your jaw unclench? Do you feel relief from finally sharing your burden? Take in their response fully. Do you feel lighter? More supported? Less alone?

Sit with your experience for 5–10 minutes. Every time the mind wanders, simply bring your inner ally's face to mind, and breathe. When you are done, notice how you feel differently about your problem.

Invoking the supportive presence of an inner ally is a vijnanamaya kosha practice in two ways: one, it reminds you that you have a social support system, and two, the inner ally is a nurturing form of witness mind. Use this practice any time you feel isolated and overwhelmed by your problems and worries.

## Chapter Summary

- Almost all clients have a support system they rely on.

- The younger the client, the more likely it is that obtaining permission and being in contact with a legal guardian is a necessity.

- Regardless of a client's age, developing alliances with key members of a client's support network can greatly support the client in their journey of healing from complex trauma.

- When a YP's services are labeled yoga therapy, more rules apply regarding interactions with clients' care teams, and whether legal consent is required. Several factors determine what rules apply to which clients.

- It is essential to learn and abide by your country and/or region's specific laws and regulations, especially if the client is a minor.

- The *age of majority* and a *client's age of consent to treatment* are not the same thing in some countries. The age of majority is when a person is legally considered an adult. The age of consent is the age at which a client can consent to their own treatment (which is younger than the age of majority in some countries like the US).

- Clients' personal health information (PHI) must be kept confidential and secure. *Confidential* means the client's information is private. *Secured* means that the client's file, whether it be in hard copy or electronic form, is stored in a secure, password-protected location.

- All information a child or adolescent client shares with you is confidential EXCEPT matters of health and safety. This can be a confusing topic for families of a minor client, so it is essential to explain this during the initial intake session.

- If a client who is a minor shares that they—or another minor—is being subjected to abuse or neglect, *or* the YP witnesses the child being subjected to circumstances that would reasonably result in abuse or neglect, the YP is legally required to report this to local authorities and/or to the local child-abuse reporting hotline.

- The YP must obtain written permission before speaking to a member of the client's care team. If the client is an adult, obtain written consent from the client. If the client is a minor (or legally/medically deemed incapable of decision making), obtain written consent from that client's legal guardian.

- Consulting and collaborating with other members of a client's care team creates integration of care and allows the YP to educate other team members about the application of yoga therapy in complex trauma treatment.

## CHAPTER 12

# Community Care and Self-Care

Now we turn our gaze to you, the YP. Working with others' pain—especially complex trauma—can have a profound impact on you as a professional caregiver. In this chapter, we examine the last and fifth component of our YTCT model—that of community care and self-care. These kinds of care, as well as prevention and intervention, are necessary to maintain one's own well-being in the field of yoga therapy. In addition, we review three of the most common symptom clusters that those in the helping and healing fields can experience: burnout, compassion fatigue, and vicarious trauma. To illustrate some of these principles let's explore how YP and community leader Mimi Felton takes care of herself.

## Mimi's Story

During our conversation with Mimi (Chapter 3), she shared the tools that help sustain her ability to provide a healing space for others by caring for herself. With regards to self-care, Mimi mentioned two important practices: eating well and creating good boundaries with others. She joked that her husband and she are real "foodies," so making time to enjoy a good meal together comes naturally to both. But creating boundaries was something she had to learn the hard way.

Mimi said her husband saw how hard she was working when she first started her wellness center in 2018. He told her she wasn't going to be able to sustain her pace if she didn't "grow a tougher skin" (M. Felton, personal communication, August 5, 2024). Mimi said she realized it's not her job to save or fix anyone. The ways she actively creates boundaries is by limiting her availability and sticking to those limits. She activates the "do not disturb" function on her phone during her downtime, days off, and vacations. Mimi added, "I listen to myself when it's time to take a break" (personal communication, August 5, 2024).

With regards to community care, Mimi said she looks to her Christian faith and has a small group of trusted friends and family she can lean on. Mimi hears a lot of tough stories from her clientele about intergenerational trauma, systemic racism, and targeted oppression. She too has experienced all these negative forces. Her social support system helps remind her it's not her job to fix others' problems, but to help them find their own solutions through self-compassion, self-awareness, and insight. Her husband's gentle admonition not to take on her clients' worries is a great example of how social support can help galvanize us as YPs to create better boundaries for ourselves, and guard against burnout and vicarious trauma.

## Community Care Versus Self-Care

Mimi's story illustrates how support from our social network is equally important to our ability and willingness to engage in self-care. In much the same way that survivors of complex trauma do better when they have social support (Exodus Health, 2024), professionals who care for CPTSD survivors also do better when they have a strong social network. This is called community care.

Many of us know the term *self-care*, the practice of engaging in activities that promote one's physical and mental health (Scott, 2024). But as Mimi's example demonstrates, equally important to our well-being as YPs is *community care*, where "the individual is seen as an integral part of a larger body of people generating care together" (Kim, 2024, "Community care" section, para. 2). Classroom educator and FuelEd™ trainer HyoYoung Minna Kim says that self-care and community care are synonymous, because "(a)n individual's wellness impacts the collective and the culture of the collective impacts the individual" (Kim, 2024, "Community care" section, para. 2).

If community and self-care are so closely related, why talk about them as if they are separate? Kim says the problem is that modern-day society often portrays self-care as do-it-yourself "self-soothing practices that come with a price tag and require free time" (2024, "Self-care industrialized complex" section, para. 1). For those who are marginalized, have limited means, or work in a war zone, the price tag and the free time required for such self-care are luxuries they just don't have. In addition, Kim (2024) astutely questions why it is that when the workplace causes stress and illness in its workers, the individual is left to treat their symptoms in isolation.

Another important reason to prioritize community care is that our emotions and feelings are not as individual as we may believe. Psychologist Amit Goldenberg says that the human brain needs social connections "just like we need water or air" (Vedantam, 2024, 39:11–39:14). In the episode 'Emotions 2.0: When I Feel What You Feel' on the podcast *Hidden Brain*, Goldenberg explained that our emotions are not independent: while we do feel emotions individually, our emotional experiences are *mostly* collective (Vedantam, 2024). As a result, Goldenberg says, "I would urge people to think about emotions… and emotion regulation much more at the collective than the individual level" (Vedantam, 2024, 39:46–39:55).

No wonder chanting, meditating, or doing yoga in a group setting can feel more powerful than on one's own. What Goldenberg is pointing out is that on a brain level, these activities *are* more powerful in a group. Thus, when a YP or anyone in the caring profession feels the stress and overwhelm of working with those who are suffering, the process of healing needs to include support from one's community, one's social network.

The question then becomes: how likely is it that a YP will feel stress because of working with traumatized individuals? The answer is very clear. The British Medical Association (BMA, 2024) states that "[a]nyone who engages empathetically with survivors of traumatic incidents, torture, and material relating to their trauma is potentially affected, including doctors and other health professionals" ("Vicarious trauma: Signs and symptoms" section, para. 2). Michelle's internship director, Shari Vanino, went further, saying that when we treat clients who have trauma our chance of experiencing vicarious trauma "is not an *if* but a *when*" (S. Vanino, personal communication, 2006). YPs working with clients with any level of trauma clearly fall within this description.

To protect against these negative outcomes, we recommend a combination of community care and self-care. By creating a strong social network as well as bolstering one's own self-care practices, the YP can minimize their risk for chronic stress and illness. Thus far, we've considered the importance of community care and self-care for YPs. At the end of this chapter, we will further divide these two types of care into prevention (that is, care tools that help prevent negative impacts) and intervention (care tools that help reduce negative impacts once they've started to occur). But now, let's review the negative impacts that YPs may experience when working with traumatized clients.

## The Cost of Caring

Opening oneself to others' pain on an ongoing basis can take a toll. Those who work in the helping and healing fields such as YPs are at a risk of burnout, compassion fatigue, and vicarious trauma (Affiliation of Multicultural Societies and Service Agencies of British Columbia [AMSSA], 2021; BMA, 2024; Tend, 2024). These terms are interrelated but are different from one another in that they were created separately by different sets of experts and/or researchers. To some extent, ranking or distinguishing among these three terms is not necessarily important (Tend, 2024).

However, these terms are useful in as much as they help you understand the factors that contribute to them, which thereby helps you to bolster your resources (Tend, 2024). With this in mind, let's define each. The WHO (2019) categorizes *burnout* as an occupational hazard and says it is "chronic workplace stress that has not been successfully managed" (para. 4). First coined in the early 1980s, "burnout" describes the physical and emotional fatigue that comes with low job satisfaction, a feeling of powerlessness, and overwhelm at work; of the three symptom clusters addressed in this section, burnout is the easiest to overcome (Tend, 2024). There are five stages of burnout (AMSSA, 2021):

- *Enthusiasm*—no burnout; this stage is characterized by excitement and energy for your role and duties

- *Stagnation*—initial stage of burnout, characterized by a slight depletion of energy and increase of stress at work; you might notice headaches and anxiety, as well as changes in appetite and sleep

- *Frustration*—in this stage you start to experience chronic stress; your job performance decreases, while feelings of powerlessness increase

- *Apathy*—this is the official stage of burnout, in which your job performance has decreased, your personal life suffers, and you may feel like you are failing

- *Intervention*—this is a stage of habitual burnout; it is sometimes referred to as the "intervention stage" because professional help is often needed to recover

*Compassion fatigue* has been described by renowned traumatologist Charles Figley as the "cost of caring" (Stoewen, 2019, para. 2). "This can occur when an individual does emotionally heavy work [by] supporting many clients through suffering or grief, [and the individual] is deeply emotionally invested in their work" (AMSSA, 2021, "Compassion fatigue" section). As the name suggests, compassion fatigue occurs over time and causes even more profound physical and emotional exhaustion than burnout, which the individual struggles to overcome (AMSSA, 2021; Stoewen, 2019; Tend, 2024).

AMSSA (2021) lists emotional, physical, and interpersonal signs of compassion fatigue on a useful online information sheet found at this link: www.amssa.org/wp-content/uploads/2021/01/Burnout-Info-Sheet-January-2021-FINAL.pdf. Emotional signs include irritability, anxiety, numbness, hypersensitivity, and lack of empathy. Physical signs include sleep issues, chronic physical symptoms like headaches, and fatigue. Interpersonal signs include isolating from others and/or increase in relational conflicts.

*Vicarious trauma*, sometimes referred to as secondary trauma (AMSSA, 2021, "Vicarious trauma" section), is the result of working for a prolonged period with others who have experienced violence, trauma, and/or acute suffering. Toward the end of her internship as a rape counselor, Michelle experienced vicarious trauma of her own: she was unable to watch shows or movies that even hinted at sex assault and felt triggered by callous jokes objectifying anyone sexually. Though she hadn't appreciated these references in the past, she knew her reactions were more hypervigilant than before. She'd be going about her day, perhaps shopping at the grocery store, and randomly feel unbearable sadness or extreme anger. Eventually these feelings passed; she graduated and forgot about these symptoms.

Then barely six months later, when Michelle was finally a newly minted yoga therapist, she was on an inpatient care team working with severely mentally ill patients. One patient with whom Michelle had worked closely, doing individual yoga therapy sessions, died suddenly and tragically. For a moment, Michelle thought perhaps she wasn't cut out for this work. Luckily, a critical incident meeting of all staff members involved in the patient's case was convened not only to discuss the death but also to support one another.

Experiencing this kind of community support reminded Michelle that she wasn't alone. She reinvigorated her own practices of yoga and meditation to continue her healing process. As a result, she became passionate about offering others the same kind of professional support through vicarious trauma trainings where she worked.

Michelle also realized she needed to practice quick self-care techniques more frequently. At her RAAP (Rape Assistance and Awareness Program) internship she'd learned some simple practices to create better boundaries for herself before and after sessions. Before client sessions, she envisioned a protective barrier—it could be as thin as a soap bubble or as thick as a brick wall. Michelle liked to visualize a car window: she could see and hear her client but was protected by the imaginary glass. After sessions, she started doing a clearing practice, such as splashing water on her face, taking a deep breath, drinking water, or going for a walk. Another effective practice after a particularly tough session is "wiping off" the session by brushing the body from head to toe with the hands.

Mimi's and Michelle's stories illustrate how each YP needs to find their own way to take care of themselves so that they can maintain and bolster well-being while doing this sometimes-challenging work. Let's look at how to minimize and perhaps even prevent the negative impacts that can occur during working with traumatized others.

## Care for the Caregiver

As noted earlier, we view care for the caregiver in terms of self-care and community care. In addition, we recommend preventive measures to guard against symptoms, as well as interventions once symptoms arise. Yoga therapist Mimi Felton used a variety of these: she listened to her husband who recommended she create better boundaries for herself. Listening to a trusted friend or family is a form of relying on community care. Felton then put the practice of boundaries in place for herself by limiting her availability—a self-care practice. Both strategies are examples of preventive measures.

Let's highlight several that are particularly important or need further explanation. First, getting in the habit before client sessions of creating an imaginary barrier between you and the client is a quick, simple way to create healthy boundaries. Two other self-care visualizations that can be done before or at the start of a session by the YP alone or with the client are Mindful Transition (Chapter 4) and Concentration on the Heart Point (Self-Care Practice at the end of this chapter).

Second, an important aspect of preventive self-care is mindfulness, which is grouped with spiritual and religious practices. In a YTCT focus group held during the writing of this book, we highlighted Kristin Neff's book *Self-Compassion: The Proven Power of Being Kind to Yourself*. In it, Neff (2011) outlines three important aspects of self-compassion: *self-kindness—* being kind to ourselves rather than harsh and judgmental (p. 40); *common humanity*—the reminder that we all suffer, and this connects us all (p. 62);

and *mindfulness*—the ability to see things clearly that fosters "nonjudgmental acceptance of what's occurring in the present moment" (p. 80). In her book and on her website (https://self-compassion.org), Neff offers a host of practices to cultivate self-compassion. We have also featured one in the Self-Care section of Chapter 10.

**Table 12.1** lists possible care options for community care and self-care, and preventive care as well as interventions.

| | Self-Care | Community Care |
|---|---|---|
| Preventive | *Before session on own*: Visualize a protective shield; Mindful Transition or Concentration on the Heart Point | *Before session with client*: Mindful Transition or Concentration on the Heart Point |
| | Create healthy boundaries | Cultivate a supportive social network |
| | Physical exercise (including yoga asana) | Join a gym, yoga studio, or other facility that encourages group support |
| | Artmaking | Join an art or music class |
| | Mindfulness, spiritual, and/or religious practices | Regularly attend meditation group, church, or other spiritual affiliations |
| | Get out in nature | Peer supervision |
| | Take mental-health days off regularly | Go on a retreat or vacation with friends or close family |
| Intervention | After session on own: clearing practice | Engage in clearing practice with colleagues or other community |
| | Take a self-assessment (ProQOL 5) | Seek out therapy for yourself |
| | Reinvigorate self-care practices listed above | Reinvigorate community care networks listed above |
| | Take time off work | Get support through your job's Employee Assistance Program |
| | Call a hotline | Join a support group |

Another important strategy listed under preventive community care is *peer supervision*. Peer supervision is when two or more professionals with similar or equal experience meet to offer one another feedback on cases, provide self-directed learning, and share resources (Lived Experience Workforce Program, 2022; McNicoll, 2008). Though peer supervision groups have an educational emphasis, they also provide a space where YPs can work through difficult cases. This increases social support in the form of professional colleagues and reduces the feelings of isolation that can come from grappling with such cases. Other YPs and care professionals know better than most what it's like to care for traumatized clients. Therefore, colleagues can offer a unique and vital level of support and compassion.

Sometimes no matter how diligently you practice preventive measures, the negative impact of working closely for an extended period with those who are suffering takes its toll. If you're concerned you have symptoms of burnout, compassion fatigue, or vicarious trauma, the best first step is to take a validated, reliable self-assessment. It's hard to see how impacted you may be by the work you're doing, and in this way, a self-assessment helps you "reality-test." We highly recommend the Professional Quality of Life measure (ProQOL 5) that measures compassion satisfaction and fatigue. It is available for free in 28 languages on the Professional Quality of Life website at https://proqol.org

Having a strong support system also serves this function: a close friend, family member, or colleague may be the first to notice and comment on differences in your behavior. Be aware of your impulses to downplay what they say and listen to your loved one's concerns. Most likely, they are seeing something that you can't. Recognize when you're too close to the situation, and heed other's loving concern—just like Mimi did when she listened to her husband's advice to create clearer boundaries.

Working with those who suffer is profoundly rewarding, even if it is also taxing. Helping others in their greatest hour of need, or when nothing else has helped, is transformative for you the YP as well as your clients. When you take care of your own well-being, and recognize the need for breaks, you can have a long career in this deeply meaningful vocation.

## Self-Care Practice: Concentration on the Heart Point

For our final self-care tool, we offer a practice our colleague Michal Orpaz-Tsipris raves about: "Therapists and teachers love it!" (personal communication, October 3, 2024). Called *Anahat Bindu Dhyan*, which roughly translates to the Concentration on the Heart Point, this practice comes from the tradition of Bhrigu Yoga as taught by Dr. Jayant K. Bhadury. Drs. Bhadury and Tsipris generously gave us permission to include this practice in our book.

You can experience the traditional practice of *Anahat Bindu Dhyan* directly from Dr. Jayant K. Bhadury (2024) in this video: https://youtu.be/DGiDS4h-NaMk. In addition, we humbly offer the following abbreviated transcription of the practice:

- Sit comfortably with a straight back and focus on a point on the back behind the heart along the spinal cord (that is in line with the xiphoid process at the tip of the sternum on the front of the body). If visualizing this point is challenging, you can place your hand on the back to feel it.

- Close your eyes if that feels comfortable and bring your attention to your breath. Feel the cool air enter the nostrils as you inhale and notice how it exits slightly warmer as you exhale. Bring all your attention to the breath for a few moments. Breathe fully and completely—breathe in deep and breathe out long.

- Now shift the attention to the Point of the Heart. See a golden light emerging from this point. The golden light is increasing. It reaches every part of your body. This golden light frees you from all negativities—mental, physical, emotional, spiritual. Allow two minutes to feel this light expanding into all areas of the body, removing any negativity. When it is large enough, you sit in a capsule of golden light. Just enjoy this state.

- After two minutes, visualize the golden light retreating very slowly. It begins to shrink and get smaller, as it goes back to its original source— the Point of the Heart, called *Anahat* in Hindi.

- Allow yourself to take another two minutes as you visualize the golden light receding back to the single point behind the heart.

- As the light merges back with the Point of the Heart, allow the eyes to remain closed (if they have been closed). Take a deep breath in, and a long, slow breath out, with the eyes still closed.

- Only when the light is fully merged—and you've taken some deep, even breaths—allow the eyes to open very slowly (if they have been closed).

- Notice how you feel differently than before the practice.

To experience *Anahat Bindu Dhyan* in action, watch Dr. Tsipris integrate this technique into her World Occupational Therapy Day lecture: www.youtube. com/watch?v=yR-CjHft7dQ

## Chapter Summary

- Community care and self-care are the last component of the YTCT model. These kinds of care, as well as prevention and intervention, are necessary to maintain one's own well-being in the caring field of yoga therapy.

- Anyone working in a caring profession, such as yoga therapy, is at risk of three kinds of negative impacts: burnout, compassion fatigue, and vicarious trauma.

- Important preventive measures include creating good boundaries, practicing self-compassion, and seeking out peer supervision from and with colleagues.

- Important interventions once a YP recognizes the signs of distress include taking a self-assessment like the ProQOL and reinvigorating one's self-care practices.

# Appendices

## Appendix 1

### Intake Form

| | |
|---|---|
| Client Legal & Preferred Name: | |
| Legal Guardian (for minor clients): | |
| DOB: | Gender/Pronouns: |
| Date of Intake: | Race/Ethnicity: |
| Address: | Client's Phone #: |
| Guardian's Phone #: | |
| Telehealth: Y/N   Length of Session: | Therapist Name: |

### Presenting Problem (Client's Chief Complaints)

| What Is the Client's Look-Feel-Sound? | |
|---|---|
| LOOK | (General appearance, body language, facial expression) |
| FEEL | (Client's report; YP observations) |
| SOUND | (Tone of voice, cadence, volume) |

**Psychiatric/Behavioral Healthcare**

**Current**

| | |
|---|---|
| Mental Health Diagnoses | |
| Psychotropic Medications | |
| Therapist | |

**Past**

| | |
|---|---|
| Previous Hospitalization | |
| Previous Suicidal Behavior | |
| Past Psychotropic Medications | |
| Past Treatment/Therapy | |

**PMK Overview**

| | |
|---|---|
| Annamaya Kosha | **Range of Motion Summary:**<br>(Jot notes from ROM tool of your choice, such as https://guthrie.tricare.mil/Portals/67/4-%20Structural%20Yoga%20Therapy.pdf):<br><br><br>**Current Injury/Illness and/or Chronic Illness:**<br><br><br>**Subjective Pain Scale:** |

**Subjective Pain Scale:**

| 0 | 1 | 2 | 3 | 4 | 5 | 6 | 7 | 8 | 9 | 10 |
|---|---|---|---|---|---|---|---|---|---|---|

No pain      Moderate pain      Worst possible pain

**Substance Use:**

.......................... / ..................... / ................

.......................... / ..................... / ................

Type(s)       Frequency       Date started

*cont.*

| PMK Overview | |
|---|---|
| Pranamaya Kosha | **Energy level:**<br>☐ Tamasic   ☐ Sattvic   ☐ Rajasic<br>**Comments:** |
| | **Sleep:** Problems getting to sleep/staying asleep |
| | **Breathing Assessment:**<br>☐ Shallow<br>☐ Irregular<br>☐ Mouth Breathing<br>☐ Reverse (Paradoxical) Breathing<br>☐ Other (specify): _____<br>**Comments:** |
| Manomaya Kosha | **Orientation ×4** (What's your name? Where are you? What is the date? What just happened to you?) |
| | **Affect:**<br>☐ Blunted (tamasic)   ☐ Calm (sattvic)   ☐ Hyperactive (rajasic)<br>**Comments:** |
| | **Highest Level of Education/Vocation:** |
| | **History of Trauma** (client's and guardian's report): |

| | |
|---|---|
| **Vijnanamaya Kosha** | Hobbies/Creative Outlets: |
| | Social Support/Important Personal Relationships (family, friends, pets): |
| **Anandamaya Kosha** | **Anchors** (activities, people, practices that bring joy, awe, peace, a sense of flow): |
| | **Community Support** (religious or spiritual affiliation, other important group associations): |

Other relevant psychosocial history, including family history of mental illness/trauma:

. . . . . . . . . . . . . . . . . . . . . . . . . . . . . . . . . . . . . . . . . . . . . . . . . . . . . . . . . . .

. . . . . . . . . . . . . . . . . . . . . . . . . . . . . . . . . . . . . . . . . . . . . . . . . . . . . . . . . . .

. . . . . . . . . . . . . . . . . . . . . . . . . . . . . . . . . . . . . . . . . . . . . . . . . . . . . . . . . . .

Client Strengths (according to client):

. . . . . . . . . . . . . . . . . . . . . . . . . . . . . . . . . . . . . . . . . . . . . . . . . . . . . . . . . . .

. . . . . . . . . . . . . . . . . . . . . . . . . . . . . . . . . . . . . . . . . . . . . . . . . . . . . . . . . . .

. . . . . . . . . . . . . . . . . . . . . . . . . . . . . . . . . . . . . . . . . . . . . . . . . . . . . . . . . . .

Barriers to Treatment (according to client and family/guardian):

. . . . . . . . . . . . . . . . . . . . . . . . . . . . . . . . . . . . . . . . . . . . . . . . . . . . . . . . . . .

. . . . . . . . . . . . . . . . . . . . . . . . . . . . . . . . . . . . . . . . . . . . . . . . . . . . . . . . . . .

. . . . . . . . . . . . . . . . . . . . . . . . . . . . . . . . . . . . . . . . . . . . . . . . . . . . . . . . . . . . . . . . . . . .

Plan (discuss with client and family/guardian—initial thoughts on target kosha, goals/objectives):

. . . . . . . . . . . . . . . . . . . . . . . . . . . . . . . . . . . . . . . . . . . . . . . . . . . . . . . . . . . . . . . . . . . .

. . . . . . . . . . . . . . . . . . . . . . . . . . . . . . . . . . . . . . . . . . . . . . . . . . . . . . . . . . . . . . . . . . . .

. . . . . . . . . . . . . . . . . . . . . . . . . . . . . . . . . . . . . . . . . . . . . . . . . . . . . . . . . . . . . . . . . . . .

Next Session:

. . . . . . . . . . . . . . . . . . . . . . . . . . . . . . . . . . . . . . . . . . . . . . . . . . . . . . . . . . . . . . . . . . . .

. . . . . . . . . . . . . . . . . . . . . . . . . . . . . . . . . . . . . . . . . . . . . . . . . . . . . . . . . . . . . . . . . . . .

. . . . . . . . . . . . . . . . . . . . . . . . . . . . . . . . . . . . . . . . . . . . . . . . . . . . . . . . . . . . . . . . . . . .

**Consent to Treatment:** I have read and understood the above information, and any questions that I had have been answered. If the client is a minor, I certify that I am legally authorized to consent to their treatment. By signing below, I certify that the information provided is accurate, and I/we freely consent to yoga therapy services:

Client Signature: . . . . . . . . . . . . . . . . . . . . . . .     Date: . . . . . . . . . . . . . . .

Guardian Signature: . . . . . . . . . . . . . . . . . . . . .     Date: . . . . . . . . . . . . . . .
(if client is a legal minor)

YP Signature: . . . . . . . . . . . . . . . . . . . . . . . .     Date: . . . . . . . . . . . . . . .

# Appendix 2

**Amy Wheeler's Mental/Emotional State Assessment Feelings Chart for Children**

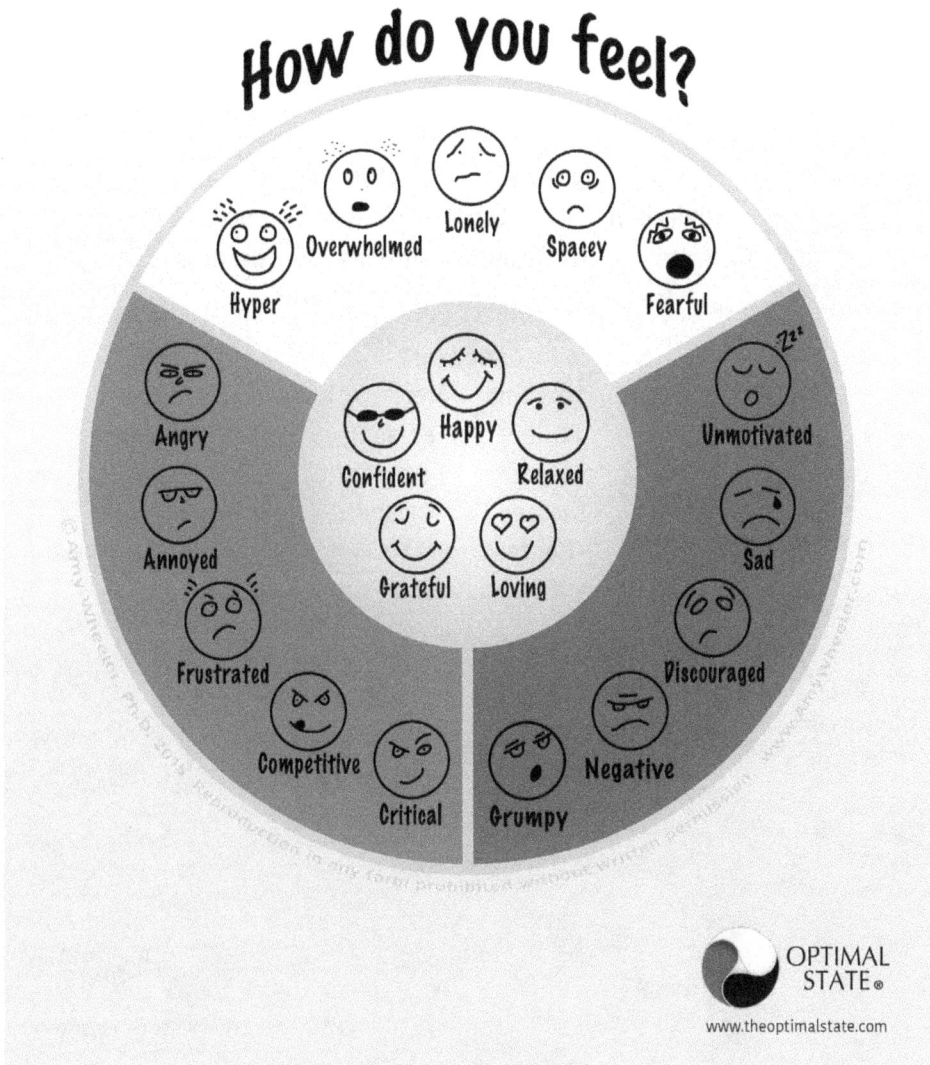

**Figure 4.8** Amy Wheeler's Mental/Emotional State
Assessment Feelings Chart for a Child.
Source: Amy Wheeler

## Appendix 3

### Amy Wheeler's Mental/Emotional State Assessment Feelings Chart for Adults

# Mental/Emotional State Assessment

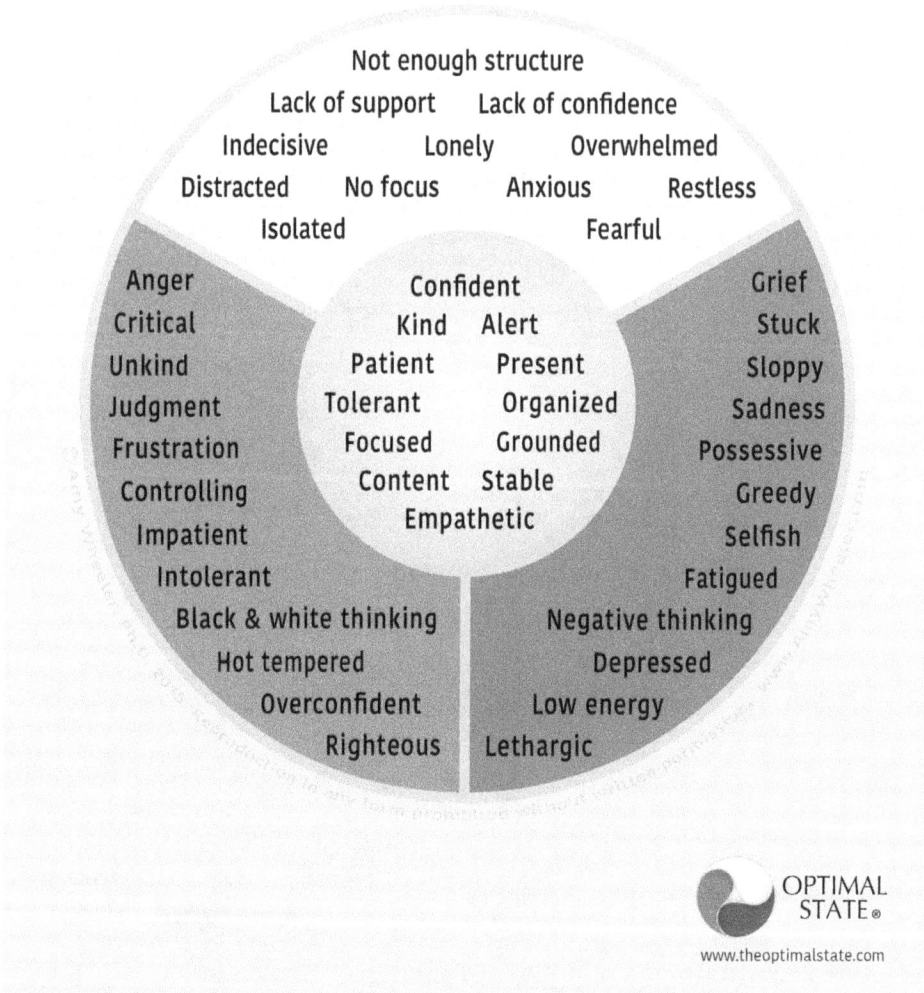

Not enough structure

Lack of support        Lack of confidence

Indecisive        Lonely        Overwhelmed

Distracted     No focus        Anxious        Restless

Isolated        Fearful

Anger                Confident                Grief

Critical            Kind    Alert            Stuck

Unkind            Patient    Present        Sloppy

Judgment        Tolerant    Organized        Sadness

Frustration        Focused    Grounded        Possessive

Controlling        Content    Stable            Greedy

Impatient            Empathetic            Selfish

Intolerant                    Fatigued

Black & white thinking        Negative thinking

Hot tempered            Depressed

Overconfident            Low energy

Righteous    Lethargic

OPTIMAL STATE®
www.theoptimalstate.com

**Figure 4.9** Amy Wheeler's Mental/Emotional State
Assessment Feelings Chart for an Adult.
Source: Amy Wheeler

# Appendix 4

## Client Information Form—Child/Adolescent

**Date Completed:** . . . . . . . . . . . . . . . . . . . . . . Telehealth?  ☐ Yes  ☐ No

*Confidentiality Notice: The information provided is confidential and will not be shared/used without written permission.*

### Client Information

Full Legal Name: . . . . . . . . . . . . . . . . . . . . . . . . . . . . . . . . . . . . . . . . . . . . . . . .

Preferred Name/Nickname: . . . . . . . . . . . . Date of Birth/Age:. . . . . . . . / . . .

Gender: . . . . . . . . . . . . . . . . . . . . . . Pronouns: . . . . . . . . . . . . . . . . . . . . . . . . .

Address: . . . . . . . . . . . . . . . . . . . . . . . . . . . . . . . . . . . . . . . . . . . . . . . . . . . . . . .

. . . . . . . . . . . . . . . . . . . . . . . . . . . . . Country: . . . . . . . . . . . . . . . . . . . . . . . .

Phone: . . . . . . . . . . . . . . . . . Email: . . . . . . . . . . . . . . . . . . . . . . . . . . . . . . .

### Parent/Guardian Information (if applicable)

Full Legal Name: . . . . . . . . . . . . . . . . . . . . . . . . . . . . . . . . . . . . . . . . . . . . . . . .

Relationship to Client: . . . . . . . . . . . . . . . . . . . . . . . . . . . . . . . . . . . . . . . . . . .

Address: . . . . . . . . . . . . . . . . . . . . . . . . . . . . . . . . . . . . . . . . . . . . . . . . . . . . . . .

. . . . . . . . . . . . . . . . . . . . . . . . . . . . . Country: . . . . . . . . . . . . . . . . . . . . . . . .

Phone: . . . . . . . . . . . . . . . . . Email: . . . . . . . . . . . . . . . . . . . . . . . . . . . . . . .

### Living Situation and School/Occupation

Who do you live with? . . . . . . . . . . . . . . . . . . . . . . . . . . . . . . . . . . . . . . . . . . . .

Friends/social support: . . . . . . . . . . . . . . . . . . . . . . . . . . . . . . . . . . . . . . . . . . .

Community involvement: . . . . . . . . . . . . . . . . . . . . . . . . . . . . . . . . . . . . . . . . . .

. . . . . . . . . . . . . . . . . . . . . . . . . . . . . . . . . . . . . . . . . . . . . . . . . . . . . . . . . . . . . .

Hobbies/interests: . . . . . . . . . . . . . . . . . . . . . . . . . . . . . . . . . . . . . . . . . . . . . . .

. . . . . . . . . . . . . . . . . . . . . . . . . . . . . . . . . . . . . . . . . . . . . . . . . . . . . . . . . . . . . .

Are you a student?  ☐ Yes  ☐ No

Grade level: . . . . . . . . . . . . . Area of Study: . . . . . . . . . . . . . . . . . . . . . . . . . . .

Extracurriculars: . . . . . . . . . . . . . . . . . . . . . . . . . . . . . . . . . . . . . . . . . . . . . . .

Physical activity/sports: . . . . . . . . . . . . . . . . . . . . . . . . . . . . . . . . . . . . . . . . . .

Do you have a job?  ☐ Yes  ☐ No

If yes, what do you do? . . . . . . . . . . . . . . . . . . . . . . . . . . . . . . . . . . . . . . . . . . . .

**Presenting Problems** (reasons for seeking yoga therapy): . . . . . . . . . . . . .

. . . . . . . . . . . . . . . . . . . . . . . . . . . . . . . . . . . . . . . . . . . . . . . . . . . . . . . . . . . . . .

**Counseling History**

Current Therapist?  ☐ Yes  ☐ No

If yes, name: . . . . . . . . . . . . . . . . . . . . . . . . . . . . . . . . . . . . . . . . . . . . . . . . . . .

Phone: . . . . . . . . . . . . . . . . . . . Email:  . . . . . . . . . . . . . . . . . . . . . . . . . . . . . .

Start Date: . . . . . . . . . . . . . . .

Previous Therapist?  ☐ Yes  ☐ No

If yes, when and duration of treatment: . . . . . . . . . . . . . . . . . . . . . . . . . . . . . .

**Medical Information**

Primary Care Physician (PCP): . . . . . . . . . . . . . . . . . . . . . . . . . . . . . . . . . . . . .

Phone: . . . . . . . . . . . . . . . . . . . Email:  . . . . . . . . . . . . . . . . . . . . . . . . . . . . . .

**Current Medications**

Medication #1: . . . . . . . . . . . . . . . . . . . . . . . . . . . . . . . . . . . . . . . . . . . . . . . . . .

Dosage: . . . . . . . . . . . . Reason: . . . . . . . . . . . . . . . . . . . . . . . . . . . . . . . . . . . .

Medication #2: . . . . . . . . . . . . . . . . . . . . . . . . . . . . . . . . . . . . . . . . . . . . . . . . . .

Dosage: . . . . . . . . . . . . Reason: . . . . . . . . . . . . . . . . . . . . . . . . . . . . . . . . . . . .

Medication #3: . . . . . . . . . . . . . . . . . . . . . . . . . . . . . . . . . . . . . . . . .

Dosage: . . . . . . . . . . . Reason: . . . . . . . . . . . . . . . . . . . . . . . . . . . . . . .

Medication #4: . . . . . . . . . . . . . . . . . . . . . . . . . . . . . . . . . . . . . . . . .

Dosage: . . . . . . . . . . . Reason: . . . . . . . . . . . . . . . . . . . . . . . . . . . . . . .

Prescriber (if different from PCP): . . . . . . . . . . . . . . . . . . . . . . . . . . . .

Allergies: . . . . . . . . . . . . . . . . . . . . . . . . . . . . . . . . . . . . . . . . . . . . . .

## Medical and Psychiatric History

Major Illness: . . . . . . . . . . . . . . . . . . . . . . . . . . . . . . . . . . . . . . . . . . .

Injuries: . . . . . . . . . . . . . . . . . . . . . . . . . . . . . . . . . . . . . . . . . . . . . . .

Surgeries/Dates: . . . . . . . . . . . . . . . . . . . . . . . . . . . . . . . . . . . . . . . . .

## Hospitalizations

Medical: . . . . . . . . . . . . . . . . . . . . . . . . . . . . . . . . . . . . . . . . . . . . . . .

Psychiatric: . . . . . . . . . . . . . . . . . . . . . . . . . . . . . . . . . . . . . . . . . . . . .

PTSD/CPTSD : . . . . . . . . . . . . . . . . . . . . . . . . . . . . . . . . . . . . . . . . . . .

Substance Use (Past and Present): . . . . . . . . . . . . . . . . . . . . . . . . . . . . .

. . . . . . . . . . . . . . . . . . . . . . . . . . . . . . . . . . . . . . . . . . . . . . . . . . . . .

## Family Psychiatric History

Family Member: . . . . . . . . . . . . . . . . . . . . . . . . . . . . . . . . . . . . . . . . . .

Mental Health Concern: . . . . . . . . . . . . . . . . . . . . . . . . . . . . . . . . . . . .

Family Member: . . . . . . . . . . . . . . . . . . . . . . . . . . . . . . . . . . . . . . . . . .

Mental Health Concern: . . . . . . . . . . . . . . . . . . . . . . . . . . . . . . . . . . . .

Family Member: . . . . . . . . . . . . . . . . . . . . . . . . . . . . . . . . . . . . . . . . . .

Mental Health Concern: . . . . . . . . . . . . . . . . . . . . . . . . . . . . . . . . . . . .

## Suicide History

Thought about suicide?   ☐ Yes   ☐ No

If yes, when: ...............................................

Attempted suicide?   ☐ Yes   ☐ No

If yes, when: ...............................................

## Client Strengths and Barriers

Strengths:................................................

Current Coping Strategies: ...............................

Barriers to Treatment: ...................................

# Appendix 5

**Client Information Form—Adult**

**Date Completed:** ...................... Telehealth?  ☐ Yes  ☐ No

*Confidentiality Notice: The information provided is confidential and will not be shared/used without written permission.*

**Client Information**

Full Legal Name: ...............................................

Preferred Name/Nickname: ............. Date of Birth/Age:........ / ...

Gender: ...................... Pronouns: .........................

Address: ......................................................

.............................. Country: .....................

Phone: .................... Email: ............................

Status:

☐ Single  ☐ Committed Relationship  ☐ Married  ☐ Divorced

☐ Other: ....................................................

**Emergency Contact**

Full Legal Name: ...............................................

Relationship to Client: .........................................

Phone: .................... Email: ............................

**Living Situation and School/Occupation**

Who do you live with? ...........................................

Friends/social support: .........................................

Community involvement: .........................................

.............................................................

Hobbies/interests: ..................................................

..................................................

## Education/Occupation

Highest Level of Education: ..................................

Area of Study: ..............................................

Occupation(s): ..............................................

## Treatment Goals

Presenting Problems (reasons for seeking yoga therapy): ...............

..................................................

What are your goals for yoga therapy?

**1.** ..............................................

**2.** ..............................................

## Counseling History

Current Therapist?   ☐ Yes   ☐ No

If yes, name: ..............................................

Phone: ................... Email: .........................

Start Date: ...............

Previous Therapist?   ☐ Yes   ☐ No

If yes, when and duration of treatment? ........................

## Medical Information

Primary Care Physician (PCP): ..............................

Phone: ................... Email: .........................

## Current Medications

Medication #1: .................................................

Dosage: ........... Reason: ...................................

Medication #2: .................................................

Dosage: ........... Reason: ...................................

Medication #3: .................................................

Dosage: ........... Reason: ...................................

Medication #4: .................................................

Dosage: ........... Reason: ...................................

Prescriber (if different from PCP): ............................

Allergies: .....................................................

## Medical and Psychiatric History

Major Illness: .................................................

Injuries: ......................................................

Surgeries/Dates: ...............................................

## Hospitalizations

Medical: .......................................................

Psychiatric: ...................................................

PTSD/CPTSD: ....................................................

Substance Use (Past and Present): .............................

................................................................

## Family Psychiatric History

Family Member: .................................................

Mental Health Concern: .........................................

Family Member: . . . . . . . . . . . . . . . . . . . . . . . . . . . . . . . . . . . . . . . . . .

Mental Health Concern: . . . . . . . . . . . . . . . . . . . . . . . . . . . . . . . . . . . .

Family Member: . . . . . . . . . . . . . . . . . . . . . . . . . . . . . . . . . . . . . . . . . .

Mental Health Concern: . . . . . . . . . . . . . . . . . . . . . . . . . . . . . . . . . . . .

**Suicide History**

Thought about suicide?　☐ Yes　☐ No

If yes, when: . . . . . . . . . . . . . . . . . . . . . . . . . . . . . . . . . . . . . . . . . . . .

Attempted suicide?　☐ Yes　☐ No

If yes, when: . . . . . . . . . . . . . . . . . . . . . . . . . . . . . . . . . . . . . . . . . . . .

**Client Strengths and Barriers**

Strengths:. . . . . . . . . . . . . . . . . . . . . . . . . . . . . . . . . . . . . . . . . . . . . .

Current Coping Strategies: . . . . . . . . . . . . . . . . . . . . . . . . . . . . . . . . . .

Barriers to Treatment: . . . . . . . . . . . . . . . . . . . . . . . . . . . . . . . . . . . . .

# Appendix 6 (Also Table 7.3)

## Case Conceptualization Form

| Client Background | Background: Client's age, stated gender, level of education, and/or vocation |
| --- | --- |
| | Look |
| | Feel |
| | Sound |
| Strengths | Review PMK Overview to identify strengths |
| | Client's stated strengths |
| Limitations | Review PMK Overview to identify limitations |

*cont.*

|  | Target kosha(s) |
|---|---|
|  | |
|  | |
|  | Fundamental movements impacted (rajasic, tamasic, sattvic) |
|  | |
| **Overall Impression** | Diagnostic impression (including DSM/ICD reported by client and/or referral source) |
|  | |
|  | Current goals and objectives (including yoga tools) and progress |
|  | |
|  | |
|  | Future directions/questions for team |
|  | |
|  | |

# Appendix 7 (Also Table 7.2)

**PMK Overview Worksheet**

| Kosha | Client's Presentation |
|---|---|
| **Annamaya Kosha** (Stability) | What are the client's strengths and imbalances in annamaya kosha? |
| | When thinking about the client's Look-Feel-Sound, what fundamental movements seem most imbalanced? Do they push their arms into their seat, revealing a rajasic relationship to *push*? Does their upper body appear collapsed, revealing a tamasic relationship to *yield*? |
| **Pranamaya Kosha** (Vitality) | What are the client's strengths and imbalances in pranamaya kosha? |
| | Do they appear calm and alert (sattvic)? Tired and collapsed (tamasic)? Restless (rajasic)? |
| | How do the gunas express in their fundamental movements to reveal imbalances of energy, vitality, and health? |
| **Manomaya Kosha** (Clarity) | What are the client's strengths and imbalances in manomaya kosha? |
| | Do they appear anxious and restless (rajasic), or collapsed and disengaged (tamasic)? |
| | What is their quality of thought? Clear (sattvic)? Overwhelmed (rajasic)? Confused/unclear (tamasic)? |
| | What characteristics or roles does the client identify with? |
| **Vijnanamaya Kosha** (Wisdom/ Intuition) | What are the client's strengths and imbalances in vijnanamaya kosha? |
| | How insightful are they about their strengths and challenges? |
| | How is the quality of their personal relationships? |
| | In relationships, does the client seem to struggle with one or a few of the fundamental movements? |
| **Anandamaya Kosha** (Joy/Awe) | What are the client's strengths and imbalances in anandamaya kosha? |
| | What brings them joy or a sense of awe? |
| | Do they have community resources (school, work, affiliations, clubs, religion)? |

# Appendix 8
## Instructions for Sa Ta Na Ma

Sit in a comfortable position and allow the hands to rest on the legs, palms face up. Each syllable of the mantra is said aloud, if possible, with a co-ordinated hand movement.

- "Sa"—touch the thumb and index finger together

- "Ta"—touch the thumb and middle finger together

- "Na"—touch the thumb and ring finger together

- "Ma"—touch the thumb and pinky finger together

The benefit of saying the mantra out loud is that it creates a vibration in the chanter's head that is peaceful, especially when chanted slowly. However, many of Michelle's clients report doing this mantra to calm anxiety when in public places like school or work, in which case the mantra can be done silently. Michelle has also found that for clients with anxiety and/or ADHD, it helps to start the mantra at a fast clip and then slow it down over the course of many (ten or more) repetitions.

**Origin:** Yogapedia (2023) says this mantra comes from the Kundalini Yoga tradition and was popularized in the US and Europe by Yogi Bhajan. The meaning of the chant's syllables are as follows: "Sa"—birth; "Ta"—life, existence, and creativity; "Na"—endings and transformation; and "Ma"—rebirth, regeneration, and joy (Yogapedia, 2023, "Yogapedia explains Sa Ta Na Ma" section). In this way, the mantra can be thought of as creating a vibrational circle that continually brings the chanter back to the present moment.

# Appendix 9
## Panchamaya Kosha Self-Assessment for Self-Care

We as caregivers often neglect ourselves. The very tools we know to offer our clients we rarely use ourselves. Here's a gentle reminder to do that now. Take a moment to consider Look-Feel-Sound for yourself. How do you look right now? How do you feel? What do the thoughts in your head sound like? Use this information to determine which of your koshas feels most out of balance.

## Annamaya Kosha

How is your annamaya kosha? What is your posture like at this moment? Are you slumped? Tense in places? Are you in physical pain?

## Pranamaya Kosha

How is your pranamaya kosha? What is your energy level? Are you exhausted? Restless?

## Manomaya Kosha

How is your manomaya kosha? Are your thoughts clear, or do you feel foggy? Are you stuck on a thought? Is there any negative self-talk going on in your head?

## Vijnanamaya Kosha

How about vijnanamaya kosha? Do you feel indecisive or confused about something in your life? Do you feel like you can detach from your worries, or do you feel entangled in them?

## Anandamaya Kosha

And how about anandamaya kosha? When was the last time you felt a sense of awe, in the positive sense, even if just briefly?

## Self-Care

Choose one kosha to focus on—it could be the one that is most out of balance, or most frequently pestering you. What yoga tool(s) would help restore balance?

# References

Ackerman, C. (2024). *What is Attachment Theory? Bowlby's 4 stages explained.* https://positivepsychology. com/attachment-theory

Affiliation of Multicultural Societies and Service Agencies of British Columbia [AMSSA]. (2021, January). *Burnout, vicarious trauma, and compassion fatigue.* www.amssa.org/wp-content/uploads/2021/01/ Burnout-Info-Sheet-January-2021-FINAL.pdf

Alegría-Torres, J. A., Baccarelli, A., & Bollati, V. (2011). Epigenetics and lifestyle. *Epigenomics, 3*(3), 267–277. doi: 10.2217/epi.11.22. PMID: 22122337. PMCID: PMC3752894.

American Psychological Association [APA]. (2017). *How long will it take for treatment to work?* www.apa. org/ptsd-guideline/patients-and-families/length-treatment

Aposhyan, S. (2007). *Natural intelligence: Body-mind integration and human development.* Now Press.

Ayre, K., & Krishnamoorthy, G. (2023). Effects of childhood trauma on brain development. In K. Ayre & G. Krishnamoorthy, *Trauma informed behaviour support: A practical guide to developing resilient learners.* University of Southern Queensland. https://socialsci.libretexts.org/Bookshelves/ Early_Childhood_Education/Trauma_Informed_Behaviour_Support%3A_A_Practical_Guide_ to_Developing_Resilient_Learners_(Ayre_and_Krishnamoorthy)/03%3A_Prevent_and_ contain/03.2%3A_Effects_of_childhood_trauma_on_brain_development

Bainbridge Cohen, B. (2023). *The difference between collapsing and yielding* [Video]. YouTube. www.youtube. com/watch?v=NQYbm1uCG7Y

Bainbridge Cohen, B. (2024). *Body-mind centering©.* https://bonniebainbridgecohen.com/pages/ body-mind-centering

Barudin, J. W. G. (2021). From breath to beadwork: Lessons learned from a trauma-informed yoga series with Indigenous adolescent girls under youth protection. *International Journal of Indigenous Health, 16*(1). https://jps.library.utoronto.ca/index.php/ijih/article/view/33220

Beltran, M., Brown-Elhillali, A. N., Held, A. R., Ryce, P., Ofonedu, M. E., Hoover, D., & Belcher, H. M. (2016). Yoga-based psychotherapy groups for boys exposed to trauma in urban settings. *Alternative Therapies in Health and Medicine, 22*(1), 39–46. https://pubmed.ncbi.nlm.nih.gov/26773320

Berger, R. (2023, November 11). *Surviving at the heart of the storm* [Video]. YouTube. www.youtube.com/ watch?v=k8LPADjIr3s

Berude, K. (2018). *Neurological/cognitive development.* www.mchkids.com/infanttoddler-program-director-blog/neurologicalcognitive-development

Beutler, S., Mertens, Y. L., Ladner, L., Schellong, J., Croy, I., & Daniels, J. K. (2022). Trauma-related dissociation and the autonomic nervous system: A systematic literature review of psychophysiological correlates of dissociative experiencing in PTSD patients. *European Journal of Psychotraumatology, 13*(2). doi: 10.1080/20008066.2022.2132599.

Bhadury, J. K. (2024, October 27). *Anahat Bindu Dhyan* [Video]. YouTube. www.youtube.com/ watch?v=DGiDS4hNaMk

Bhavanani, A. B., Sullivan, M., Taylor, M. J., & Wheeler, A. (2019). Shared foundations for practice: The language of yoga therapy. *Yoga Therapy Today,* Summer, pp. 44–47.

Bidzan-Bluma, I., & Lipowska, M. (2018). Physical activity and cognitive functioning of children: A systematic review. *International Journal of Environmental Research and Public Health, 15*(4), 800. https:// doi.org/10.3390/ijerph15040800

Blackmore, A. (2020). *What is "midline" and why is "crossing the midline" important for your child's brain development?* www.centreofmovement.com.au/what-is-midline-and-why-is-crossing-the-midline-important-for-your-childs-brain-development/

Blue Knot. (2021). *What is complex trauma?* https://blueknot.org.au/resources/understanding-trauma-and-abuse/what-is-complex-trauma

Bornstein, M. H., & Esposito, G. (2023). Coregulation: A multilevel approach via biology and behavior. *Children, 10*(8), 1323. doi: 10.3390/children10081323. PMID: 37628322. PMCID: PMC10453544.

Brach, T. (2019). *Radical compassion: Learning to love yourself and your world with the practice of RAIN.* Penguin Life.

British Medical Association [BMA]. (2024, June 28). *Vicarious trauma: Signs and strategies for coping.* www.bma.org.uk/advice-and-support/your-wellbeing/vicarious-trauma/vicarious-trauma-signs-and-strategies-for-coping

Brockman, R. M. (2024). *Epigenetics and a paintbrush.* www.psychologytoday.com/us/blog/a-map-of-the-mind/202401/epigenetics-and-a-paintbrush-0

Brook, A. (n.d.). *Free downloads: The satisfaction cycle* [Video]. www.anniebrook.com/pdf-library

Buczynski, R. (2023). *Mastering the treatment of trauma: A quickstart guide; Module 1—How to identify and treat the invisible wounds of neglect* [Webinar]. www.nicabm.com/confirm/mastering-the-treatment-of-trauma-cwzsb

Casey, B. J., Jones, R. M., & Hare, T. A. (2008). The adolescent brain. *Annals of the New York Academy of Sciences.* www.ncbi.nlm.nih.gov/pmc/articles/PMC2475802

Cavell, T. A., & Quetsch, L. B. (2023). A framework for working with parents of aggressive children. In T. A. Cavell & L. B. Quetsch, *Working with parents of aggressive children: A practitioner's guide* (2nd ed., pp. 29–64). American Psychological Association. https://doi.org/10.1037/0000355-002

Centeio, E., Whalen, L., Thomas, E., & Kulik, N. (2017). Using yoga to reduce stress and bullying behaviors among urban youth. *Health, 9*(3), 409–424. doi: 10.4236/health.2017.93029.

Centers for Disease Control and Prevention [CDC]. (2021). *About the CDC-Kaiser ACE study.* www.cdc.gov/violenceprevention/aces/about.html

Centers for Disease Control and Prevention [CDC]. (2023). *Early brain development and health.* www.cdc.gov/ncbddd/childdevelopment/early-brain-development.html

Centers for Disease Control and Prevention [CDC]. (2024). *About adverse childhood experiences.* www.cdc.gov/aces/about/?CDC_AAref_Val=www.cdc.gov/violenceprevention/aces/fastfact.html

Chaya, M. S., Nagendra, H., Selvam, S., Kurpad, A., & Srinivasan, K. (2012). Effect of yoga on cognitive abilities in schoolchildren from a socioeconomically disadvantaged background: A randomized controlled study. *Journal of Alternative and Complementary Medicine, 18*(12), 1161–1167. https://doi.org/10.1089/acm.2011.0579

Children's Hospital of Orange County [CHOC]. (2016). *Sleep hygiene for teens.* https://choc.org/wp-content/uploads/2016/04/Sleep-Hygiene-Teen-Handout.pdf

Cleveland Clinic. (2022, March 29). *EMDR therapy.* https://my.clevelandclinic.org/health/treatments/22641-emdr-therapy

Cleveland Clinic. (2023, April 4). *CPTSD (complex trauma): What it is, symptoms & treatment.* https://my.clevelandclinic.org/health/diseases/24881-cptsd-complex-ptsd

Cleveland Clinic. (2024). *Yoga therapy.* https://my.clevelandclinic.org/health/treatments/24889-yoga-therapy

Colorado Department of Human Services. (2024). *Mandatory reporting of child abuse and neglect in Colorado.* https://co4kids.org/child-abuse-prevention/mandatory-reporters

Colorado General Assembly. (2019). *Youth mental health education and suicide prevention.* https://leg.colorado.gov/bills/hb19-1120

Complex Trauma Resources. (2024). *Co-regulation.* www.complextrauma.org/glossary/co-regulation

Cook, T. (2024). *Yoga and the koshas—the layers of being.* www.ekhartyoga.com/articles/practice/yoga-and-the-koshas-the-layers-of-being

Corrigan, K. (Host). (2022, August 23). *Parenting and the brain with neuroscientist Lisa Feldman Barrett* [Audio podcast episode]. In *Kelly Corrigan wonders.* PRX. www.kellycorrigan.com/podcast/lisafeldmanbarrett?rq=Lisa%20Feldman%20barrett

Courtois, C., & Ford, J. (2016). *Treatment of complex trauma: A sequenced, relationship-based approach.* Guilford Press.

Cover Three. (2020). *Kids' brain development: The factors & stages that shape kids' brain.* https://coverthree.com/blogs/research/kids-brain-development

Daly, L. A., Haden, S. C., Hagins, M., Papouchis, N., & Ramirez, P. M. (2015). Yoga and emotion regulation in high school students: A randomized controlled trial. *Evidence-Based Complementary and Alternative Medicine.* https://doi.org/10.1155/2015/794928

Darcy, A. M. (2023). *Emotional awareness—What it is and why you need it.* www.harleytherapy.co.uk/counselling/emotional-awareness.htm

Dariotis, J. K., Chen, F. R., Park, Y. R., Nowak, M. K., French, K. M., & Codamon, A. M. (2023). Parentification vulnerability, reactivity, resilience, and thriving: A mixed methods systematic literature review. *International Journal of Environmental Research and Public Health*, 20(13), 6197. https://doi.org/10.3390/ijerph20136197

Dean, K. (2023, April 13). *6 steps to understand and address grief and trauma in your core.* https://thetummyteam.com/6-steps-to-understand-and-address-grief-and-trauma-in-your-core

Deoni, S. C., O'Muircheartaigh, J., Elison, J. T., Walker, L., Doernberg, E., Waskiewicz, N., Dirks, H., Piryatinsky, I., Dean, D. C., III, & Jumbe, N. L. (2016). White matter maturation profiles through early childhood predict general cognitive ability. *Brain Structure & Function*, 221(2), 1189–1203. https://doi.org/10.1007/s00429-014-0947-x

Diamond, A., & Lee, K. (2011). Interventions shown to aid executive function development in children 4 to 12 years old. *Science*, 333(6045), 959–964. https://doi.org/10.1126/science.1204529

D'Onofrio, B., & Emery, R. (2019). Parental divorce or separation and children's mental health. *World Psychiatry: Official Journal of the World Psychiatric Association (WPA)*, 18(1), 100–101. https://doi.org/10.1002/wps.20590

Downie, S., Walsh, J., Kirk-Brown, A., & Haines, T. P. (2023). How can scope of practice be described and conceptualised in medical and health professions? A systematic review for scoping and content analysis. *International Journal of Health Planning & Management*, 38(5), 1184–1211. doi: 10.1002/hpm.3678. PMID: 37434288.

Eagleman, D. (2017). *The brain: The story of you.* Vintage Books.

Emmons, A. E. R., Chan, D. V., & Burker, E. J. (2021). Yoga therapy as an innovative treatment for complex trauma. *Journal of Applied Rehabilitation Counseling*, 52(4). doi: 10.1891/JARC-D-20-00019.

Employee Assistance Program Association—South Africa [EAPA-SA]. (2023, August 15). *What is the difference between trauma therapy and trauma-informed care?* www.eapasa.co.za/what-is-the-difference-between-trauma-therapy-and-trauma-informed-care

Exodus Health. (2024, May 1). *Role of social support in long-term PTSD recovery.* https://newexodushealth.com/role-of-social-support-in-long-term-ptsd-recovery

Farhi, D., & Stuart, L. (2022). *Pathways to a centered body: Gentle yoga therapy for core stability, healing back pain, and moving with ease.* Embodied Wisdom Publishing.

Feldman Barrett, L. (2017). *How emotions are made: The secret life of the brain.* Harper.

Feuerstein, G., Kak, S., & Frawley, D. (1995). *In search of the cradle of civilization.* Quest Books.

Fierce Calm. (2024). www.fierce-calm.com

Finlayson, D. (2018, December 20). *A yoga therapy perspective on the human system: The panchamaya model.* https://yogatherapy.health/2018/12/20/a-yoga-therapy-perspective-on-the-human-system-the-panchamaya-model

Fishman, S. (2023). *Piaget's 4 stages of cognitive development.* https://psychcentral.com/health/piaget-stages-of-development#piaget-history

Flaherty, S. C., & Sadler, L. S. (2011). A review of Attachment Theory in the context of adolescent parenting. *Journal of Pediatric Health Care*, 25(2), 114–121. www.jpedhc.org/article/S0891-5245(10)00046-5/abstract

Foo, S. (2022). *What my bones know: A memoir of healing from complex trauma.* Ballantine Books.

Ford, J. D. (2020). Developmental neurobiology. In J. D. Ford & C. A. Courtois (Eds.), *Treating complex traumatic stress disorders in adults: Scientific foundations and therapeutic models* (2nd ed., pp. 35–61). Guilford Press.

Ford, J. D., & Courtois, C. A. (2020). Defining and understanding complex trauma and complex trauma stress disorders. In J. D. Ford & C. A. Courtois (Eds.), *Treating complex traumatic stress disorders in adults: Scientific foundations and therapeutic models* (2nd ed., pp. 3–34). Guilford Press.

Formosa, J. (2017, September 1). *Discover your dosha to find mind–body harmony.* www.back2health.net.au/discover-your-dosha-to-find-mind-body-harmony

Frank, J. L., Kohler, K., Peal, A., & Bose, B. (2017). Effectiveness of a school-based yoga program on adolescent mental health and school performance: Findings from a randomized controlled trial. *Mindfulness*, 8(3), 544–553. https://doi.org/10.1007/s12671-016-0628-3

Frank, R. (2001). *Body of awareness: A somatic and developmental approach to psychotherapy.* GestaltPress.

Frank, R. (2013, May 29). *Developmental Somatic Psychotherapy™: An introduction* [Video series]. https://vimeo.com/ondemand/dspintroduction

Frank, R. (2024). *Ruella Frank, PhD: Bio.* https://somaticstudies.com/ruella-frank

Frawley, D. (1999). *Yoga and ayurveda: Self-healing and self-realization.* Lotus.

Fritscher, L. (2023, September 20). *What is a presenting problem?* verywellmind.com. www.verywellmind.com/presenting-problem-2671638

Fury, M. (2015). *Using yoga therapy to promote mental health in children and adolescents.* Handspring.

Gaines, J. (2022). *How to write a case conceptualization.* https://positivepsychology.com/case-conceptualization-examples

Germer, C. (2009). *Mindful path to self-compassion: Freeing yourself from destructive thoughts and emotions.* Guildford Press.

Germer, C. (2021, April). *Dr. Chris Germer on shame and self-compassion* [Video]. YouTube. www.youtube.com/watch?v=UaI-uAqohmU&ab_channel=ChristopherGermer%2CPh.D

Gibbs, B. (2021, January 22). *Increasing self-awareness—and healing—through panchamaya kosha.* https://yogatherapy.health/2021/01/22/increasing-self-awareness-and-healing-through-panchamaya-kosha

Goldberg, L. (2016). *Classroom yoga breaks: Brief exercises to create calm.* W. W. Norton & Company.

Goldstein, E. (2023). *What is "parts" therapy? Internal family systems explained.* https://integrativepsych.co/new-blog/what-is-parts-work-therapy-ifs

Gothe, N., Pontifex, M. B., Hillman, C., & McAuley, E. (2013). The acute effects of yoga on executive function. *Journal of Physical Activity and Health, 10*(4), 488–495. https://doi.org/10.1123/jpah.10.4.488

Granger, T. (2019). *Draw breath: The art of breathing, mindfulness & meditation.* Summersdale.

Greenberg, T. M. (2022, September 7). *What is complex PTSD?* www.newharbinger.com/blog/self-help/what-is-complex-ptsd

Greene, R. W. (2014). *Lost at school: Why our kids with behavioral challenges are falling through the cracks and how we can help them.* Scribner.

Guber, T., Kalish, L., & Fatus, S. (2005). *Yoga pretzels: 50 fun yoga activities for kids and grownups* [Cards]. Barefoot Books.

Harvard Health Publishing. (2024, July 24). *Blue light has a dark side.* www.health.harvard.edu/staying-healthy/blue-light-has-a-dark-side

Herman, J. (1992a). Complex PTSD: A syndrome in survivors of prolonged and repeated trauma. *Journal of Traumatic Stress, 5*(3), 377–391.

Herman, J. (1992b). *Trauma and recovery: The aftermath of violence—From domestic abuse to political terror.* Basic Books.

Hillman, C. H., Erickson, K. I., & Kramer, A. F. (2008). Be smart, exercise your heart: Exercise effects on brain and cognition. *Nature News.* www.nature.com/articles/nrn2298

HM Government. (2023). *Working together to safeguard children.* https://assets.publishing.service.gov.uk/media/65797f1e0467eb000d55f689/Working_together_to_safeguard_children_2023_-_statutory_framework.pdf

Holzer, A. (2022, December 5). *How yoga helps with trauma,* [with] *Dr. Bessel van der Kolk* [Video]. YouTube. www.youtube.com/watch?v=TAGzGXBYBsI

Homossany, A., & Calo-Henkin, D. (2015). *Enchanted wonders A–Z cards: Inspiring yoga activities to elevate your child's self-expression.* Self-published.

Huang, Y. (2021). Comparison and contrast of Piaget and Vygotsky's theories. *Atlantis Press, 554,* 28–32. http://creativecommons.org/licenses/by-nc/4.0

International Classification of Diseases [ICD-11]. (2018). *6B41 Complex post traumatic stress disorder.* https://icd.who.int/browse/2024-01/mms/en#585833559

Isobel, S., Goodyear, M., Furness, T., & Foster, K. (2019). Preventing intergenerational trauma transmission: A critical interpretive synthesis. *Journal of Clinical Nursing, 28*(7–8), 1100–1113. https://doi.org/10.1111/jocn.14735

Iyengar, B. K. S. (1979). *Light on yoga.* Schocken.

Iyengar, B. K. S. (1993). *Light on the Yoga Sutras of Patanjali.* Aquarian Press.

Jeyasundaram, J., Cao, L. Y. D., & Trentham, B. (2020). Experiences of intergenerational trauma in second-generation refugees: Healing through occupation. *Canadian Journal of Occupational Therapy / Revue Canadienne d'Ergotherapie, 87*(5), 412–422. https://doi.org/10.1177/0008417420968684

Kabat-Zinn, J. (2005). *Wherever you go, there you are: Mindfulness meditation in everyday life.* Hatchette Books.

Kaley-Isley, L., & Fury, M. (2018). Children and adolescents. In H. Mason & K. Birch (Eds.), *Yoga for mental health.* Handspring.

Kalm Kids. (2024, February 6). *I spy with my little eye* [Video]. YouTube. www.youtube.com/watch?v=HMp2Aj7Z9uc

Keith, J., & Skidmore, C. (2024). *Sexual assault experienced as an adult.* www.ptsd.va.gov/professional/treat/type/sexual_assault_adult

Keller, D. (2016). *The therapeutic wisdom of yoga: Workbook.* Self-published.

Keller, D. (2021). *The therapeutic wisdom of yoga: Volume 2: Applications.* Self-published.

Kelly-Irving, M., & Delpierre, C. (2019). A critique of the adverse childhood experiences framework in epidemiology and public health: Uses and misuses. *Social Policy and Society, 18*(3), 445–456. doi: 10.1017/S1474746419000101.

Keltner, D. (2023). *Awe: The new science of everyday wonder and how it can transform your life.* Penguin Press.

Kemble, H. K. (Producer). (2018). *The moving child III: Developmental movement in the first year* [Film]. The Movement Arc. https://themovementarc.com/product/film-the-moving-child-iii-developmental-movement-in-the-first-year-personal-use

Kempton, S. (2020, November 17). *Getting to know you.* www.sallykempton.com/getting-to-know-you

Khalsa, M. K., Greiner-Ferris, J. M., Hofmann, S. G., & Khalsa, S. B. (2015). Yoga-enhanced cognitive behavioural therapy (Y-CBT) for anxiety management: A pilot study. *Clinical Psychology & Psychotherapy, 22*(4), 364–371. https://doi.org/10.1002/cpp.1902

Kim, H. M. (2024). *Self-care versus community care.* https://fueledschools.org/blog/communitycare

Klaus, C. (2023, November 23). *Ayurvedic clock: Stages of life.* www.carrieklaus.yoga/blog/ayurvedic-clock-stages-of-life

Konrad, K., Firk, C., & Uhlhaas, P. J. (2013). Brain development during adolescence: Neuroscientific insights into this developmental period. *Deutsches Arzteblatt International, 110*(25), 425–431. https://doi.org/10.3238/arztebl.2013.0425

Kornfield, J. (2008). *A Path with heart: A guide through the perils and promises of spiritual life.* Bantam Books.

Kornfield, J. (2017, August 7). *A mind like sky meditation* [Audio]. https://jackkornfield.com/a-mind-like-sky

Krentzman, R. (2016). *Yoga for a happy back: A teacher's guide to spinal health through yoga therapy.* Singing Dragon.

Kumar, V., Pavitra, K., & Bhattacharya, R. (2024). Creative pursuits for mental health and well-being. *Indian Journal of Psychiatry, 66*(Suppl 2), s283–s303. https://doi.org/10.4103/indianjpsychiatry.indianjpsychiatry_781_23

Lanius, R. A., Terpou, B. A., & McKinnon, M. C. (2020). The sense of self in the aftermath of trauma: Lessons from the default mode network in posttraumatic stress disorder. *European Journal of Psychotraumatology, 11*(1). https://doi.org/10.1080/20008198.2020.1807703

L'Engle, M. (1972). *A circle of quiet.* Farrar, Straus and Giroux.

Levine, P. A. (1997). *Waking the tiger: Healing trauma.* North Atlantic Books.

Levine, P. A., & Kline, M. (2006). *Trauma through a child's eyes: Awakening the ordinary miracle of healing.* North Atlantic Books.

Liberzon, I. (2018). Searching for intermediate phenotypes in posttraumatic stress disorder. *Biological Psychiatry, 83*(10), 797–799. https://pubmed.ncbi.nlm.nih.gov/28648648

Lived Experience Workforce Program [LEWP]. (2022). *Mental health peer supervision framework.* https://mhcsa.org.au/wp-content/uploads/2022/02/LEWP-Peer-Supervision-Framework-140222.pdf

Lundgren, T., Dahl, J., Yardi, N., & Melin, L. (2008). Acceptance and commitment therapy and yoga for drug-refractory epilepsy: A randomized controlled trial. *Epilepsy & Behavior, 13*(1), 102–108. https://doi.org/10.1016/j.yebeh.2008.02.009

MacGregor, J. (2008). *Introduction to the anatomy and physiology of children: A guide for students of nursing, child care and health.* Routledge.

May, J. (2022, September 25). *Our 5 developmental movements & their psychological significance* [Video series]. YouTube. www.youtube.com/watch?v=3115sM76KgM

McCleod, S. (2024). *Vygotsky's theory of cognitive development.* www.simplypsychology.org/vygotsky.html

McFarlane, A. C. (2010). The long-term costs of traumatic stress: Intertwined physical and psychological consequences. *World Psychiatry: Official Journal of the World Psychiatric Association (WPA), 9*(1), 3–10. https://doi.org/10.1002/j.2051-5545.2010.tb00254.x

McNicoll, A. (2008, October 22). *Peer supervision: No-one knows as much as all of us.* www.coachingmentoring.co.nz/articles/peer-supervision-no-one-knows-much-all-us

Mehrabian, A. (1972). *Nonverbal communication.* Routledge.

Merriam-Webster. (2024). *Risk factor.* www.merriam-webster.com/dictionary/risk%20factor

MindRemapping Academy. (2023, June 7). *Difference between trauma aware, trauma sensitive, trauma informed, and trauma responsive: Understanding the nuances.* www.linkedin.com/pulse/difference-between-trauma-aware-sensitive-informed-responsive

Mirtz, T. A., Chandler, J. P., & Eyers, C. M. (2011). The effects of physical activity on the epiphyseal growth plates: A review of the literature on normal physiology and clinical implications. *Journal of Clinical Medicine Research, 3*(1), 1–7. doi: 10.4021/jocmr477w. PMID: 22043265. PMCID: PMC3194019.

Mittelmark, M. B., & Bauer, G. F. (2016, September 3). The meanings of salutogenesis. In M. B. Mittelmark, S. Sagy, & M. Eriksson (Eds.), *The handbook of salutogenesis.* Springer. www.ncbi.nlm.nih.gov/books/NBK435854/doi: 10.1007/978-3-319-04600-6_2

Mohan, A. G., & Mohan, I. (2004). *Yoga therapy: A guide to the therapeutic use of yoga and ayurveda for health and fitness.* Shambhala.

Moore, C. (2019, April 8). *What is eudaimonia? Aristotle and eudaimonic wellbeing.* https://positivepsychology.com/eudaimonia/#3-examples-of-eudaimonic-wellbeing

Mualem, R., Leisman, G., Zbedat, Y., Ganem, S., Mualem, O., Amaria, M., Kozle, A., Khayat-Moughrabi, S., & Ornai, A. (2018). The effect of movement on cognitive performance. *Frontiers in Public Health*, 6. www.frontiersin.org/articles/10.3389/fpubh.2018.00100

Narayanan, M., Owers-Bradley, J., Beardsmore, C. S., Mada, M., Ball, I., Garipov, R., Panesar, K. S., Kuehni, C. E., Spycher, B. D., Williams, S. E., & Silverman, M. (2012). Alveolarization continues during childhood and adolescence: New evidence from helium-3 magnetic resonance. *American Journal of Respiratory and Critical Care Medicine*, 185(2), 186–191. https://doi.org/10.1164/rccm.201107-1348OC

National Association of Social Workers. (2024). *Read the code of ethics*. www.socialworkers.org/About/Ethics/Code-of-Ethics/Code-of-Ethics-English

National Center for Complementary and Integrative Health. (2024, February 15). *Ayurvedic medicine: In depth*. www.nccih.nih.gov/health/ayurvedic-medicine-in-depth

National Child Traumatic Stress Network [NCTSN]. (2023). *Complex trauma*. www.nctsn.org/what-is-child-trauma/trauma-types/complex-trauma

National Health Service [NHS]. (2022a). *Children and young people: Consent to treatment*. www.nhs.uk/conditions/consent-to-treatment/children/

National Health Service [NHS]. (2022b). *Complex PTSD: Post-traumatic stress disorder*. www.nhs.uk/mental-health/conditions/post-traumatic-stress-disorder-ptsd/complex

National Institute for the Clinical Application of Behavioral Health [NICABM]. (2019). *How to help your clients understand their window of tolerance*. www.nicabm.com/trauma-how-to-help-your-clients-understand-their-window-of-tolerance

National Institute of Health. (n.d.). *Tummy time for a healthy baby*. https://safetosleep.nichd.nih.gov/reduce-risk/tummy-time

Neff, K. (2011). *Self-compassion: The proven power of being kind to yourself*. William Morrow.

Nhat Hanh, T. (2017). *Happy teachers change the world: A guide for cultivating mindfulness in education*. Parallax Press.

Ogden, P., & Fisher, J. (2015). *Sensorimotor psychotherapy: Interventions for trauma and attachment*. W.W. Norton & Company.

Ogden, P., & van der Kolk, B. (2023). *Power of the body in treating trauma* [Webinar]. Sensorimotor Psychotherapy Institute. https://sensorimotorpsychotherapy.org/the-power-of-the-body-in-treating-trauma

Ong, I. (2020). Treating complex trauma survivors: A trauma-sensitive yoga (TSY)-informed psychotherapeutic approach. *Journal of Creativity in Mental Health*, 16(2), 182–195. https://doi.org/10.1080/15401383.2020.1761498

Pangari, M. (2022). *The satisfaction cycle*. https://moniquepangari.com/the-satisfaction-cycle-basic-neurocellular-patterns

Parker, G. (2020). *Restorative yoga for ethnic and race-based stress*. Singing Dragon.

Parker, G. (2021). *Transforming ethnic and race-based traumatic stress with yoga*. Singing Dragon.

Pascoe, M. C., Thompson, D. R., & Ski, C. F. (2017). Yoga, mindfulness-based stress reduction and stress-related physiological measures: A meta-analysis. *Psychoneuroendocrinology*, 86, 152–168. https://doi.org/10.1016/j.psyneuen.2017.08.008

Patrinos, N. (2021). Cultivating resilience and safety in yoga therapy practice. In D. Finlayson & L.C.H. Robertson (Eds.), *Yoga therapy: Foundations, tools, and practice*. Singing Dragon.

Penman, D. (2012). *Mindfulness for creativity: Adapt, create and thrive in a frantic world*. Piatkus.

Perlman, S. B., & Pelphrey, K. A. (2010). Regulatory brain development: Balancing emotion and cognition. *Social Neuroscience*, 5(5–6), 533–542. https://doi.org/10.1080/17470911003683219

Perry, B. D. (2020a, April 2). *Regulate, relate, reason (Sequence of Engagement): Neurosequential network stress & trauma series* [Video]. YouTube. www.youtube.com/watch?v=LNuxy7FxEVk

Perry, B. D. (2020b, August 25). *Stress, trauma and the brain: Insights for educators* [Video]. YouTube. www.youtube.com/watch?v=nqW2Xv16bWw&ab_channel=ThinkTVPBS

Perry, B. D., & Szalavitz, M. (2007). *The boy who was raised as a dog; And other stories from a child psychiatrist's notebook: What traumatized children can teach us about loss, love, and healing*. Basic Books.

Perry, B. D., & Winfrey, O. (2021). *What happened to you? Conversations on trauma, resilience, and healing*. Flatiron Books.

Petrow, S. (2021, September 11). Words describing mental health can stigmatize: That's painful and dehumanizing. *The Washington Post*. www.washingtonpost.com/health/mental-health-words-stigma/2021/09/10/1aaefb02-0b3b-11ec-9781-07796ffb56fe_story.html

Pondisco, R. (2020, April 22). *Researchers warn about misuses of a common measure of childhood trauma*. https://fordhaminstitute.org/national/commentary/researchers-warn-about-misuses-common-measure-childhood-trauma

Porges, S. W. (2011). *The polyvagal theory: Neurophysiological foundations of emotions, attachment, communication, and self-regulation*. W. W. Norton & Co. https://psycnet.apa.org/record/2011-04659-000

Practical Psychology. (2023). *Magical thinking: Definitions + examples.* https://practicalpie.com/magical-thinking

PsychCentral. (2021). *Symptoms of complex post-traumatic stress disorder (C-PTSD).* https://psychcentral.com/ptsd/complex-posttraumatic-stress-disorder-symptoms#next-steps

Psychology Today. (2024). *Neuroplasticity.* www.psychologytoday.com/us/basics/neuroplasticity

Qina'au, J., & Masuda, A. (2020). Cultural considerations in the context of establishing rapport: A contextual behavioral view on common factors. In L. T. Benuto, F. R. Gonzalez, & J. Singer (Eds.), *Handbook of Cultural Factors in Behavioral Health.* Springer. https://doi.org/10.1007/978-3-030-32229-8_7

Riegler, A., Bumb, J. M., Wisch, C., Schuster, R., Reinhard, I., Hoffmann, S., Frischknecht, U., Enning, F., Schmahl, C., Kiefer, F., & Koopmann, A. (2023). Does the augmentation of trauma informed hatha yoga increase the effect of dialectical behavior therapy for substance use disorders on psychopathological strain of patients with borderline personality disorder and comorbid substance use disorder? Results of a quasi-experimental study. *European Addiction Research, 29*(1), 1–8. https://doi.org/10.1159/000526670

Rothenberg, R. L. (2020). *Restoring prana—A therapeutic guide to pranayama and healing through the breath of yoga therapist, yoga teachers, and healthcare practitioners.* Singing Dragon.

Rothschild, B. (2000). *The body remembers: The psychophysiology of trauma and trauma treatment.* W. W. Norton & Company.

Rothschild, B. (2017). *The body remembers, Volume 2: Revolutionizing trauma treatment.* W. W. Norton.

Salzberg, S. (2018). *Lovingkindness: The revolutionary art of happiness.* Shambhala.

Sample, R. J., Lee, J., Rosa, D., & Miller, L. F. (2010). A randomized trial of mindfulness-based cognitive therapy for children: Promoting mindful attention to enhance social-emotional resiliency in children. *Child and Family Studies, 19,* 218–229.

Santos, E., & Noggle, C. A. (2011). Synaptic pruning. In S. Goldstein & J. A. Naglieri (Eds.), *Encyclopedia of child behavior and development.* Springer. https://doi.org/10.1007/978-0-387-79061-9_2856

Saraswati, S. S. (2003). *Yoga education for children.* Yoga Publications Trust.

Schwartz, A. (2018). *Somatic psychology and the satisfaction cycle: Dr. Arielle Schwartz.* https://drarielleschwartz.com/somatic-psychology-satisfaction-cycle-dr-arielle-schwartz

Schwartz, A. (2021). *The complex PTSD treatment manual: An integrative, mind–body approach to trauma recovery.* PESI Publishing.

Scott, E. (2024, March 6). *5 types of self-care for every area of your life: How are you caring for yourself today?* www.verywellmind.com/self-care-strategies-overall-stress-reduction-3144729

Shafir, H. (2024, May 2). *Adoption trauma: What it is & how to cope.* www.choosingtherapy.com/adoption-trauma

Sharma, H., & Keith Wallace, R. (2020). Ayurveda and epigenetics. *Medicina (Kaunas), 56*(12), 687. doi: 10.3390/medicina56120687. PMID: 33322263. PMCID: PMC7763202.

Siegel, D. J. (2014). *Brainstorm: The power and the purpose of the teenage brain.* TarcherPerigee.

Siegel, D. J., & Bryson, T. P. (2012). *The whole-brain child.* Random House Publishing Group.

Silver, G. (2018). *Metta (loving-kindness) meditation for kids.* www.lionsroar.com/metta-loving-kindness-meditation-for-kids

Silvernale, C., Garcia-Fischer, I., & Staller, K. (2024). Relationship between psychological trauma and irritable bowel syndrome and functional dyspepsia in a joint hypermobility syndrome/Ehlers–Danlos syndrome patient population. *Digestive Diseases and Science, 69,* 870–875. https://doi.org/10.1007/s10620-023-08201-y

Sincero, S. M. (2012, May 17). *Bowlby Attachment Theory.* https://explorable.com/bowlby-attachment-theory

Smith, T. O., Easton, V., Bacon, H., Jerman, E., Armon, K., Poland, F., & Macgregor, A. J. (2014). The relationship between benign joint hypermobility syndrome and psychological distress: A systematic review and meta-analysis. *Rheumatology, 53*(1), 114–122. https://doi.org/10.1093/rheumatology/ket317

Sperry, J., & Sperry, L. (2020). *Case conceptualization: Key to highly effective counseling.* www.counseling.org/publications/counseling-today-magazine/article-archive/article/legacy/case-conceptualization-key-to-highly-effective-counseling#

Sprouts. (2018, August 1). *Piaget's theory of cognitive development* [Video]. YouTube. www.youtube.com/watch?v=IhcgYgx7aAA

Stapella, A. (2023, September 12). *Everything you need to know about crossing the midline.* https://kidsgrooveandgrow.com/crossing-the-midline

Stewart-Henry, K., & Friesen, A. (2018, August/September). *Promoting powerful interactions between parents and children.* www.naeyc.org/resources/pubs/tyc/aug2018/promoting-powerful-interactions

Stiles, M. (2000). *Structural yoga therapy™ charts.* Samuel Weiser, Inc. https://guthrie.tricare.mil/Portals/67/4-%20Structural%20Yoga%20Therapy.pdf

Stiles, M. (2012). *Structural yoga therapy.* Goodwill Publishing House.

Stoewen, D. L. (2019). Moving from compassion fatigue to compassion resilience, Part 2: Understanding compassion fatigue. *Canadian Veterinary Journal / La revue veterinaire canadienne*, 60(9), 1004–1006.

Stubbe, D. E. (2018). The therapeutic alliance: The fundamental element of psychotherapy. *Focus*, 6(4), 402–403. https://doi.org/10.1176/appi.focus.20180022

Sullivan, M. (with Hyland Robertson, L. C.) (2020). *Understanding yoga therapy: Applied philosophy and science for health and well-being*. Routledge.

Swenson, D. (1999). *Ashtanga yoga: The practice manual*. Ashtanga Yoga Productions.

Teicher, M., Samson, J., Anderson, C., & Ohashi, K. (2016). The effects of childhood maltreatment on brain structure, function and connectivity. *Nature Reviews Neuroscience*, 17, 652–666. https://doi.org/10.1038/nrn.2016.111

Tend. (2024). *What is compassion fatigue?* www.tendacademy.ca/what-is-compassion-fatigue

Therapistaid. (2024). *Trauma narratives*. www.therapistaid.com/therapy-guide/trauma-narratives

Thornton-Hardy, S. (2023). *Yoga therapy for children and teens with complex needs*. Singing Dragon.

Tiwari, S., Sangate, S., Kanojiya, S., Naz, M., Patidar, A., Sangate, M., Prajapat, M., Saste, M., Siddiqui, A., Sahu, R., Tiwari, V., Brahme, A., & Solanki, J. (2024). Investigating the impact of prolonged sitting and lack of physical activity on the musculoskeletal health of school students. *International Journal for Multidisciplinary Research*, 6(4). https://doi.org/10.36948/ijfmr.2024.v06i04.24562

Tohoku University. (2022, November 2). *Glial cells eating synapses may enhance learning and memory*. https://medicalxpress.com/news/2022-11-glial-cells-synapses-memory.html

The Trauma Conscious Yoga Institute. (2024). *Empowerment, embodiment and evolution in trauma healing*. https://traumaconsciousyoga.com

Treleaven, D. A. (2018). *Trauma-sensitive mindfulness: Practices for safe and transformative healing*. W. W. Norton & Company.

Tull, M. (2024, July 26). *What is distress tolerance? How easily do your feathers get ruffled?* www.verywellmind.com/distress-tolerance-2797294

UK Trauma Council. (2024). *Complex trauma*. https://uktraumacouncil.org/trauma/complex-trauma?cn-reloaded=1

Ullah, H., Ahmad, H., Tharwani, Z. H., Shaeen, S. K., Rahmat, Z. S., & Essar, M. Y. (2023). Intergenerational trauma: A silent contributor to mental health deterioration in Afghanistan. *Brain and Behavior*, 13(4), e2905. https://doi.org/10.1002/brb3.2905

United Kingdom Department of Education. (2024). *Working together to safeguard children*. www.gov.uk/government/publications/working-together-to-safeguard-children--2

US Department of Health and Human Services. (2023). *Surgeon General issues new advisory about effects social media use has on youth mental health*. www.hhs.gov/about/news/2023/05/23/surgeon-general-issues-new-advisory-about-effects-social-media-use-has-on-youth-mental-health.html

van der Kolk, B. (2014). *The body keeps the score: Brain, mind, and body in the healing of trauma*. Penguin Books.

Vandekerckhove, M., & Wang, Y. L. (2017). Emotion, emotion regulation and sleep: An intimate relationship. *AIMS Neuroscience*, 5(1), 1–17. https://doi.org/10.3934/Neuroscience.2018.1.1

Vedantam, S. (Host). (2024). *Hidden brain* [Audio podcast]. NPR. https://hiddenbrain.org/podcast/emotions-2-0-when-i-feel-what-you-feel

Villines, Z. (2017, November 5). *What is paradoxical breathing?* www.medicalnewstoday.com/articles/319924

Vygotsky, L. S. (1978). *Mind in society: Development of higher psychological processes* (M. Cole, V. John-Steiner, S. Scribner, & E. Souberman, Eds.). Harvard University Press.

Wamboldt, M. Z., Kaley-Isley, L. C., Fury, M., & Hansen, P. (2019). A manualized yoga intervention for adolescents with co-occurring physical and psychiatric conditions shows improvements in mental and physical health. *Journal of Yoga and Physiotherapy*, 6(5). doi: 10.19080/JYP.2019.06.555698.

Warren, S. (2022, April 21). *What is pandiculation?* https://somaticmovementcenter.com/pandiculation-what-is-pandiculation

WebMD. (2024, March 7). *What is proprioception?* www.webmd.com/brain/what-is-proprioception

Wheeler, A. (2021). Foundations of yoga as therapy: Assessment and healing approach. In D. Finlayson & L. C. Hyland Robertson (Eds.), *Yoga therapy: Foundations, tools, and practice* (pp. 60–77). Singing Dragon.

Wikipedia. (2023, November 15). *Protective factor*. https://en.wikipedia.org/wiki/Protective_factor

Winnicott, D. W. (1953). Transitional objects and transitional phenomena: A study of the first not-me possession. *International Journal of Psychoanalysis*, 34, 89–97. https://psycnet.apa.org/record/1954-02354-001

World Health Organization [WHO]. (1994, January 1). *Life skills education for children and adolescents in schools. Part 1: Introduction to life skills for psychosocial competence* (2nd revision). https://iris.who.int/handle/10665/63552

World Health Organization [WHO]. (2019, May 28). *Burn-out an "occupational phenomenon": International Classification of Diseases.* www.who.int/news/item/28-05-2019-burn-out-an-occupational-phenomenon-international-classification-of-diseases

The Yoga Sanctuary. (2024). Vijnanamaya kosha. www.theyogasanctuary.biz/vijnanamaya-kosha

Yoga Service Council. (2015). Relationship building: Communicate with and respect school staff. In T. Childress & J. Cohen-Harper (Eds.), *Best practices for yoga in schools* (Vol. 1, pp. 53–69). Omega Publications.

YogaFit. (2024). *Yoga for intergenerational and collective trauma.* https://catalog.yogafit.com/product/yogafit-yoga-for-intergenerational-and-collective-trauma-live-online

Yogapedia. (2023, December 21). *Sa Ta Na Ma: What does Sa Ta Na Ma mean?* www.yogapedia.com/definition/10781/sa-ta-na-ma

Young, K. S., Sandman, C. F., & Craske, M. G. (2019). Positive and negative emotion regulation in adolescence: Links to anxiety and depression. *Brain Sciences, 9*(4), 76. https://doi.org/10.3390/brainsci9040076

Zarbo, C., Tasca, G. A., Cattafi, F., & Compare, A. (2016). Integrative psychotherapy works. *Frontiers in Psychology, 6.* https://doi.org/10.3389/fpsyg.2015.02021

Zerotothree. (2024). *Why 0–3?* www.zerotothree.org/why-0-3

# Subject Index

Page numbers followed by f relate to figures; page numbers followed by t relate to tables.

# Author Index